European Collaboration:
Towards Drug Development and Rational Drug Therapy

Proceedings of the Sixth Congress of the European Association for Clinical Pharmacology and Therapeutics
Istanbul, June 24 – 28, 2003

Springer
*Berlin*
*Heidelberg*
*New York*
*Barcelona*
*Hong Kong*
*London*
*Milan*
*Paris*
*Singapore*
*Tokyo*

F. C. Tulunay M. Orme (Eds.)

# European Collaboration: Towards Drug Development and Rational Drug Therapy

## Proceedings of the Sixth Congress of the European Association for Clinical Pharmacology and Therapeutics

## Istanbul, June 24 – 28, 2003

With 3 Figures and 22 Tables

Springer

Professor Cankat Tulunay
Clinical Pharmacology Society
Department of Pharmacology and Clinical Pharmacology
Ankara University Medical School
Merkez Bina
SIHHIYE
6100 Ankara
TURKEY

Professor Michael Orme
EACPT
Dept. of Pharmacology and Therapeutics
The University of Liverpool
Ashton Street, PO Box 147
Liverpool
GREAT BRITAIN

Cataloging-in-Publication data applied for

A catalog record for this book is available from the Library of Congress.

Bibliopgraphic information published by Die Deutsche Bibliothek
Die Deutsche Bibliothek lists this publication in the Deutesche Nationalbibliografie;
detailed bibliographic data is available in the Internet at http://dnb.ddb.de

ISBN 3-540-14010-7 Springer-Verlag Berlin Heidelberg New York



Springer-Verlag Berlin Heidelberg New York
a member of BertelsmannSpringer Science+Business Media GmbH

http://www.springer.de



Cover design: Erich Kirchner, Heidelberg

Printed on acid-free paper SPIN: 10929346 14/3109 - 5 4 3 2 1 0

# Preface

"European Collaboration: Towards Drug Development and Rational Drug Therapy" is the title of the 6th Congress of the European Association for Clinical Pharmacology and Therapeutics ( EACPT )being held in Istanbul, Turkey from June 24th -28th 2003. Istanbul has been chosen as the venue for this congress as a unique city bridging two continents and bringing together scientists from a large number of countries.

This volume has been edited by Prof Cankat Tulunay ( the President of the Congress ) and Prof Michael Orme ( co-ordinator of the Scientific Committee and Hon. Secretary of EACPT. The volume contains details of the 21 symposia and 3 workshops that are taking place in Istanbul together with the abstracts from the more than 400 submitted and being presented in Istanbul.

The organisers hope that you will enjoy both the scientific and cultural aspects of this Congress.

# Table of contents

# Abstracts of lectures

23 June 2003 Whole Day Course

**Introduction to the Methodology of Clinical Trials**

Paola Antonini
Medical Affairs Director, Merck Sharp & Dohme
Italy

The 2 principles of GCP are Ethics, as protection of human rights, and Science, as integrity and reproducibility of data produced from clinical trials. GCP responsibilities are shared among sponsor, monitor and investigator: methodology of clinical trial means the actuation by all the above actors of those behaviors that grant data reliability, worldwide regulatory acceptance and public credibility. Performance in routine clinical practice should not be confused with performance in clinical trials: the adopted methodologies are different except for the ultimate attention to the patient's well-being. But while in the routine clinical practice the physician follows his best discretional medical behaviour, in clinical trials the investigator is called to follow a number of rules and procedures, to ensure proper documentation, to respect established timelines, to maintain written records, to accept the need for periodic monitoring and auditing. On the other side, the sponsor and the monitor must work with the investigator in order to ensure that each single produced data is reliable, accurate and adequately collected and analyzed. All above and much more can be synthesized as the methodology of clinical trial. This methodology is now a new branch of the science, the branch of Clinical Research.

23 June 2003 Whole Day Course

**The Drug Development Process**

Domenico Criscuolo
President of IFAPP

The drug development process is considered one of the most complex process in industrial organizations: in fact, many divisions are working simultaneously on the same New Chemical Entities (NCEs), in order to explore their potential advanteges for the final benefit of patients. We usually divide this process into Phases; from Preclinical Phases into Clinical Phases (from I to IV): indeed it is important to stress that this process in a continuum, with useful information coming from different departments contributing day by day to the final product profile. Key areas of Preclinical Development are Pharmacology, Toxicology, Pharmacokinetics and Chemistry and Pharmacy. The Clinical Development represents the moment of the truth for NCEs: only clinical data can finally support the supposed benefits coming from preclinical investigations. The four Phases of clinical development must provide clear answers about efficacy and safety of the NCEs; however, because of the limited number of patients included in pre-registration studies, only the post marketing observation studies (Phase IV) will give a final answer to the benefit/risk ratio of the new drug.

23 June 2003 Whole Day Course

**Ethics First!**

Domenico Criscuolo
President Of IFAPP

The present methodology to perform Clinical Trials makes reference to Good Clinical Practice; it is a series of obligations and recommendations to Investigators and Sponsors, prepared to safeguard the Ethics principles and to give public reassurance about the study conduct. While starting a clinical study, the Investigator bears significant responsibilities concerning Ethical issues. In fact, She/He is responsible of two key aspects: to inform the Ethics Committee of the Institution, for the approval of the study; and to explain the study to the patients, in order to obtain the signed Informed Consent. This universal approach to the implementation of a clinical study is indeed of high social and scientific value: the Clinical Investigator is in fact the only person in contact with patients. She/he has the critical task to evaluate the study and finally to talk with the patients about study procedures, and its supposed benefits and potential risks. However, in this delicate task she/he is supported by the scientific and ethical review of the Ethics Committe, who represents an active body following the Investigator during all study duration, and providing advice and answers when necessary.

23 June 2003 Whole Day Course

## The Role and Responsibilities of Sponsors

G. Nell
Novartis Pharma GmbH, Austria

The roles and responsibilities of sponsors are defined in international guidelines (ICH: Harmonised Tripartite Guidelines for Good Clinical Practice) and in international or regional laws (eg. EC Directive 2001 / 20 / EC) and national laws and ordinances (eg FDA GCP Regulations).

A sponsor is an individual, company, institution or organisation which takes responsibility for the initiation, management and for financing of a clinical trial (ICH Definition).

Sponsors are usually pharmaceutical companies performing drug development. Part of the duties and responsibilities of a sponsor may be delegated to CROs (Contract Research Organisations) but the ultimate responsibility resides with the sponsor.

In case of socalled „academic" research the investigator has to take over the responsibilities of a sponsor in addition to his duties as investigator („sponsor-investigator").

The main responsibilities of a sponsor are to provide appropriate personnel for trial design and conduction, quality assurance in order to ensure uniformity of performance, to carry out audits to evaluate compliance with protocol and regulatory requirements, to cover administrative aspects of trial management, data handling and record keeping, to obtain all necessary approvals by Ethics committees and competent authorities, to provide the investigationial drugs and to monitor its handling and to supervise closely all safety aspects.

23 June 2003 Whole Day Course

## The Role and Responsibilities of the Investigators

Ádám Vas
Gedeon Richter Ltd., Budapest, Hungary

By definition the investigator of a clinical trial is the person responsible for the conduct of the trial at the trial site .If the trial is conducted by a team at the trial site, then the investigator is the leader of the team.If there are more trial sites and teams then the leader of the whole trial is generally called as the Principal Investigator.The investigator should be thoroughly familiar with all the informations necessary for the trial and supplied by the sponsor and others officially involved with the conduct of the trial (investigational product(s),Investigator's Brochure,experience in the therapeutic area etc.) and must comply with GCP. The investigator should have all the adequate resources (number of qualified staff, number of recruitable patients, equipments etc.). The investigator should communicate with the representatives of the sponsor,the authorities and ethical boards. The investigator should comply with the trial protocol, has the responsibility of notification on any deviations,unawaited events and adverse drug reactions according to the rules defined by the trial protocol. The investigator bears responsibility for the recountibility, storage and administration of the invesigational product(s) and is responsible for the health and human rights of the investigational subjects. The investigator should obtain the relevant informed consents. The investigator is responsible for the adequate documentation of the trial, the safe storage of the documents generated at the site during the trial. The investigator has the task of reporting and compiling the final clinical report towards the sponsor. Practice and pitfalls will be discussed during the course presentation of the topic.

23 June 2003 Whole Day Course

## The Role and Responsibilities of the Clinical Research Monitor

Juan Lahuerta
Secretary, International Fedaration of Associations of Pharmaceutical Physicians, Spain

The role of the clinical research monitor, as part of the clinical trial team, is discussed under the light of the current legal framework (ICG Guideline for GCP, 1996; WHO Guideline for GCP, 1995).

A description of the background, qualifications, training and expertise of these professionals is presented, as well as career development expectations and various particular roles they can take on as part of a clinical research group, within and without the pharmaceutical industry.

The main responsibilities of the clinical research monitor; ensuring that the rights and well-being of clinical trial participants are protected; that the reported data are accurate, complete and verifiable; and that the clinical trial is conducted in compliance with the protocol, Good Clinical Practice and the applicable regulatory requirements, are highlighted.
The activities carried out by the clinical research monitor before study initiation (including investigator and site selection), during the study and following closure of the centres are described.
Finally, questions related to managerial issues, including productivity and quality of clinical research, are discussed.

Key Words: Clinical research monitor. Clinical research associate. Functions. Responsibilities. Good Clinical Practice.

23 June 2003 Whole Day Course

**The Importance of Drug Surveillance**

Mirela Barbu, MD
Specialist in Pharmaceutical Medicine, Head Medical Department, Eli Lilly (Suisse), SA Secretary of the Swiss Society of Clinical Pharmacology and Toxicology (SKPT/SPTC)

Pharmacovigilance is the discipline responsible for collecting, monitoring, evaluating, and communicating information regarding adverse events of investigational and marketed products worldwide in order to maximize the safe use and comply with local laws and regulations as well as GCP guidelines.
The goal of pharmacovigilance is to ensure the safe use of pharmaceutical products by identifying, quantifying, and reporting the associated risks.
The entire process of drug development, from initial discovery through clinical trials to product launch, takes an average of 2,500 days or 6.8 years. The pharmacovigilance process covers the entire life cycle of a drug. This ongoing process begins during clinical trials and extends throughout the postmarketing period.
Adverse Drug Event (ADE): is any untoward medical occurrence in a patient or clinical investigation subject administered a pharmaceutical product and which does not have to have a causal relationship with this treatment.
Serious Adverse Drug Event (SAE) is an event who has possibly caused death, hospitalization or prolonged hospitalization, is life-threatening, causes congenital anomaly, disability or overdose.
In clinical trials, ADEs and SAEs must be reported within different timelines which will be described in further details during the presentation.
A brief description of Safety Mailings and Periodic Safety Update Reports will be provided

24 June 2003 Whole Day Course

**The Nature-nurture Controversy. Concepts and Methods. Twin-studies in Pharmacogenetics**

Kirsten Kyvik
Institute of Public Health, University of Southern Denmark

Studies of twins have been used for several decades to disentangle the relative importance of genetic and environmental variance for diseases and quantitative phenotypes.
While a clustering of a phenotype in a family is often attributed to genes shared within the family this could just as well be caused by the shared environment. Twin studies is a good means to circumvent this problem.
Dizygotic twin pairs share approximately 50% of their genes like ordinary siblings, while monozygotic twin pairs are genetically identical. Both types of twins share intrapairwise environment to the same degree despite the twofold difference in genetic similarity.
This means (1) that discordance in monozygotic pairs can be attributed to environmental effects
(2) that a greater phenotypic similarity among monozygotic than dizygotic twins must be caused by the greater genetic similarity, i.e. the trait of disease or a disease is influenced by genetic factors.
In addition to this so-called classical twin study twins can be used as a mean to demonstrate the presence of gene/environment interaction to identify important environmental exposures and as a mean to identify important genes or genetic

markers for interesting phenotypes. This means that twin studies are also important for pharmacogenetics.
In the lecture the basics of genetic epidemiology and twin study will be taught with a demonstration of cases from pharmacologic and -genetic areas.

24 June 2003 Whole Day Course

**The Pharmacogenetics of Cytochrome P450 2C9**

Umit Yasar
Department of Pharmacology, Faculty of Medicine, Hacettepe University. Ankara, Turkey

Cytochrome P450 2C9 (CYP2C9) is one of the most important drug metabolizing enzymes in human liver. It catalyses the metabolism of a wide range of different drugs such as S-warfarin, acenocoumarol, phenytoin, losartan, irbesartan, numerous oral antidiabetics, non-steroidal anti-inflammatory drugs and some endogenous compounds such as arachidonic acid. Single nucleotide polymorphisms in the coding region of the CYP2C9 gene give rise to enzyme variants with different amino acid residues and enzymatic properties. Twelve distinct genetic polymorphisms have been identified in different populations (www.imm.ki.se/cypalleles/cyp2c9.htm). The most common enzyme variants originate from the CYP2C9*2 and CYP2C9*3 alleles (approximately 35% of Caucasian individuals) that code for enzymes with amino acid substitutions RR144C and I359L, respectively. These alleles are significantly less prevalent in African and Asian populations. There is accumulating evidence that this genetic polymorphism gives rise to clinically important interindividual differences in drug metabolism are related to this genetic polymorphism. The clinical consequences of these genetic polymorphisms can be serious. Patients with these variant genotypes appear to be more susceptible to side effects during the treatment with the narrow therapeutic index drugs such as warfarin and phenytoin. It is of interest to clarify the potential clinical use of genotyping and phenotyping of CYP2C9 prior to initiation of therapy with these drugs.

24 June 2003 Whole Day Course

**The Pharmacogenetics of CYP2C19**

Marja-Liisa Dahl
Dept of Medical Sciences, Clinical Pharmacology, University Hospital, Uppsala, Sweden

The CYP2C19 polymorphism, originally described as the mephenytoin hydroxylation polymorphism, influences the metabolism of a number of drugs from different therapeutic and chemical groups. These include proton pump inhibitors, diazepam, phenytoin, the antimalarial proguanil and certain antidepressants. About 3% of Caucasians but as many as 15-25 % of Orientals are classified as poor metabolisers (PM). The hydroxylations of S-mephenytoin and omeprazol co-segregate, and omeprazole has been validated as an alternative probe for CYP2C19 phenotyping. The major *CYP2C19* gene variant associated with the PM phenotype is *CYP2C19*2*, with an allele frequency of about 13% in Caucasians and 32% in Orientals. Another major variant is *CYP2C19*3*, found at a frequency of about 12% in Orientals, but very rarely in Caucasians. Up to now, further six defect variants (*CYP2C19 *4* to **8*) associated with no enzyme activity have been described. The clinical impact of CYP2C19 polymorphism on drug pharmacokinetics and pharmacodynamics is best described for proton pump inhibitors, PM having greater drug exposure, suppression of acid secretion, and better ulcer healing compared to extensive metabolisers (EM). CYP2C19 is the major enzyme activating proguanil to cycloguanil, but it has not been established whether PM are at a higher risk for treatment failure compared to EM.

24 June 2003 Whole Day Course

**Genetic Polymorphisms and Drug Dosing**

Julia Kirchheiner
Institute of Clinical Pharmacology, Charité, Humboldt University of Berlin

In many cases, drug therapy is characterized by a high rate of therapeutic failure and difficulties in predicting drug response and adverse drug effects. Genetic factors are known to cause high inter-individual variability in drug efficacy and adverse events. A great impact of genetic polymorphisms in cytochrome P450 drug metabolizing enzymes has been demonstrated for many drugs such as ß-blockers, antidepressants, antipsychotics, antiemetic drugs etc. Due to polymorphisms in the CYP2D6 gene, oral clearances of drugs which are CYP2D6 substrates might differ up to ten-fold; however, genetic factors are not yet considered in every-day clinical practice. If pharmacogenetic diagnostics is to be used for optimizing individual drug therapy, concise recommendations for selecting therapeutic strategies and dosages have to be derived from pharmacogenetic data. Dose adaptations could be calculated from pharmacokinetic studies according to the principles of bioequivalence. However, non-linear kinetics, enantioselective metabolism, and pharmacological activity of metabolites have to be taken into account. The final aim is, to study the genetic variability not only in drug pharmacokinetics but also in drug transport and drug action to develop valid predictors of drug response. However, most results from studies of polymorphisms in molecular receptors, transporters and molecules of signal transduction cannot yet be translated into treatment recommendations. This is partly due to difficulties in replication of data found in explorative trials but as well due to the complexity of the gene-gene and gene-environment interactions involved: rather than simple influences of single polymorphisms, complex systems have to be considered. Haplotype-analyses, consideration of multiple genes and multiple environmental factors and their interactions might reveal the best and worst responder genotype and the overall susceptibility to adverse drug effects.

---

24 June 2003 Whole Day Course

**Pharmaco-economics of Losartan in Type 2 Diabetic Patients with Nephropathy; Comparing the Within-trial Analysis and Markov Modelling**

MJ Postma, J At Thobari

Groningen University Institute for Drug Exploration / university of Groningen Research Institute of Pharmacy (GUIDE/GRIP), Groningen, Netherlands

Background The RENAAL (Reduction of End Points in type 2 Diabetes with the Angiotensin II Antagonist Losartan) clinical trial has shown that losartan confers health gains to diabetes type 2 patients with nephropathy beyond mere blood pressure control only. Particularly, in addition end-stage renal disease (ESRD) is delayed. RENAAL provides the first hard-endpoint evidence for any drug on renal protection for this patient group. Whether savings on expensive care for ESRD outweigh the costs of long-term pharmacotherapy with losartan (net cost savings) is the core pharmaco-economic question addressed here.

Objective To estimate the pharmaco-economic profile of losartan in type 2 diabetic patients with nephropathy in the Netherlands.

Methods Both a within-trial analysis of RENAAL, based on bootstrapping and a Markov-model approach were used. Any within-trial analysis is based directly on the data from the randomised clinical trial and this averts the necessity of making many assumptions. Furthermore it enables derivation of formal 95%-confidence intervals for pharmaco-economic profiles to be elaborated. Drawbacks of the method refer to inflexibility with regard to sensitivity analysis and limited time horizon of the analysis corresponding with follow-up in the trial only. Markov-modelling allows analysis beyond the clinical trial horizon and extensive variation in assumptions in sensitivity analysis. In particular, we varied assumptions regarding progression of disease (nephropathy ↓ ESRD) as representativeness of RENAAL for the specific Dutch patient population remains unclear. For the Markov-model these assumptions were derived from (i) the RENAAL-trial and (ii) the assumptions used for the development of the Dutch treatment guideline for diabetes type 2.

Results (i) Drawing the assumptions for the Markov-model directly from RENAAL, the model confirms findings from the within-trial analysis of potential net cost savings. Furthermore, net cost savings remain if the time horizon for analysis is extended beyond that of RENAAL (4 years ↓ 10 years). (ii) Factoring in the assumptions of the Dutch treatment guideline, still potential cost savings are suggested, however only on the long term (starting from 5 years follow-up and beyond).

Discussion & Conclusions We performed a combined approach to the pharmaco-economics of losartan using both a within-trial analysis on

RENAAL and a Markov model to extend the analysis beyond the clinical trial. We estimated a favorable long-term pharmaco-economic profile using both methods of analysis and various assumptions.

25 June 2003 08:30 – 11:00

## Genetic Factors in the Response to Treatment for Hypertension

Morris J. Brown
University of Cambridge, UK

Hypertension is the commonest cause of serious morbidity in the West, and there is a higher genuine choice of drug classes for hypertension than for most other diseases. Antihypertensive drugs lend themselves therefore to an investigation of genetic variation in drug response. We undertook a series of drug rotations in which patients received in random order each of the main classes. The results of these studies confirmed systematic variation in patients' response to different classes, but did not support the existence of discrete groups of patients responding best to each of the main classes.[1,2] Drug classes fell into two main classes, those working by suppression of the renin system – ACE inhibitors, Angiotensin blockers, β blockers – and those which lower blood pressure through natriuresis and vasodilatation – Calcium blockers and Diuretics. This recognition led to our AB/CD rule now adopted as part of the British Hypertension Society guidelines for treatment of hypertension.[3] This rule recognises that, within a population, the over-riding influence on type of hypertension and response to treatment is not genetic variation but age as a surrogate for the level of plasma renin.[4] The results are concordant with recent genome scans that have failed to find consistent genetic loci for hypertension with LOD scores >3.[5-7] We conclude from these two types of study that in the typical hypertensive patient a large number of genes are each making a small contribution, that will be hard to detect. By contrast, in patients who are atypical for their age group – particular young low-renin patients with $Na^+$ dependent hypertension – a number of rare monogenic syndromes are recognised which are profoundly sensitive to particular diuretics.[8,9] Within essential hypertension, we now recognise resistant hypertension as a clue to the presence of spironolactone sensitive hypertension,[9,10] and predict that in this population and their offspring we will find genetic variants increasing secretion or response to aldosterone.[9]

1. Dickerson JE, Hingorani AD, Ashby MJ, Palmer CR, Brown MJ. Optimisation of antihypertensive treatment by crossover rotation of four major classes. *Lancet* 1999;**353**:2008-2013.
2. Deary A, Schumann A, Murfet H, Haydock S, Foo R, Brown M. Double-blind, placebo-controlled crossover comparison of five classes of antihypertensive drugs. *Journal of Hypertension* 2002;**20**:771-777.
3. Brown MJ, Cruickshank JK, Dominiczak AF, et al. Better blood pressure control: how to combine drugs. *J Hum Hypertens* 2003;**17**:81-6.
4. Laragh JH, Letcher RL, Pickering TG. Renin profiling for diagnosis and treatment of hypertension. *JAMA* 1979;**241**:151-6.
5. Sharma P, Fatibene J, Ferraro F, et al. A genome-wide search for susceptibility loci to human essential hypertension. *Hypertension* 2000;**35**:1291-5.
6. Kardia SLR, Rozek LS, Krushkal J, et al. Genome-wide linkage analyses for hypertension genes in two ethnically and geographically diverse populations. *American Journal of Hypertension* 2003;**16**:154-157.
7. Caulfield M, Pembroke J, Dominiczak A, et al. The MRC British Genetics of Hypertension Study: genome-wide screen results. *J Hum Hypertens* 2002;**16**:18.
8. Lifton RP. Molecular Genetics of Human Blood Pressure Variation. *Science* 1996;**272**:676-680.
9. Mackenzie IS, Brown MJ. Genetic profiling versus drug rotation in the optimisation of antihypertensive treatment. *Clin Med* 2002;**5**:465-473.
10. Lim PO, Jung RT, MacDonald TM. Raised aldosterone to renin ratio predicts antihypertensive efficacy of spironolactone: a prospective cohort follow-up study. *Br J Clin Pharmacol* 1999;**48**:756-60.

25 June 2003 08:30 – 11:00

## Consequences of the Lack of Drugs for Children. The Situation in Europe

H. W. Seyberth
Department of Pediatrics, University of Marburg

For long children has been considered as small adults, who can be treated with adult medicines just by deviding the dose by simple rules. However, children are in a dynamic process of development and they differ from adults by anatomy, physiology, pathophysiology, and pschology and therefore certainly also by pharmacotherapy! Now at least five phases of development have been defined by the ICH guidelines: the preterm newborn infant, the term newborn infant, the infant and toddler, the child, and the adolescent. Nevertheless many medicines used in children by pass the licensing process. Already in the early 80's we showed that 89 % of 41 standard drugs used in the ICU for newborns, 68 % for infants, and 43 % for children were not licensed or labeled for the use in these age groups. This observation has been cooperated in the last few years in many other European countries. As a consequence of unlabeled drug use no dosage recommendation, warning for adverse drug reactions (ADRs) and drug interactions nor pediatric preparations are available. Therefore it is not suprising that ADRs have been observed about twice as often in children when medicines are prescribed outside the marketing authorization. It is hoped that the long expected European Regulation Better-Medicines-for-Children will close the gap in drug tehrapy for European children!

---

25 June 2003 08:30 - 11:00

**Pediatric Medicine Availability in Europe**

Ceci A.[1], Baiardi P.[2], Felisi M.[2]
[1]Dipartimento di Farmacologia e Fisiologia Umana, Università degli Studi di Bari, Italy
[2]Consorzio per le Valutazioni Biologiche e Farmacologiche, Fondazione "S. Maugeri" - Università di Pavia, Italy

The lack of specific drugs for the paediatric population is a problem known for time. In the past years to reduce the gap in paediatric medicine availability in Europe, the EU Institutions developed a number of initiatives that have led to limited results. In front of this situation, the European Commission - Enterprise Directorate has recently taken specific actions to promote research and development of paediatric medicines (economic incentives, legal requirements, etc).

In order to evaluate if the taken measures are leading to real benefits in the field of paediatric pharmaceutical products at European level and to provide proper information on rational use of medicines in children, a monitoring electronic system of the drugs - authorised under Centralised and Mutual Recognition procedures in the European Community - has been set up. The database - organised by active ingredient and medicinal product – collects: paediatric indications, formulations, dosages, contraindications, timing and typing of the studies which have allowed paediatric uses and it is intended to monitor and possibly compare paediatric medicine availability among different Member States.

Currently, the database collects information either on 144-CP and 143-MR drugs respectively. Availability of medicines for children significantly differs among the two considered, groups varying from 13 to 32 %, as well it's different the number of paediatric studies which have led to the product authorisation.

---

25 June 2003 08:30 - 11:00

**Drug Evaluation in Children**

Gerard Pons
Paris, France

Specific problems have to be overcome during drug evaluation in children : invasiveness, difficulties in measuring the effect of drugs, ethical issues in when to expose children for the first time to a new chemical entity, in the use of placebo, patients recruitment due to the low incidence of some diseases, the dispersion of patients, the parent's reluctance to chidren's involvement in clinical studies.

Some methodological approaches are proposed to overcome these difficulties:

- The population pharmacokinetic approach, less invasive than the classical approach
- The Continual Reassessement Method, a sequential Bayesian approach aiming with about 20 patients at screening the dose to be used in phase III trials.
- Sequential approaches such as the Triangular test in phase III comparative trials allowing to stop the study as soon as the collected informations are sufficient to reach the conclusion Treatment responder population enrichment before randomization allowing a smaller number of patients
- Post-marketing long term prospective follow-up studies for late toxicity not predicted on developing organs and side effects that occur far beyond the period of drug exposure.

An appropriate strategy in the onset of drug development in children has been proposed by ICH E11.

25 June 2003 08:30 – 11:00

**Legislative Incentives in Europe – Current Status**

Kalle Hoppu
Medical Director, Poison Information Centre, Helsinki University Central Hospital, Helsinki, Finland

The development of modern pharmaceutical regulations was to a large extent the result of drug catastrophes, mainly involving children. However, children have not been able to fully profit from new therapeutic advantages since. The problem of paediatric drugs, although known for decades, has seriously been approached first in the late 1990.ies in the US.

The present EU Orphan Regulation (EU 141/2000) in effect since 16.12.1999, provides incentives for development of medicinal products intended for rare disorders. These incentives can, and have been used also to develop and bring to market medicinal products for paediatric diseases. However, the Orphan Regulation is not enough to solve the problem of paediatric drugs.

During the French EU Presidency, in July 2000, a Memorandum on Paediatric Medicinal products was presented for the Health Council of the EU. The Council adopted a Resolution on Paediatric Medicinal Products on 14.12.2000, requiring the EU Commission to take action. The EU Commission released a Consultation document "Better Medicines for Children" on 28.2.2002. The Commission is currently drafting a new Paediatric Regulation. The first legislative proposal was expected before the end of last year (2002) and the regulation was expected to be operational in 2003-2004. However, as of April 2003 legislative proposal it has and not yet been presented.

25 June 2003 08:30 – 11:00

**Progress in the Nutritional Treatment of Diabetes**

Prof. Nicholas Katsilambros, MD
Medical Director, 1st Department of Propaedeutic Medicine of the Athens University

The field of nutrition and diabetes is generally very controversial. One reason for that is that the scientific evidence presented in the literature often suffers from major flaws due to inadequate-sometimes unavoidable – study methodology.

The prescription of a diet for a diabetic patient is influenced from a variety of factors including sex, age, degree of obesity, level of activity, cultural and ethnic aspects and the presence or not of diabetic complications.

The goals of nutrition therapy can be summarized as follows:

- maintenance of as near-normal glucose levels as possible
- achievement of optimal serum lipid levels
- provision of adequate calories for maintaining or attaining reasonable weights for adults and normal growth and development rates in children and adolescents
- prevention and treatment of the diabetic complications
- improvement of overall health through optimal nutrition.

It should be noted that energy restriction even in the absence of weight loss improves the metabolic abnormalities.

It is reminded that the vast majority of diabetic persons belong to type 2 of the disease and most of them are over-weight. Therefore, a reduction in energy intake is recommended.

According to the most recent recommendations of the Nutrition Study Group of the European Association for the Study of Diabetes, 60 to 70% of the total daily energy should be covered form a combination of carbohydrates and monounsaturated fatty acids with a cis-configuration. The percentage of energy contributed by each may vary according to individual preferences and clinical characteristics. It is, also, important to reduce the intake of saturated and trans unsaturated fatty acids (< 10% total energy). Protein intake should not exceed 20% total energy intake. Rich in fibre and/or antioxidant carbohydrate containing foods (fruits, vegetables, legumes) or those with a low glycaemic index are strongly recommended. Moderate amounts of foods rich in ω3-fatty acids (mainly oily fish) should be regularly consumed.

25 June 2003 14:30 – 17:00

**Role of Drug Transporters at Blood-Tissue Barriers**

Alfred H Schinkel, Johan W Jonker, Maarten T Huisman, Antonius E van Herwaarden, Corina MM van der Kruijssen, Ellen CM Bolscher, Els Wagenaar
Div. Experimental Therapy, The Netherlands Cancer Institute, Amsterdam, The Netherlands

Our research focuses on genes and proteins that cause multidrug resistance in tumors and influence the pharmacological behavior of anticancer, anti-HIV/AIDS and many other drugs. Insight into these systems may improve chemotherapy approaches for cancer and HIV/AIDS, as well as pharmacotherapy in a broader sense. To study the physiological, pharmacological and toxicological roles of the proteins involved and their interactions, we generate and analyze knockout or transgenic mice lacking or overexpressing the relevant genes.

We have established that the murine ABC transporters P-glycoprotein (Abcb1a) and Breast Cancer Resistance Protein (Bcrp1/Abcg2) have important roles in limiting the oral availability of a range of substrate drugs, toxins and carcinogens, in mediating their hepatobiliary and intestinal excretion, and in restricting the penetration of these compounds in a range of critical tissues, including brain, testis, and fetus. Data obtained by others in Mrp2 (Abcc2) mutant rats indicate that Mrp2 has similar functions with respect to oral availability and hepatobiliary, and possibly intestinal and renal excretion of substrate compounds. There is extensive overlap between the transported substrates of P-glycoprotein, BCRP and MRP2, suggesting that the concerted action of these transporters will have a profound impact on the general pharmacokinetics of such shared substrates. Moreover, the modulation of the activity of each of these transporters with various other co-administered compounds can markedly affect the in vivo pharmacokinetic and toxicological behavior of substrate compounds. The challenge for the future will be to investigate whether such pharmacological modulation of transporter activity can be used to advantage in order to improve pharmacotherapy. Compound knockout mouse strains with deficiencies in two or more of the drug transporters will be valuable tools to study such transporter modulation strategies in vivo.

25 June 2003 14:30 – 17:00

**P-glycoprotein and Antiretroviral Therapy**

David J Back
Dept of Pharmacology & Therapeutics, University of Liverpool, Liverpool, UK

P-gp is a 170 kDa membrane glycoprotein. Two closely related genes, *ABCB1* (*MDR1*) and *ABCB4* (*MDR2* or *MDR3*), encode P-gps. The *ABCB1* gene product encodes for the transporter implicated in efflux of many xenobiotics. P-gp is distributed in liver, colon, jejunum, kidney, the blood-brain barrier and blood-testis barrier and this has implications for both the bioavailability of some antiretroviral drugs (particularly protease inhibitors, PIs) and limiting penetration to these organs, with the resultant formation of sanctuary sites for the virus. In addition, human lymphocytes express P-gp with different cell subsets expressing variable levels of the protein (CD56+ cells > CD8+ > CD4+). P-gp expression in the lymphocyte alters the *in vivo* accumulation of PIs, raising the possibility that P-gp expression may impact on treatment outcome. These issues have fuelled the investigation of the role of genetic variations in the *ABCB1* gene on P-gp, drug exposure and immune recovery in HIV and a correlation between the C3435T single nucleotide polymorphism (SNP) was recently observed. The C3435T SNP is a non-coding, non-promoter SNP in exon 26. It is unlikely to affect *ABCB1* gene expression *per se*, but may be linked to functionally important SNPs in the promoter or enhancer regions of the *ABCB1* gene. Further investigations are required to determine haplotypes in relation to both pharmacokinetics and virological and immunological outcome. Also since PIs are substrates for MRP1/2 it is important to delineate the role of these transporters in PI pharmacokinetics/pharmacodynamics.

25 June 2003 14:30 – 17:00

## Functional Interaction of Intestinal CYP3A4 and P-glycoprotein

Martin F. Fromm
Dr. Margarete Fischer-Bosch-Institute of Clinical Pharmacology, Stuttgart, Germany

Many drugs are substrates of both CYP3A4 and P-glycoprotein. The gut wall mucosa is the first barrier, which limits access of orally administered drugs to the systemic circulation. Enterocytes express the efflux transporter P-glycoprotein in their apical membrane, which pumps its substrates back into the gut lumen. Moreover, the major drug metabolizing enzyme CYP3A4 is localized in enterocytes and can cause considerable prehepatic extraction of certain drugs. Recent human data generated with a multilumen perfusion catheter will be shown, indicating that intestinal CYP3A4 and P-glycoprotein act in a coordinate fashion and determine plasma concentrations after oral administration of its substrates (e.g. the antiarrhythmic quinidine). Moreover, direct measurements of intraluminal drug concentrations indicate that intestinal P-glycoprotein is a major determinant of drug absorption in humans. Taken together, intestinal CYP3A4 and P-glycoprotein are major determinants of variable pharmacokinetics of orally administered drugs.

25 June 2003 14:30 – 17:00

## Drug Transporters and Hepatotoxicity

Peter Meier-Abt
Clinical Pharmacology and Toxicology, University Hospital, Zurich, Switzerland

Hepatic uptake and excretion of drugs is mediated by distinct transport systems at the sinusoidal and canalicular membrane domains of hepatocytes. Drug uptake is mediated predominantly by members of the superfamily of organic anions transporting proteins (Oatps/OATPs; gene symbol, SLC21A) (BBA 1609, 1-18, 2003).They include Oatp1 (Slc21a1), Oatp2 (Slc21a5) and Oatp4 (Slc21a10) in rodent and OATP-C (SLC21A6) and OATP8 (SLC21A8) in human liver. Drug induced Oatp/OATP inhibition (e.g. rifampicin, cyclosporine A) as well as genetic polymorphisms leading to downregulation of OATP-C expression (Pharmacogenetics 13, 189-198, 2003) can increase the oral bioavailability and systemic toxicity of certain drugs (e.g. statins), but also reduces the hepatotoxicity of certain hepatotoxins (e.g. phalloidin, microcystins). - On the canalicular side hepatocytes express an array of ABC (ATP-Binding Cassette) transporters including the multidrug resistance P-glycoprotein MDR1 (ABCB1), the phospholipid translocase MDR3 (ABCB4), the bile salt export pump Bsep/BSEP (ABCB11), the multi-organic anion pump MRP2 (ABCC2), the breast cancer resistance potein BCRP (ABCG2), and the cholesterol flippase ABCG5/G8 (ABCG5,ABCG8). Hereditary defects in expression of MDR3 and BSEP result in severe familial intrahepatic cholestasis. Lack of MRP2 expression is the cause of Dubin-Johnson syndrome. Drug induced inhibition of BSEP or stimulation of MRP2 can cause drug induced cholestatic liver disease.

25 June 2003 14:30 – 17:00

## Pharmacological Treatment of Cancer Pain

Vittorio Vetafridda

The analgesic drug treatment of cancer pain is based on recommendation of WHO which in 1986 published the Cancer Pain Relief. This method relied on the use of the three step ladder. On the first step, N.S.A.I.D; second step, weak opioids; third step, strong opioids. Adjuvant drugs (anticonvulsant, psychotropic, steroids) are added for particular pain situation.

The author revise up to date this method, in particularly on the use of opioids and on the existing problem for availability, administration and information regarding the their use. The morphine consumption is regarded as an attitude of care givers on the issue of Cancer pain Relief, which is nowadays very low or non existing in several Countries. This problem is responsible of the severe pain on advanced cancer patients. Governments should applied new rules for the facilitation of the use of opioids drugs and great campaign on education and on modality of Cancer Pain Relief.

25 June 2003 14:30 – 17:00

## Development, Evaluation and Validation of Biomarkers: Mechanism-Based PK/PD Modelling

Meindert Danhof, PharmD, PhD
Leiden/Amsterdam Center for Drug Research, Division of Pharmacology, Leiden, The Netherlands

In recent years important progress has been made in the field of pharmacokinetic/ pharmacodynamic (PK/PD) modelling. Key elements in this development have been the incorporation of receptor theory and dynamical systems analysis. This has resulted in an entirely new class of mechanism-based PK/PD models with much improved properties for extrapolation and prediction. An important feature of mechanism-based PK/PD models is that they contain specific expressions for processes on the causal path between drug administration and response. This has implications for the development, evaluation and validation of biomarkers. In this context the COST-B15 Working Group 'Markers of Pharmacological and Toxicological Action' of the European Union has proposed a mechanism-based classification of biomarkers: 0. Phenotype/genotype, 1. Concentration, 2. Target occupancy, 3. Target activation, 4. Physiological measures, 5. Disease processes and 6. Clinical scales. In addition strategies for the evaluation and validation of biomarkers are proposed, which are based on the application of mechanism-based PK/PD modelling concepts. The importance of developing biomarkers very early in drug development (i.e. in the pre-clinical phases) is emphasised.

25 June 2003 14:30 – 17:00

## Clinical Pharmacology = Disease Progress + Drug Action

Nicholas HG Holford
MBChB, FRACP

Clinical pharmacology is based on an understanding of diseases and drugs. The action of drugs on health can be understood in terms of models for disease progress. Drug action covers all aspects of pharmacology – including in particular pharmacokinetics (dose-time-concentration) and pharmacodynamics (dose-concentration-effect). Drug action can be described in terms of its mechanism e.g. at a receptor, patho-physiological responses (biomarker), and clinical outcome. Disease process can be described in terms of the time course of a disease status. Disease status defines the activity of the disease at a point in time. The status may be a biomarker e.g. blood pressure or a clinical outcome e.g. pain intensity.

Typically there is little or no theoretical basis for predicting the time course of disease progress therefore we must resort to descriptive, empirical models. If disease progress is slow then over an appropriately short interval a linear function of time can provide an adequate model for description, interpolation and some limited extrapolation. The slope of the line describes the rate of disease progression. Disease time profiles may be known to have an asymptote that suggests exponential models as a basis for description and the convenient parameterisation of progress in terms of a disease progress half-life.

Chan PLS and Holford NHG (2001) Drug treatment effects on disease progression. Annual Review of Pharmacology and Toxicology 41:625-659.
Holford NHG, Mould DR and Peck CC (2001) Disease Progress Models, in Principles of Clinical Pharmacology (Atkinson A ed) pp 253-262, Academic Press, San Diego.

25 June 2003 14:30 – 17:00

## Development and Application of Biomarkers for Safety, Focussing on the Toxicological Aspects

Munir Pirmohamed
Department of Pharmacology, The University of Liverpool, Ashton Street, Liverpool, UK

Drug safety issues are an important consideration for both healthcare systems and the pharmaceutical industry. For the former, adverse drug reactions cause a considerable degree of morbidity and mortality, and unnecessary costs, while for the industry, drug withdrawal due to the occurrence of adverse reaction represents a major economic burden. The identification of biomarkers that predict both the potential of a drug to cause toxicity, and the susceptibility of an individual, would be a major advance. Biomarkers in this regard can be defined as indicators signalling events in biological systems and samples that can be used to clarify the relationship, if any, between exposure to a xenobiotic substance and disease. The US National Research Council has suggested that biomarkers can be divided into three different categories:

- Biomarkers of exposure, e.g. the measurement of low-level toxic metabolites important in the pathogenesis of an adverse reaction.
- Biomarkers of effect, e.g. the measurement of parameters that indicate that the drug is having an effect, which may be adverse, on an organ.
- Biomarkers of susceptibility, e.g. indicators that suggest an unusual sensitivity of an individual to a xenobiotic.

In this presentation, these three areas will be considered in further detail, in particular to highlight the current state of knowledge, the problems with existing biomarkers, and how the use of the new technologies may allow the identification of novel biomarkers, which in turn may be used to reduce the burden of toxicity caused by prescription medicines and environmental toxicants.

---

25 June 2003 14:30 - 17:00

**Advanced Modelling and Simulation Technologies with Emphasis on the Modelling from Biomarkers to Clinical Outcome**

Oscar Della Pasqua
Division of Pharmacology, LACDR,University of Leiden, The Netherlands, Clinical Pharmacology & Discovery Medicine, GlaxoSmithKline, United Kingdom

Biomarkers have been used as surrogate endpoints in medical research when the end-point of primary interest is difficult to observe. For example, in HIV research viral load or CD4 cell-count may be used as surrogate for progression to AIDS. The literature on the use of biomarkers in the analysis of data from clinical trials is rather extensive, and, quite apart from its technical variety, displays a wide range of theoretical positions concerning the aims of the data analysis in establishing the significance of a treatment effect. However, extrapolation from drug effect on biomarkers to clinical efficacy remains one of the most controversial aspects of clinical drug development, particularly when the clinical effect is a time-to-event measurement or linked to a categorical scale. This debate is greatly explained by biomarker validation issues and uncertainty about disease mechanisms.

Computer-assisted modelling and simulation has been introduced as a tool to predict and characterise drug response and variability in treatment, becoming an important component of decision-making strategy in drug development. The use of non-linear mixed effects models allow exploration of scenarios to assessing the magnitude of interindividual variability and separating intrinsic from extrinsic variability factors (e.g., disease status vs. compliance). In addition, pharmacostatistical models also enable the user to ask 'What if...?' questions for future scenarios.

Recent advances in mechanism-based modelling have resulted in new approaches for addressing uncertainty and for incorporating biomarker parameter distributions as link between drug exposure and treatment efficacy. In contrast to empirical data mining and conventional statistical hypothesis testing, modelling and simulation technologies can be applied to prospectively optimise clinical trial design. It can lead to further understanding of disease processes and explanation of time-dependencies in the relationship between surrogate and clinical endpoints.

---

26 June 2003 08:30 - 11:00

**The Doping Problem in Sports – New Directions in Prevention**

Arne Ljungqvist

Any anti-doping program should be based on for corner stones - education, information, doping controls and research. Doping controls and their results constitute the most spectacular part of such a program, particularly when great sports stars are found doped. But as in drug misuse in general, prevention should be priority one. This is best achieved by proper information and education. To that effect a joint initiative has recently been taken by the Stockholm University College of Physical Education and Sports, the International Association of Athletic Federations (IAAF), the Union des Associations Européens de Football (UEFA), Ligue Européenne de Natation (LEN) and International Doping Tests & Management (IDTM). A web-based Anti-Doping Education program was developed for young athletes in Europe (YAADIS) in order to make information and education easily accessible and affordable. This education program will be presented in detail.

26 June 2003 08:30 – 11:00

**Detection of Doping by Analytical Methods**

Jordi Segura
Municipal Institute for Medical Research IMIM-UPF, Barcelona, Spain

The presence of a prohibited substance in a biological fluid of an athlete is recognized as the strongest evidence of doping in sport. Reliable and accurate methods of analyses are required to warranty total fairness for the subjects involved.

Analytical methods used are designed to identify in a first step any suspicious sample (screening) and subsequently to unambiguosly demonstrate the presence of a prohibited substance (confirmation), if present. Sample preparation usually requires solid or liquid phase extractions and enzymatic hydrolysis of metabolite's conjugates. Separation of analytes is usually carried out by gas and liquid chromatography. Final identification makes use of different types of mass spectrometry (low and high resolution, tandem MS, isotopic ratio measurements, etc).

When the prohibited substance is identical to a body hormone (eg. erythropoietin or growth hormone), either indirect (measure of some surrogate physiological markers) or direct (attempt to differentiate the endogenous natural hormone from the externally administered prohibited analogue) methods are used.

The accredited anti-doping laboratories are tightened by severe controls by the ISO system (ISO 17025) and sport accreditation bodies (International Olympic Committee and the World Anti-doping Agency) regulations.

26 June 2003 08:30 – 11:00

**Genetic Confounders in Androgen Metabolism and Doping Tests**

Jenny Jakobsson, Lena Ekström, Mats Garle, Ingemar Björkhem and Anders Rane
Department of Laboratory Medicine at Karolinska Institutet, Division of Clinical Pharmacology, Huddinge University Hospital, SE-141 86 Stockholm, Sweden

The testosterone/epitestosterone urinary concentration ratio (T/EpiT) is one of the mainstays in the testing program for doping with anabolic androgenic steroids (AAS). Epitestosterone (EpiT) is a naturally occurring 17α-hydroxy epimer of testosterone (T). To detect T abuse the urinary T/EpiT ratio is measured. According to the International Olympic Committee, aA urinary ratio above 6 is considered an indication of abuse of certain androgens including Ttestosterone. However, large inter-individual and inter-ethnic differences in this ratio have been detected. Orientals generally have lower T/EpiT ratios (< 0.5) than Caucasians (around 1). Constitutional T/EpiT ratios >6 have been found in Caucasian individuals.

Androstenedione is a weak androgen that is converted to T in the body. Whereas androstenedione administration has beenis associated with an increase of urinary EpiT levels in the majority of Asians (Catlin, et al., 2002; own observations) this occurs only rarely in Caucasians. The enzyme responsible for this conversion has not yet been identified. We are searching for the enzyme catalysing the T → EpiT conversion in order to investigate the genetic basis of the variation in excretion.

We have investigated the presence of SNPs in genes of importance for androgen turnover and urinary excretion of androgens. Based on previously published information 3α-hydroxysteroid dehydrogenase (3α-HSD) is a likely candidate for this reaction. There are three human types of 3α-HSD with different substrate specificities and different tissue distribution. in the body.

We have identified 4 polymorphisms in the 3α-HSD II gene, of which one is in the coding region and non-synonymousexon . The allele frequency of this mutation is different in Caucasians and in

Asians. The different phenotypes are currently investigated in bioassays and may be related to the observed difference in formation of EpiT and in urinary T/EpiT ratios.
Genetic differences are important to investigate since it has major implications for the interpretation of anti-doping test results.

Reference: Catlin et al, Steroids 2002, 67: 559-564.

26 June 2003 08:30 – 11:00

**Challenges in the Design and Evaluation of Bioequivalence Studies in the 21st Century**

Henning H. Blume
SocraTec R&D, Feldbergstr. 59, Oberursel, Germany

The assessment of efficacy and safety as well as the documentation of pharmaceutical quality are essential premises for drug registration in most countries. For this purpose the potential impact of formulation properties on rate and extent of drug absorption has to be evaluated. Bioequivalence studies play an important role in this context, not only for generic products but also for innovator drugs to demonstrate their consistent quality during the clinical development process, from batch to batch during production and until end of shelf life.
In the last 15 years significant progress was achieved concerning the harmonisation of the existing (national or regional) guidelines on the requirements for bioavailability/bioequivalence studies. Nevertheless, some important questions are still unresolved, e.g.

- BA/BE: properly «controlled» by formulation properties or strongly dependent on gastro-instestinal parameters?
- Dose dumping: phantom caused by physiology or product-related reality?
- In-vitro/in-vivo-Correlations: acceptable conditions for extrapolation from dissolution findings to bioequivalence?
- Subject-related factors: terra incognita and uncontrollable?

These aspects should be carefully considered for study design and appropriate interpretation of results obtained in BA/BE investigations.

26 June 2003 08:30 – 11:00

**Epidemiology of the Abuse of Anabolic Steroids**

Ingemar Thiblin
Department of Forensic Medicine, Karolinska Institute, Stockholm

The fact that the use of non-prescription anabolic steroids (AS) is illegal in most countries imposes serious difficulties in designing epidemiological studies concerning mortality and morbidity among abusers of these substances. Prospective randomised controlled studies regarding the long-term effects of supraphysiological doses of AS on human health are, for obvious reasons, impossible to perform. Consequently, most epidemiological studies of this nature have consisted of cross-sectional surveys documenting the life-time prevalence of abuse in a certain region, sometimes supplemented with personal profiles of the abusers and/or the perceived complications of abuse. To date, there is only one published report concerning mortality among AS users or, more precisely, among power weight lifters who were presumed to have used AS earlier. The risk of death was 4.6 times higher among the power lifters compared with the mortality of population controls. At our department of forensic medicine we have recently conducted a cohort study of morbidity and mortality among confirmed users of AS, which showed a standardized mortality ratio of 17.3.

In general, cross-sectional investigations have demonstrated that the life-time prevalence of AS abuse among adolescents or young adults in several Western societies is between 1 and 12%. In addition, consistent associations between such abuse and certain personality traits or disorders and psychiatric or somatic disease have been described in case studies, case series studies or survey studies involving selected populations. Furthermore, longitudinal studies have revealed highly elevated mortality rates among both presumed and confirmed AS abusers.

However, at present the general applicability of these findings and the basic causal relationship are still open questions. There are indications that the majority of heavy AS abusers are difficult to achieve contact with using the conventional methods employed in investigations of prevalence. Thus, more reliable quantitative data regarding the prevalence of AS abuse, as well as both quantitative and qualitative data concerning related morbidity and mortality are needed. Strategies for obtaining acceptably conclusive data in these areas will be discussed, as well as the relevance of the concept "life-time prevalence" in this connection.

26 June 2003 14:00 – 16:00

### Optimal Antibiotic Prescribing: Who Should be Educated

FM Haaijer-Ruskamp
Dept of Clinical Pharmacology, Univ Groningen, The Netherlands

Antibiotic use is high on the agenda. Multi- resistant germs are a worldwide problem, asking for a more restrictive and rational use. Much effort has focussed on supporting doctors to prescribe less. The doctor, however, doesn't only react to research evidence or policy documents, but also to patients' expectations and demands. Moreover, antibiotic use without prescription occurs. Therefore, in recent years more attention has been given to the patient perspective. The perception of the illness that patients have is one of the most important aspects. Patients often feel antibiotics are necessary to speed up recovery or to prevent the illness from getting worse[1]. Patients show different coping strategies to deal with their symptoms which vary from 'nursing one's illness' to using antibiotics[2] Attitudes vary from 'better safe then sorry', to'antibiotics, if there is no alternative', 'rather not but accepting' and 'refusing'. Antibiotic use should be understood against the background of a general ambivalence but also pragmatic considearions. Finally, the general cultural context seems to be relevant. Deschepper[3] provides a convincing argument that the dimensions 'uncertainty avoidance' and 'individualis may help us to understand the different antibiotic levels in Europe. Targeting patients, their beliefs and expectations may be even more important than what has been thought so far, in the effort to rationalise the use of antibiotics and limit resistance.

[1] Duijn H van et al. Patients' views on respiratory tract symptoms. Scan J Prim health Care 2002201-202

[2] Deschepper R et al. Cross-cultural differences in lay attitudes and utilisation of antibiotics in a Belgian and Dutch city. Patient education and counselling 2002;48:191-169

[3] Deschepper R. Verschillen in antibioticagebruik tussen Belgie en Nederland. Shaker Publishing 2002

26 June 2003 14:00 – 16:00

### Drug Utilisation of Antibiotics Versus Development of Resistance

J. Gulbinovic
Centre of Pharmacology, Vilnius University, Lithuania

Antibiotic-resistant bacteria were soon identified after the introduction of these agents into medical practice. While new antibiotics were beeing discovered at a steady rate, little attention was paid to the consequences of resistance. During the last decades very few new agents have been introduced into clinical practice, at the same time the frequency and spectrum of antibiotic resistance were steadily growing. Today the problem of antibiotic resistance is fast escalating into global health crisis. Several lines of evidence suggest that there is a causal association between the use of antimicrobial agents and the prevalence of drugs resistance in microorganisms. This relationship was demonstrated between the use of macrolides and the resistance of group A streptococci to macrolides, between the use of beta-lactams and macrolides and the resistance of S. pneumoniae to penicillin. Existing data relates the resistance of Pseudomonas aeruginosa to fluoroquinolones or to carbamenems to overuse of these agents. However, the results of other studies do not support this. It seems that the problem is more complex and depends not only on amount of antibacterial agents used, but also on other factors, e.g. underdosing, spread of resistant bacteria, lack of infection control.

26 June 2003 14:00 - 16:00

## The Emerging Problem of Therapy Resistant Tuberculosis

Kiivet R.
University of Tartu, Estonia

Despite the effectiveness of antimicrobial chemotherapy, tuberculosis (TB) remains a leading infectious cause of death worldwide. Mycobacterium tuberculosis strains, resistant to antituberculosis drugs have been found in all geographic sites studied. Whereas the median prevalence of multi-drug-resistance (MDR) among new cases of TB has been estimated as 1%, the prevalence in Estonia during the 1990's has been considerably higher - 14-16%.

The aim of the present study was to evaluate adherence of in-patient and out-patient treatment of TB in Estonia to the WHO treatment guidelines in the 1990's - i.e prior to the implementation of the National Programme Against Tuberculosis in 1998. Data for in-patient tuberculosis treatment was obtained from the medical records of in-patients and data on all filled anti-tuberculosis drug prescriptions for out-patient treatment was obtained from the National Health Insurance databases.

Results. Treatment with a single antituberculosis drug or treatment with non-standardised combinations accounted for one-quarter of all treatment days. The individual anti-tuberculosis drugs were consumed in suboptimal daily doses, as defined by less than one third of the recommended dose, on more than half of all treatment days. Thus, the optimal treatment of tuberculosis - minimum of two antituberculosis drugs in adequate daily doses - was used only on minority of treatment days.

Conclusions. Anti-tuberculosis drugs were prescribed by the doctors and purchased by patients in combinations and quantities, which were not adherent to the WHO standardised treatment regimens. Irregular use of anti-tuberculosis treatment in Estonia can be associated with high rate of MDR Mycobacterium tuberculosis.

26 June 2003 14:00 - 16:00

## What is the Rational Use of Medicines?

Hans V. Hogerzeil
MD, PhD, FRCP Edin, World Health Organization, Department of Essential Drugs and Medicines Policy, Geneva

Rational use of medicines implies that patients receive medicines appropriate to their clinical needs, in doses that meet their own individual requirements, for an adequate period of time, and at the lowest cost to them and their community. However, world-wide more than 50% of medicines are prescribed, dispensed or sold inappropriately. Moreover, about one third of the world's population lacks access to essential medicines. Common types of irrational medicines use are poly-pharmacy, inappropriate use of anti-microbials, over-use of injections, failure to prescribe in accordance with clinical guidelines, and inappropriate self-medication.

Twelve core interventions to promote a more rational use of medicines are:

1. A mandated multi-disciplinary national body to coordinate medicines use policies
2. Evidence-based clinical guidelines
3. Essential medicines lists based on treatments of choice, for reimbursement
4. Drug and Therapeutics Committees in districts and hospitals
5. Problem-based pharmacotherapy teaching in undergraduate curricula
6. Continuing in-service training as licensure condition
7. Supervision, audit and feed-back
8. Independent information on medicines
9. Public education about medicines
10. Avoidance of perverse financial incentives
11. Appropriate and enforced regulation
12. Sufficient government expenditure to ensure availability of medicines and staff

Although originally intended for developing countries, an increasing number of developed countries use key components of the essential medicines concept as a means to ensure the rational selection of efficacious, safe and cost-effective medicines for reimbursement. This development was triggered by increasing drug costs and the introduction of many new and often expensive medicines. For example, in the USA annual medicine expenditure rose by 18% in 1999, 16% in 2000 and 17% in 2001; this rise is much higher than the increase in GNP or the consumer price index over the same period. Much of this increase is related to the introduction of new, often expensive medicines.

26 June 2003 14:00 – 16:00

**Does Problem-Based Learing (PBL) Improve Rational Drug Prescribing?**

Vries de ThPGM., Richir M., Vollebregt J.
VU Medical Centre, Vrije Universiteit Amsterdam, The Netherlands

PBL addresses the essential needs of students: involvement and acceptance in their future working surrounding. It enhances the deep approach of learning aimed at understanding the meaning of what they are studying, in contrast to the surface approach aimed at merely reproduce what they learn or copy what they are told. In medical education it has been shown that gaining or revising basic science knowledge during the clinical phase leads to a qualitative change in the knowledge of students rather than a quantitative one. They learn for example that knowledge gained in one area could be applied in others. The level of medical PBL is determined by the concreteness of the problem. It varies from (physiological/pharmacological) concepts of diseases, written clinical cases, video presentations, role-play/simulated patients sessions, to actual clinical experience: the so-called Context Learning(CL). Interestingly, researchers know intuitively that the highest level of CL applies highly for learning how to do research. PBL in clinical pharmacology/therapeutics at various levels is more effective regarding rational drug prescribing than traditional knowledge-based teaching A recent study shows that pre-clinical students who followed a CL program with role-play/simulating patients sessions reach the same level of rational drug choice as graduates! The effect of postgraduate/continuing RUD training is limited due to several factors.

26 June 2003 14:00 – 16:00

**The Rational Use of Medicines**

David Barnett
University of Leicester, Dept of Medicine, Leicester, UK

The Influence of Governmental Institutions on Rational Drug Use : the NICE experience The National Institute for Clinical Excellence (NICE) was established to address the widespread variation in access to health technologies and the need for clear standards of evidence based health care within the NHS. NICE's technology appraisals programme has been established for 3 years and has produced 58 sets of guidance for the NHS in England and Wales. The methodology paradigm for the appraisals programme is based on an independant advisory committee that reviews an inclusive research evidence base of the clinical and cost effectiveness of the technology, as well as written and oral submissions from both specialist health care professionals and patient/carer organisations. The process is fully consultative and transparent at all stgaes. The final guidance feeds directly into NHS policy making and health care commissioners are mandated to make funds available for its implementation at local level. NICE guidance has generally been favourably received despite concerns expressed by the ABPI of restrictions to marketing. The views of health care workers have been variably enthusiastic but all accept the need for rational use of drugs based upon both the best evidence of clincal effectiveness and the rational use of available resources within the NHS. The effects of the NICE programme are becoming evident internationally and a number of countries are considering instituting similar approaches for the rational use of medicines.

26 June 2003 14:00 – 16:00

**The Efficacy of Herbal Medicines**

Edzard Ernst
Director, Complementary Medicine, Peninsula Medical School, Universities of Exeter & Plymouth, Exeter, UK

Herbal medicines are more popular then ever before. This clearly begs the question whether or nor a given herbal remedy is effective in treating a given condition. It is best answered on the basis of randomised (preferably placebo-controlled, double-blind) clinical trials. Where such evidence exists, it is often contradictory, i.e. one trial may show a positive finding while another comes to a negative conclusion. In this situation the best evidence is provided by a systematic review or meta-analysis, i.e. an evaluation of the totality of the available data on a specific topic. More than 40 such articles are available today. They relate to a range of herbal medicines (from aloe vera to peppermint). Examples of some of these systematic reviews will be briefly summarised. Overall conclusions are not possible, as every herbal medicine has to be judged on its own merit. Nevertheless, the data leave little doubt that some (not all) herbal medicines are effective in treating some (not all) clinical conditions.

26 June 2003 14:00 – 16:00

## Herb-Drugs Interactions

Angelo A. Izzo
Department of Experimental Pharmacology, University of Naples Federico II, Naples, Italy

Herbal medicines are mixtures of more than one active ingredient. In many cases it is uncertain which or how many constituents are pharmacologically important. Obviously, the multitude of active ingredients increases the likelihood of interactions. Importantly, the majority of people who use herbal medicine do not reveal this use to their physician or pharmacist, thereby greatly increasing the risk of side-effects from the interactions between herbal components and concurrent pharmacotherapy.

Despite many uncertainties in commercial preparations, herbal medicines adhere to modern pharmacological principles. Hence, herb-drug interactions are based on the same pharmacokinetic and pharmacodynamic principles as drug-drug interactions [1]. Herbal medicines may thus affect absorption (e.g. gum guar reduces digoxin absorption), metabolism (St John's wort may increase the metabolism of a number of drugs including indinavir, warfarin, and cyclosporin) or excretion (St John's wort increases renal excretion of digoxin) of concomitantly administered synthetic drugs [2-3]. Examples of pharmacokinetic herb-drug interaction include the ability of kava to reduce the activity of the antiparkinsonian drug levodopa [2-3].

Interactions between herbal medicines and synthetic drugs pose a serious threat for human health and represent an important issue to be tackled sooner rather than later. Healthcare professionals need to be aware of potential herb-drug interactions and researchers should strive to fill the numerous gaps in our present understanding of this problem.

References

1. Izzo AA, Borrelli F, Capasso R (2002) Herbal medicine: the dangers of drug interaction. Trends Pharmacol Sci;23:358-91.
2. Fugh-Bergman A, Ernst E (2001) Herb-drug interactions: review and assessment of report reliability. Br J Clin Pharmacol 52:587-595.
3. Izzo AA, Ernst E (2001) Interactions between herbal medicines and prescribed drugs. A systematic review. Drugs 61:2163-2175.

26 June 2003 16:15 – 18:15

## The Rational Use of Psychotherapeutic Agents in Primary Care

Rihmer Z.
Natl. Inst. Psychiat. Neurol., Budapest, Hungary

Depression and anxiety are the most frequent psychiatric disorders either in the community or in the general practice. The point-prevalence of these disorders in primary care are 15-25 percent'. A vast majority of depressed and anxious patients visit their general practitioners (GPs), and these two disorders account for more than 80 percent of all psychiatric diagnoses in primary caré. Recent findings indicate that GPs underdiagnose depression and overdiagnose anxiety. Consequently, GPs underutilize antidepressants and overutilize anxiolytics. Particularly depressions with predominantly somatic presentation (masked depression) and with significant somatic comorbidity are not recognized by GPs. There are some evidences that repeated and well-focused postgraduate training for GPs increases their ability to diagnose and treat depressive and anxiety disorders. The rational use of antidepressants and anxiolytics in primary care means to prefer newer (less toxic) compounds, to use them in adequate dose for a sufficient period of time and to avoid polypharmacy.

Lecrubier Y,Hergueta T. Int.Clin.Psychopharmacol.,1998, 13: (. Suppl.2 ) 7-11.
Üstün TB, Gater R. Curr. Opin. Psychiat. 1994,7:173-180.
Rutz W. et al. Acta Psychiat.Scand. 1992, 85: 83-88.

---

26 June 2003 16:15 - 18:15

**Newer Versus Older Antipsychotics: Comparison of Efficacy and Tolerability Profile**

Olav Spigset
Department of Clinical Pharmacology, St. Olav's University Hospital, Trondheim, Norway

In contrast to what is often claimed, it is not unequivocally demonstrated that newer antipsychotic drugs (clozapine, olanzapine, risperidone, ziprasidone, quetiapine and sertindole) are generally more effective and have fewer adverse effects than older antipsychotics. Possible methodological reasons for the discrepancies between the numerous studies and meta-analyses comparing older, first generation, drugs with newer, second generation drugs, will be presented. Focus will be given on issues related to efficacy, both with regard to positive and negative symptoms, as well as on safety, in particular the risk of extrapyramidal symptoms. In addition, specific adverse drug reactions related to newer antipsychotics, including metabolic effects (body weight gain, diabetes, hyperlipidemia) and cardiovascular effects (myocarditis, cardiomyopathy, thromboembolism, long QT syndrome), will be discussed.

---

26 June 2003 16:15 - 18:15

**Drug Interactions with New Psychotropic Drugs**

Edoardo Spina
Section of Pharmacology, Department of Clinical and Experimental Medicine and Pharmacology, University of Messina, Italy

In recent years new psychotropic drugs were introduced in clinical practice including antidepressants, such as selective serotonin reuptake inhibitors (SSRI) and "third generation" antidepressants, and atypical antipsychotics. These agents are extensively metabolised in the liver by cytochrome P450 (CYP) enzymes and are susceptible to metabolically-based drug interactions with other psychotropic medications or with compounds used for the treatment of concomitant somatic illnesses. New antidepressants differ in their potential for metabolic drug interactions. Fluoxetine and paroxetine are potent inhibitors of CYP2D6, fluvoxamine markedly inhibits CYP1A2 and CYP2C19, while nefazodone is a potent inhibitor of CYP3A4. Other new antidepressants, i.e. sertraline, citalopram, venlafaxine, mirtazapine and reboxetine are weak in vitro inhibitors of the different CYP isoforms and appear to have less propensity for important metabolic interactions. The new atypical antipsychotics do not affect significantly the activity of CYP isoenzymes and are not expected to impair the elimination of other medications. Conversely, coadministration of inhibitors or inducers of the CYP isoenzymes involved in metabolism of the various antipsychotic compounds may alter their plasma concentrations, possibly leading to clinically significant effects. Knowledge about the CYP enzymes responsible for the metabolism of any new psychotropic agent and about its effect on the activity of these enzymes may guide selection of an appropriate compound which is less likely to interact with already taken medication(s).

---

26 June 2003 16:15 - 18:15

**Conflicts of Interest in Carrying out a Clinical Trial: Focus on Non-Inferiority and Equivalence Trials**

Silvio Garattini
Mario Negri Institute, Milan, Italy

The latest declaration of Helsinki has reinforced the concept that clinical trials should not use placebo unless no treatment is available for a given indication. Unfortunately, however, European legislation requires that new drugs demonstrate their quality, efficacy and safety as if they were in a therapeutic vacuum. Therefore, new drugs do not need to be compared with existing drugs to obtain approval. Furthermore, for comparative trials there is an increasing tendency to adopt an "equivalence" or "non-inferiority" design. Frequently the trial has "margins" of equivalence too large to obtain any meaningful comparison. The author will discuss when comparative trials with equivalence design are acceptable and when they are ethically unacceptable. Examples will be given that illustrate the tendency to give the market priority over patients' interests.

26 June 2003 16:15 - 18:15

**Conflicts of Interest in Drug and Therapeutics Committees**

Folke Sjöqvist
Department of Clinical Pharmacology, Huddinge University Hospital Stockholm, Sweden

Drug and Therapeutics Committees (DTC:s) play an important tole in promoting the rational use of drugs in many European countries. In Sweden DTC:s are instituted by law at the countylevel (1). The members (clinicians, clinical pharmacologists and pharmacists) make recommendations of the drugs of choice for common disorders and also participate in the purchase of drugs for hospital use from the manufacturers. The committees also have important roles in organizing postgraduate education and information about drugs applying the philosophy - the right drug for the right patient in the right dosage at an affordable price and with the right (unbiased) information. Obviously drug experts involved in this effort have to be free from conflicts of interest vis á vis the pharmaceutical industry. They therefore are obliged to declare of conflicts of interest on an annual basis. While scientific collaboration with industry is encouraged (if transparent) participation (directly or indirectly) in the marketing of individual drug products is considered to be highly inappropriate.

Referens:

1. Sjöqvist F, Bergman U, Dahl M-L, Gustafsson LL, Hensjö L-O. Drug and therapeutics committees: a Swedish experience. WHO Drug Information 2002;16(3):207-13.

27 June 2003 08:30 - 11:00

**Cardiovascular Implications of Inhibition of Cyclooxygenases**

G.A.FitzGerald
Center for Experimental Therapeutics, University of Pennsylvania, Philadelphia, USA

Cylooxygenase (COX) - 2 accounts largely, but not exclusively for prostaglandin (PG) generation in inflammatory syndromes and in cancer. Nonsteroidal anti inflammatory drugs (NSAIDs) are competitive, active site inhibitors of both COX isozymes and their GI adverse effects have been ascribed to inhibition of COX-1 dependent PGE2 and PGI2, which afford cytoprotection. Aspirin uniquely inhibits COXs irreversibly, via acetylation of Ser530 close to the active site, rendering the anucleate platelet a preferred target for cumulative inhibition by chronic administration of low doses. Inhibition of COX-1 derived, platelet TxA2 is sufficient to explain cardioprotection by aspirin. However, the effects of COX inhibition on the cardiovascular system are complex. Rofecoxib, a selective COX-2 inhibitor caused a reduction in important GI events when compared to the NSAID naproxen at equi inflammatory doses in the VIGOR study , whereas celecoxib failed to exhibit such discrimination from NSAID comparators in the CLASS study. A 5 fold divergence in the incidence of myocardial infarction in the VIGOR study groups has focused attention on the possibility of a cardiovascular hazard from coxibs. More recently, newer inhibitors have been evaluated and mPGE synthase has emerged as a downstream alternative target to COX - 2.

27 June 2003 08:30 - 11:00

**NO-NSAIDS : Potent Anti-Inflammatory, Analgesic and Cardioprotective Agents with Markedly Reduced Toxicity**

John L. Wallace
Mucosal Inflammation Research Group, University of Calgary, Alberta, Canada

While nonsteroidal anti-inflammatory drugs (NSAIDs) are extremely useful drugs for the treatment of a number of inflammatory conditions as

well as for reducing pain and fever, they also exert significant toxic effects, particularly in the gastrointestinal tract and kidney. In an effort to circumvent such toxicity, a new class of agents called nitric oxide-releasing NSAIDs (NO-NSAIDs) were developed. We have extensively characterized the effects of these drugs in various inflammatory and pain models, and for toxicity in the GI tract and kidney. NO-NSAIDs inhibit prostaglandin synthesis as effectively as the parent drugs, without having to first undergo metabolism. However, NO-NSAIDs have substantially reduced ulcerogenic effects in the stomach and intestine. Moreover, while conventional NSAIDs interfere with renal blood flow and contribute to the generation of hypertension, the NO-NSAIDs do not. Particularly interesting is the observation that NO-NSAIDs exhibit anti-inflammatory and analgesic effects beyond those of the parent drug. This appears to be attributable to the nitric oxide released from the NO-NSAIDs, since a similar increase in efficacy can be seen when NO donors are given together with an NSAID. NO-NSAIDs also exhibit significant anti-hypertensive and cardioprotective effects.
NO-NSAIDs represent a significant advance in anti-inflammatory and analgesic therapy, not only because of the markedly reduced toxicity, but because of a significant enhancement of efficacy.

---

27 June 2003 08:30 – 11:00

**Pharmacokinetic Guided Anti-Cancer Treatment**

Martínková J., Chládek J., Grim J.
Charles University in Prague, Faculty of Medicine in Hradec Králové, the Czech Republic

Most anticancer drugs are characterized by a narrow pharmacotherapeutic window and large interindividual variability in both response to drug therapy (PD) and pharmacokinetic parameters (PK). The achievement of therapeutic benefit is particularly important in patients with curable disease (ALL in children, Hodgkin´s lymphoma or testicular carcinoma, and in the setting of adjuvant chemotherapy), therefore, an individualised dosage is required. The analysis of dosing strategies for most cytostatics have shown commonly used morphometric measures (BSA, weight and height) to be inappropriate predictors for individualised dosage regimens. It indicates that other variables or clinical factors may be important in explaining the high variability in PK and PD observed (e.g. genetic factors, age, gender, disease conditions, chronobiology, concomitant drugs and other conditions). Knowledge of the PK of each agent is the most accurate method to establish its effect. Pharmacokinetic monitoring is already routinely employed to reduce the toxicity of high-dose chemotherapy, which includes methotrexate (MTX). The current standard of MTX monitoring is based on the use of plasma drug levels to predict both MTX efficacy and toxicity, and determines leucovorin rescue. Methods of monitoring PK parameters have also been explored for various other drugs, including continuous infusion of etoposide and 5-fluorouracil, and others.
Pharmacokinetic guided therapy in oncology
Dosing strategies based on photometric measures (BSA, weight and height) have shown that these measures are inappropriate predictors for individualised dosage regimens of most cytostatics

---

27 June 2003 08:30 – 11:00

**Added Value of Population Analysis during Oncological Drug Development**

Mats O Karlsson
Div. Pharmacokinetics and Drug Therapy, Dept of Pharmaceutical Biosciences, Uppsala University, Sweden

Population pharmacokinetic (PK) analysis of (sparse) concentration-time data have for about a decade provided useful and sometimes crucial information during oncological drug development. There are far fewer reports on the use of population pharmacodynamic (PD) models describing the relationship between drug concentration-time profiles and responses to drug therapy. Based on a recently published population pharmacodynamic model for haematological toxicity (J Clin Oncol, 20:4713-21;2002), the added value of population pharmacodynamic models will be discussed and illustrated. The mechanism-based model describes the system in terms of a pool of proliferative cells, which are capable of self-replication and if not victims of drug-induced cell death will generate non-proliferative cells that after maturation will be released to the systemic circulation and subsequently taken up by tissues. As the system-related parameters are the same across drugs, such a model may be used in drug development in order to analyse particularly small and/or sparse data sets. It may also find advantages in making early (preclinical) predictions of the clinical toxicity profile, to predict consequences of drug combinations or new dosing schedules, in aiding prodrug development, incorporate and predict the effect of modifying agents like G-CSF and find covariates that may influence the haematological toxicity profile across many anti-cancer agents.

---

27 June 2003 08:30 - 11:00

**New Targets in the Field of Cancer Chemotherapy**

Jacques Robert
Institut Bergonié and Université Victor Segalen, Bordeaux, France

The anticancer drugs that have been discovered and developed in the past 50 years were all aimed at the destruction of proliferative cells, whatever the mechanism of the malignant transformation leading to oncogenesis. These drugs targeted DNA itself (alkylating agents), DNA synthesis (antimetabolites), DNA supercoiling (topoisomerase inhibitors) or tubuline polymerisation (mitotic spindle poisons), but the ultimate target was always cell proliferation. As a consequence, general and common toxicities to all normal proliferating cells were encountered, especially haematopoietic cells and cells of the digestive mucosas.

Continuous progress in the understanding of oncogenesis has led to the conception of new anticancer drugs targeted at the precise molecular mechanisms involved in malignant transformation and in tumour invasion and metastasis. A large number of potential targets have been identified and intensive research has been implemented for the discovery and development of drugs able to reach and inhibit these targets. Some drugs have already been successfully developed and many other should rapidly join the anticancer armamentarium. However, some targets may appear of poor relevance and there will probably be more failures than successes as was the case for the former anticancer agents. Among the potential molecular targets which may bring a renewal in cancer chemotherapy, one can mention :

- the tyrosine kinase receptors which transmit growth factor proliferation signals
- the adaptive proteins between proliferation signals and the implementation of cell proliferation (e.g. RAS proteins and those of the MAP kinase pathway) ;
- the cell cycle regulatory proteins, especially cyclin-dependent kinases ;
- the mitochondrial apoptotic machinery, mainly BCL-2 family proteins ;
- the telomerase immortalisation protein , which is one of the hallmarks of cancer ;
- the angiogenic signalling pathway which is required for tumour nutrition and growth.

After the validation of each new target that can be defined from the knowledge of the molecular alterations involved in oncogenesis, one of the most difficult steps is the design of molecules able to interfere with this target. The resources of big pharmaceutical companies provide a large number of potential drugs, and high-throughput screening techniques must be implemented to identify drug leads. At the next step, the refinements of combinatorial chemistry will help the design of the most active molecules. Preclinical and clinical evaluation of these new therapeutic strategies have thereafter to follow the usual rules for drug development. Considering the facts that these new targeted therapies may not be cytotoxic and may be only active for the patients exhibiting the molecular alteration targeted, the clinical evaluation of these new agents may be more difficult than that of the former cytotoxic drugs. The challenging hope of opening new avenues in cancer chemotherapy may be at this cost.

---

27 June 2003 08:30 - 11:00

**Pharmacogenetics and Cancer Treatment**

JHM Schellens
TM Bosch, I Meijerman, PHM Smits, JH Beijnen,Amsterdam/Utrecht, The Netherlands

After standard dosing patients encounter wide variation in exposure to the applied drug. This is largely due to wide interpatient variation in the activity of enzyme systems involved in drug elimination. Especially for anticancer drugs pharmacokinetic variability is troublesome, because these drugs are generally dosed close to the "maximum tolerated dose" and show steep exposure-toxicity relationships. Several enzyme systems contribute to drug elimination, in particular dug oxidation by cytochrome P450 (CYP), drug conjugation by uridine-glucuronosyl transferase (UGT), glutathion S-transferase (GSH), N-acetylation and ABC transporters, including P-glycoprotein, BCRP (ABCG2) and MRPs. Specific other enzymes play a role, for example dihydropyrimidine dehydrogenase for 5FU and thiopurine methyl transferase for azathioprine and 6-mercaptopurine detoxification. Genetic polymorphism in genes coding for these enzymes contributes largely to the observed interpatient variation in activity of these enzyme systems. Single nucleotide polymorphisms (SNPs) can be screened using PCR and sequencing or RFLP. In current clinical studies main SNPs are routinely determined in patients treated with anticancer agents to explore relationships between genetic variation and likelihood of toxicity and anticancer activity. The results of these studies may serve as a template to design individualized treatment regimens with anticancer agents.

---

27 June 2003 08:30 – 11:00

**Combined Therapy in Hypercholesterolemia**

Dieter Lütjohann
The Department of Clinical Pharmacology, University of Bonn, Germany

The recent success of many combination drugs for hypertension has accelerated the interest in combination drugs for treatment of hypercholesterolemia and reduction of cardiovascular risk.
The nonlinear dose-response relation of statins, bile acid sequestrants, and niacin and their additive LDL cholesterol-lowering effect when used together suggest a strategy for treating hypercholesterolemia that may optimize effectiveness while minimizing adverse effects and cost. Ideally, the combination of an agent that specifically targets cholesterol absorption and promotes sterol excretion with a statin, simultanueosly decreasing endogenous cholesterol synthesis, may provide the greatest therapeutic benefit. The recent development of selective cholesterol inhibitors, including ezetimibe, provides an approach to lowering LDL that has significant potential both as monotherapy and in combination therapy. More research will be needed to determine the full clinical potential of such approaches to the management of hypercholesterolemia.

---

27 June 2003 08:30 – 11:00

**Pharmacoeconomic Aspects of Treatment with Lipid-Lowering Agents**

Marina Chauvenet, MD
A.C. Economics and La Pitié Hospital, Paris, France

Coronary heart disease is a major cause of morbi/mortality and the leading source of health expenditure in industrialised countries (hospital care, drug treatment, prevention cost...).
The first economic evaluations of a lipid-lowering intervention or agent (cholestyramine) were carried out almost 20 years ago. Cholesterol reduction cost-effectiveness studies with non-statin treatments (bile acid resins, fibrates, niacin and diet) were performed.
Model-based cost-effectiveness studies of statins were published before mega-trials based on clinical endpoints were made available.
The role of prediction versus observation in pharmacoeconomic assessments is discussed, as the cost of primary versus secondary prevention programmes in the clinical perspective of broader target-populations who may benefit from statin therapy.

---

27 June 2003 08:30 – 11:00

**Guidelines for the Treatment of Hyperlipidemia**

Mats Eriksson, MD, PhD

All over the world guidelines have been published regarding the treatment of hyperlipdemia. The latest guideline in Europe regarding the prevention of coronary heart disease in clinical practice including lipid treatment, was published 1998.

These guidelines stressed that the priority for physicians is to concentrate on patients with overt coronary heart disease (CHD), or other atherosclerotic disease, as well as high-risk individuals. For calculation of risk for primary prevention of CHD, coronary risk charts were presented taking in consideration systolic blood pressure, smoking, diabetes mellitus, gender and age. A risk between 20% to 40 % for the development of a CHD event during a ten year period is defined as high. The "Third report of the national cholesterol education program (NCEP) expert panel on detection, evaluation and treatment of high blood cholesterol in adults (adult treatment panel III) presented in USA in 2001. The expert panel pointed out that the primary goals of therapy and the cutpoints for initiating treatment are stated in terms of LDL (low density lipoprotein) cholesterol. In patients at the highest risk with CHD or CHD risk equivalents the LDL goal is 2.6 mmol/L. The panel also focused upon treatment of the metabolic syndrome, a condition characterised by abdominal obesity, atherogenic dyslipidemia, raised blood pressure, insulin resistance and prothrombotic and proinflammatory states. ATP III recommends a multifaceted lifestyle approach to reduce risk for CHD. These lifestyle changes include: reduced intake of saturated fats and cholesterol, the use of therapeutic options for LDL cholesterol reduction as plant sterols and increased viscous fiber, weight reduction and increased physical activity.
The results from two great trials in patients with multiple risk factors (high risk individuals) and treatment with LDL cholesterol lowering HMG CoA reductase inhibitors (statins) have to some extent complicated the situation. The studies are the Heart Protection Study and the lipid lowering arm of the ASCOT trial. In those two trials it is clearly shown that 1 mmol/L of LDL lowering gives significant benefits in CHD events despite low levels of LDL cholesterol.
Conclusion: Several trials with LDL cholesterol lowering drugs have shown beneficial effects on CHD events even in cases with apparent low levels of LDL cholesterol. This makes it to some extent much more difficult to construct guidelines. The number of side effects from statin treatment is low. However, there are dose dependent muscle problems and other side effects apart from the cost for the treatment. Therefore, the work on guidelines for the correct management of high-risk individuals for CHD is even more important.

---

27 June 2003 14:30 – 17:00

## Are Surrogate Endpoints Informative Enough for the Risk-Benefit Assessment of the Treatment of Hepatitis with Interferon?

Zahariy Krastev
Clinic of Gastroenterology, St. Ivan Rilsky University Hospital, Sofia Medical University, Sofia, Bulgaria

IFN-alpha is the most effective drug for treatment of chronic viral hepatitis, but this therapy is associated with several problems: limited number of patients, suitable for IFN and high rates of non-responders and relapsers. The current surrogate endpoints of treatment include achievement of both biochemical and virological response. However, the main treatment goal is improvement of long-term outcome of chronic liver disease and the following factors have to be taken into account: achievement of prolonged remission of liver disease, prevention of hepatic decompensation and/or HCC, reduction of liver related deaths and improvement of the patients' survival. The term «sustained treatment response» needs to be clarified, because the longer post-treatment follow-up have been performed the lower rates of «sustained response» have been found. Furthermore, the introduction of PCR technique for measurement of serum HBV DNA in hepatitis B points a question about the real virological response in chronic hepatitis B. It seems that the reported differences in virological response rates to IFN in chronic HBV and HCV infections, are due to the different sensitivity of techniques used for response assessment. The surrogate markers are important milestones in management of patients with chronic viral hepatitis, but the clinical approach should be adapted also according to patients' age, co-morbid conditions, viral replication and severity of liver histology. The decision for treatment should weigh the likelihood of a long-term response against the risk of lack of response or relapse after the treatment as well as of developing the serious adverse events and complications.

27 June 2003 14:30 – 17:00

## Interferon-lamivudine Combination Therapy

HLA Janssen, SW Schalm
Dept. of Hepatology & Gastroenterology, Erasmus Medical Center Rotterdam, The Netherlands.

It is logical to assess whether combination therapy of interferon and lamivudine is effective since the two drugs appear to complement each other in antiviral and immunomodulatory activities. The first pilot studies showed no pharmacological interaction, good tolerability (similar to interferon monotherapy), but also no striking efficacy in non-responders to interferon. Two large randomized controlled trials in 226 and 238 predominantly Caucasian patients with HBeAg positive chronic hepatitis B have been carried out subsequently. In the study in 238 interferon non-responders the HBeAg seroconversion rate for placebo, lamivudine and combination therapy was between 12 and 18 % without a statistical significant difference. However, in the study in 226 previously untreated patients the HBeAg seroconversion rate for combination therapy was 29% and for the two monotherapies 19 and 20%, respectively. The difference between the response with combination and those with monotherapy was not significant in the intention-to-treat analysis, but in the 180 patients who adhered to the study protocol the rate of response with combination therapy (36%) was significantly higher than the response with lamivudine (19%) or interferon (22%).
Recently the results of a new large randomized controlled trial comparing 24 weeks of interferon combination therapy with 52 weeks of lamivudine monotherapy in 151 patients with HBeAg positive chronic hepatitis B were presented; 20 patients were non-responders to a previous course of interferon therapy. Strong elements in the trial design are the longer duration of combination therapy (24 weeks), the assessment at the end of therapy (24 or 52 weeks) and at the end of follow-up (48 weeks later). The study was completed by 94-96 % of the patients, indicating also an excellent tolerance of combination therapy. HBeAg seroconversion with undetectable levels of serum HBVDNA by a solution-hybridization test was observed in 35% at the end of treatment for the combination therapy versus 19% for lamivudine monotherapy. Relapse of detectable HBeAg and HBVDNA was observed in 7% for combination therapy and 21% for lamivudine therapy. The sustained HBeAg seroconversion rate of 33% for combination therapy was - on an intention to treat basis- significantly different from 15% for lamivudine monotherapy.
These results from an independent trial strongly support the concept of combining lamivudine and interferon for the treatment of HBeAg positive chronic hepatitis B.

27 June 2003 14:30 – 17:00

## Is Combination Treatment of Chronic Hepatitis C Beneficial for Society? Results of a Health Technology Assessment

Kim Krogsgaard
Clinical Research Unit, Copenhagen University Hospital, Hvidovre; DK Denmark

Chronic HCV infection affects 15.000 persons in Denmark. Fifty per cent of patients with chronic HCV infection will probably never develop symptoms or a liver disease. Fifty per cent will develop a liver disease and perhaps symptoms hereof in the course of a great many years. However, in a minority of the patients chronic hepatitis C may develop into a life threatening chronic liver disease. Many of these patients are unknown to the health care system, and amongst the patients with a diagnosis not all will be able to benefit from treatment. The combination treatment with PEG IFN and ribavirin can permanently eliminate HCV from the blood and thus cure and prevent a liver disease in approx. 50% of all treated patients. The combination treatment has quite a few side effects, some of which can be serious or permanent, viz. interference with thyroid function. The treatment and being offered treatment are considered to be unambiguously good by the patients. Despite the side effects the patients will recommend the treatment to other patients. A decision to offer the combination treatment to all patients who could

possibly benefit from the treatment can be implemented within the framework of the existing Danish health care system. A decision to offer treatment is not considered to require organisational changes in the individual departments/clinics, between departments or at the hospital level. With the present rather high price of PEG IFN and ribavirin and with the conservative estimates of costs related to health care services offered to patients with advanced liver disease, the health economic analysis shows that treatment with combination of IFN and ribavirin from a health economic point of view will be beneficial for society after a 10 year period of time.
Based upon all the stated considerations the Danish working group will recommend that the combination treatment with IFN and ribavirin should be offered to patients with chronic hepatitis C who fulfil the criteria for treatment.

---

27 June 2003 14:30 – 17:00

**European Surveillance of Antimicrobial Consumption : Quality Indicators**

Vander Stichele RH, MD,
European Drug Utilization Research Group, Heymans Institute of Pharmacology, Ghent University, Gent

Rising resistance to antibiotics, few new antibiotic drugs and low tolerance for unjustified expenditures will force the health authorities and prescribers to enhance appropriateness of prescribing. But how can a core set of health indicators can be developed for a data-driven, evidence-based, research-sustained health policy with regard to appropriate antibiotic usage ?
Can key quality indicators be selected, within the limits of validity for aggregated administrative data (lacking indication, prescriber and patient information) by linking to resistance data ? Is it possible to establish limits of appropriate use of specific antimicrobial classes, based upon prevalence data for specific infectious diseases and guidelines ? What promises do population-based databases hold ? These questions will be adressed with the following examples:

- EuroDURG data collection initiative (1994-1999 data from 16 countries)
- ESAC (European Surveillance of Antimicrobial Consumption) : a continuous surveillance project (1997-2001 data from 25 countries).
- Farmanet (Belgium) with prescribing profiles of medical specialists providing care to outpatients
- A Belgian Feedback Program to local quality circles of general practitioners

---

27 June 2003 14:30 – 17:00

**Quality Indicators of Drug Prescribing in Croatia**

Vera Vlahovic-Palcevski
Department of Clinical Pharmacology, Karolinska Institutet, Huddinge University Hospital, Stockholm, Sweden

Quality of prescribing has become an important issue in assessing the quality of health care. The quality of drug prescribing has been measured through indicators which are defined as measurable elements of practice performance for which there is evidence or consensus that they can be used to asses quality. However, prescribing remains a controversial area of quality assessment with only a few validated quality indicators existing. There are considerable variations in prescribing standards in various countries, and indicators should be based on them. After defining what indicators are intended to measure and what conclusions can be made, they may help identify potential problems. For indicators to be useful for quality assessment, consistent and comparable data must be available across the relevant healthcare organizations. With this benchmarking approach, best practices could be found and implemented. In Croatia, several quality indicators have been in use to audit prescribing both in hospitals and primary care. Adherence to recommendations in prescribing nonsteroidal antinflammatory drugs and antimicrobials, using DU90% methodology, has been used as an indicator of prescribing appropriateness. Recently we have been investigating the incidence of potential drug interactions when drugs are coprescribed. These indicators may provide a starting point for developing a common set of prescribing indicators.

27 June 2003 14:30 - 17:00

### Implementing Quality Indicators of Drug Prescribing in Sweden

Ulf Bergman
Sweden

Quality of care has become an important issue in health care. As drug therapy is an integral part of health care, quality assurance programmes for drug prescribing are needed. In 1999, the Swedish Medical Quality Council published "Quality indicators for drug use and drug handling". Indicator 1) focused on the number of drugs constituting 90% of the volume - DU90% - and adherence to drug committee guidelines within this segment. Indicator 2) quantified correctly given prescriptions in hospital wards. Indicator 3) was designed to stimulate the reporting of clinically important pharmacological adverse drug reactions (type A, thus theoretically preventable) by providing feed back of spontaneously reported adverse reactions to each clinic. All three indicators are using currently available health care data and they can all be quantified.

The credibility and usefulness of each indicator was evaluated by questionnaires. These three indicators also formed the basis of a "Quality account report".

Five clinics, representing cardiology, internal medicine, psychiatry and surgery, participated in this pilot implementation.

Although these indicators neither examine the appropriateness nor give the outcome data, preliminary results suggest that this is a useful tool for the implementation of high quality evidence based prescribing.

27 June 2003 14:30 - 17:00

### Quality Indicators Derived from Prescription Databases; Can They Be Trusted?

Jesper Hallas, MD, PhD
Department of Clinical Pharmacology, University of Southern Denmark, Denmark

The emergence of high-quality population-based prescription registers has allowed us to describe the population's drug use with a so far unseen richness of detail and to assess its adherence to prescribing guidelines. However, the validity of such quality indicators is controversial.

The validity issue can be separated into questions about internal validity, i.e., the quality of prescription data and about external validity, i.e., to what extent the quality indicators - given the data are correct - truly reflect prescribing quality. Studies of internal validity are hampered by the inherent absence of good data on patients' actual drug ingestion. Although the patients' own account may seem obvious as the gold standard, there are examples of gross discrepancies with valid data from other sources. Studies of external validity are hampered by problems in translating the quality of a prescriber's performance into meaningful measures. To be useful, a quality indicator should measure pertinent problems with a limited number of preventable causes, be comprehensible and generally accepted by the prescribers.

Finally, some examples of intervention studies are presented that were based on use of quality indicators.

27 June 2003 14:30 - 17:00

### Treatment of Behavioral Symptoms and Dementia in Parkinson's Disease

Murat Emre, M.D., Professor of Neurology
Istanbul Faculty of Medicine, Department of Neurology, Çapa, Istanbul, Turkey

A variety of behavioral symptoms and cognitive impairment can occur in patients with Parkinson's disease. The prevalance of psychotic symptoms was reported to be up to 80%, when minor forms were included. Behavioral symptoms and cognitive impairment are often a more significant source of distress for patients and families than the motor symptoms, they significantly impair the quality of life and are often the main reason for nursing home placement. Personality changes, agitation, agression, affective disorders, psychotic features such as hallucinations and delusions, sleep disturbances can all occur.. Dementia is also frequently associated with Parkinson's disease, the incidence is increased up to six fold compared to controls and the prevalance is close to 40%. The first step in the management of behavioral and cognitive symptoms involves assessment of potential underlying causes. Acute confusion due to systemic disorders such as dehydratation or infections, drug-induced confusion, psychosis or cognitive impairment, psychodynamic factors due to conflicts in social or interpersonal relations should all be considered. The symptoms may spontaneously abate once exogenous reasons are identified and managed. These symptoms, however, may also be due to the underlying disease pathology and may necessitate pharmacological intervention. Several clinical trials suggest that choline-esterase inhibitors may effectively control behavioral symptoms and cognitive impairment in patients with PD. Atypical anti-psychotics such as quetiapine or clozapine, anti-depressants, anti-epileptics with affect-stabilizing properties are other drugs which can be considered. In choosing drugs the whole symptom profile should be considered, if possible several symptoms should be targeted with one drug. The treatment should be iniatated with low doses and slowly titrated. After effective symptom control is achieved dose reduction and discontinuation of treatment should be attempted.

---

27 June 2003 14:30 - 17:00

**Use of fMRI as a Tool to Study Drug Responsiveness in Alzheimer's Disease**

SHD Jackson
Department of Health Care of the Elderly , Kings College, London

Magnetic resonance (MR) imaging relies on the magnetic properties of atoms. The MR signal from hydrogen nuclei (ie protons, the majority of which are found in the form of water) is used in most clinical applications to image both structure and function. Functional magnetic resonance imaging (fMRI) uses blood oxygen level dependent (BOLD) contrast to map brain activity under conditions of experimentally controlled stimuli. This endogenous contrast arises from the rise in oxyhaemoglobin : deoxyhaemogloblin ratio seen after brain activation. The mechanism underlying the coupling of brain activity and blood flow is not yet clear. Using fMRI the activation maps of motor, sensory and cognitive paradigms can be assessed. The effect of drug treatment on such activation can therefore be studied without ionising radiation exposure. BOLD fMRI involves multislice T2* weighted brain images acquired using a pulse sequence capable of imaging the entire brain in under three seconds. Data acquisition is continuous throughout a five minute paradigm where the stimulus is presented for 30 seconds alternating with an "off" state for 30 seconds. Image analysis involves a movement correction algorithm, time series analysis, transformation of the activation map into standard (Talairach) space and the generation of generic brain activation maps.

We have applied the technique of fMRI to the study of anticholinesterase therapy in AD. The hypothesis under test was that differences in brain activation resulting from cognitive and sensory paradigms would be seen during treatment versus baseline. Eighteen patients with mild to moderate AD underwent cognitive assessment and fMRI. A high resolution structural scan, an auditory and visual stimulation paradigm and a working memory task were performed within the scanner. Patients then received donepezil at a dosage of 5 mg titrated up to 10 mg daily. At 3 months patients were reassessed. Differences in activation of a variety of brain areas were seen. An additional technique - chemical shift imaging (CSI) - uses the chemical environment of atoms to identify the compounds in which they are bonded. Proton CSI allows the identification of a number of metabolites: the neuronal marker, N-acetyl aspartate (NAA), creatine and non-cell membrane ("free") choline containing compounds. Until recently it has only been possible to acquire these data over large regions. CSI allows the construction of metabolite maps with voxel sizes of around 1.5ml. CSI holds great promise as a method of measuring drug response in conditions such as Alzheimer's disease. Using appropriate hardware it is also possible to measure concentrations of drugs with paramagnetic properties. The newest generation of MR machines will be able to image such substances over a sufficiently short time period to enable concentration time data to be obtained. Thus pharmacokinetic modelling at different brain sites will be possible and could be combined with pharmacodynamic data sets obtained from fMRI studies conducted concurrently enabling pharmacokinetic pharmacodynamic modelling to be performed.

---

27 June 2003 14:30 – 17:00

**Treatment of Osteoarthritis**

J. C. Frölich
Dept. Of Clin Pharm, Hannover Medical School, Hannover, Germany

Osteoarthritis is by far the most frequent joint disorder leading to drug therapy. Guidelines for treatment have been established and reflect evaluation of efficacy and safety. Interestingly, guidelines vary considerably from country to country in Europe. Thus, in Great Britain first line therapy is paracetamol while in other European countries it is NSAR. A recent survey by the Arthritis Action Group covering patients with long lasting joint or muscle disorders brought to light that many of them are not treated adequately and that their quality of life is severely impaired. Major obstacles to adequate drug treatment include the belief that NSAR cause drug dependence and that they will loose their effect, if used regularly. Risk is severely underestimated as many patients think that NSAR are absolutely safe when taken as prescribed. The risk awareness on the part of medical doctors surprisingly is unsatisfactory as many do not ask for the most common major risk factors (previous ulcers, asthma, hypertension) and share the belief, that NSAR cause drug dependence. The safety of the new COX-inhibitors and NSAR will be critically reviewed and a reassessment of paracetamol presented.

---

27 June 2003 14:30 – 17:00

**The Use of Placebo in Clinical Trials**

Domenico Criscuolo
Director of Int'l Operations, CRC, Milano, Italy

The implementation of the placebo controlled trial represents a milestone in the scientific process to develop new drugs. After the historical placebo controlled trial of the use streptomycin in the treatment of pulmonary tuberculosis, sponsored by the Medical Research Council and published in the British Medical Journal in 1948, placebo controlled trials were considered the necessary tools to assess the therapeutic value of new medicines: this pragmatic approach was on one side very useful to Investigators, who got clear answers from the studies where a placebo group was present, and was also corroborated by the attitude of many Regulatory Agencies, who liked the evidence provided by placebo controlled trials. It is also true that for many years the lack of a standard therapy for many diseases represented an additional support to the implementation of placebo controlled trials. However, in recent years, this approach in under critical revision; the availability of therapies for many diseases makes more difficult to accept the placebo arm, even if this treatment is foreseen for short periods. In addition, ethical concerns are growing, and the attitude towards the indiscriminate use of placebo is under critical revision. Mankind had the benefits of placebo controlled trials for about fifty years; time is now mature for alternative approaches to the clinical development of new drugs.

---

27 June 2003 14:30 – 17:00

**The Ethical Issues of Controlled Randomised Double Blind Clinical Trials**

Janos Borvendég
National Institute of Pharmacy, Budapest, Hungary

Controlled randomised double blind clinical trials (CRT) are widely accepted as a most proper method of scientific evaluation. The Evidence based medicine relies mostly on the results of CRT-s. Despite of its wide use, CRT-s remain the fiercely argued aspect of clinical research. The question is frequently raised, wether it is ethical to subject patients to invalidated procedures random and to keep both the physicians and the volunteers blinded during the trial. Strictly speaking the randomisation can only be ethical if the clinician is being in »equipoise», or alternatively uncertain about the best treatment for the patient. The principle of controlled trials is that the results produced by the investigational product are compared with those obtained by placebo or with a selected reference drug. Is it ethical to use placebo or an active drug selected not by the physician but by the sponsor? Is the use of double blind technique ethical keeping the applied therapy secreet from the doctors as well as from the patients? In which way and extent can a physician acts ethically in his/her double role, namely from one hand as a doctor, working only in the patient's interest and from the other hand as an investigator fulfilling the strict scientific requirements of the protocol.

28 June 2003 08:30 – 11:00

**Rational Prescribing in Primary Care**

Tom Walley
University of Liverpool L69 3GF UK

Most prescribing occurs in primary care, about 90% by volume in the UK for instance. But this is where the doctor is least supported in this vital role and open to many pressures which may lead to irrational prescribing: difficulties in keeping up to date, professional isolation, pharmaceutical company detailing, inappropriate demands by patients, excessive workload. There are many examples of where this leads to irrational i.e. wasteful and dangerous prescribing, or fails to make best use of prescribed drugs in all European countries. The definition of what is irrational prescribing in primary care is important, and a purely pharmacologically oriented definition is inadequate if it does not also consider the psychosocial aspects of prescribing also.

Many ways have been tried to improve prescribing in primary care: they require a combination of approaches, educational and structural, and sustained effort, to achieve change. These will be considered in more depth. Clinical Pharmacologists need to be careful not to condemn prescribing in primary care but to understand its context more fully and work with general practitioners and other health professionals to try to improve it.

28 June 2003 08:30 – 11:00

**Is it Possible to Influence GPs' Prescribing habits?**

Jens Sondergaard
Research Unit of General Practice, Aarhus University and General Practice Research Unit, University of Southern Denmark, Aarhus, Denmark

There is an increasing focus on the need for improving GPs' performance, but most quality improvement initiatives are based on the unfounded beliefs of those responsible for the interventions rather than on solid evidence for effect. For instance, it has often been assumed that suboptimal performance is mainly due to lack of knowledge and that GPs may be unaware that they are not living up to standards. Inexpensive strategies like prescriber-feedback or simple provision of information through guidelines and newsletters have been believed to be effective. However, the decision to prescribe and what to prescribe is complex and GPs take into account many factors including medical, social, economic and logistic ones. Furthermore, many barriers must be overcome. This is not achieved by simple interventions, and many resources have been wasted on ineffective interventions.
Strategies aimed at improving performance should be based on theoretical and empirical knowledge about the effectiveness of different kinds of interventions and an understanding of the components influencing the process of care, the goals and the setting. Achieving change should be seen as interplay between motivation, competence and barriers. Change strategies should be tailored and targeted and include combinations of different kinds of interventions.
This presentation will outline the effects of frequently used interventions aimed at improving GPs' performance. Different barriers and facilitators for impact will be discussed and a model for planning quality improvement will be presented. Finally, a widely accepted Danish quality improvement method will be shown.

28 June 2003 08:30 – 11:00

## Is the WHO Model List of Essential Medicines relevant for industrialized countries?

*Hans V. Hogerzeil*, MD, PhD, FRCP Edin
World Health Organization, Department of Essential Drugs and Medicines Policy, Geneva

The WHO Model List of Essential Drugs has been updated every two years since 1977 and is one of WHO's most powerful tools to promote equity in public health. The 2002 Model List contains 325 active ingredients, including 12 antiretroviral medicines for the treatment of HIV/AIDS. By the end of 1999 156 countries had developed their own national list of essential drugs, using it for drug supply in the public sector, reimbursement schemes, training and local production.

The selection of essential drugs is a two-step process: (1) review of efficacy, safety and quality prior to market approval; (2) review of comparative efficacy, safety and cost-effectiveness, used for procurement or reimbursement decisions. The WHO List is a model for the second step. It is now part of the WHO Essential Medicines Library, a web-based information resource combining the Model List of Essential Medicines with summaries of WHO clinical guidelines, the WHO Model Formulary, key evidence supporting the selection of essential medicines, price information and normative information regarding nomenclature and quality assurance.

Although originally intended for developing countries, an increasing number of developed countries use key components of the essential drugs concept as a means to ensure the rational selection of efficacious, safe and cost-effective medicines for reimbursement. This development was triggered by increasing drug costs and the introduction of many new and often expensive drugs. For example, in the USA annual medicine expenditure rose by 18% in 1999, 16% in 2000 and 17% in 2001; this rise is much higher than the increase in GNP or the consumer price index over the same. Much of this increase is related to the introduction of new, often expensive medicines.

The systematic evaluation of comparative efficacy, safety and cost-effectiveness, together with information on the underlying treatment guidelines and evidence-base, make the WHO Model List of Essential Drugs into a process which is universally applicable. This is equally relevant for industrialized countries.

28 June 2003 08:30 – 11:00

## Upper Gastrointestinal Bleeding and Non-Steroidal Anti-Inflammatory Drugs

Ibáñez L, Laporte JR, Leone R, Vendrell L, Vidal X.
Fundació Institut Català de Farmacologia, Hospital Universitari Vall d'Hebron, Universitat Autònoma de Barcelona (Spain) and Servizio di Farmacologia Medica, Università di Verona (Italy)

Background/Aims. Drug-induced upper gastrointestinal haemorrhage (UGIB) is one of the most frequent adverse drug reactions (ADRs) leading to hospital admission. The contribution of individual old and newer non-steroidal anti-inflammatory drugs (NSAIDs) is unknown.
Methods. Population-based case-control study in several areas in Spain and Italy with 2,813 cases of UGIB from a peptic lesion leading to hospital admission, and 7,193 sex-, age, and centre-matched controls.
Results. The annual incidence of UGIB was 401 per 106 older than 15 years. Thirty-eight percent of cases were attributable to NSAIDs. Individual relative risks for NSAIDs ranged from 1.39 (0.58-3.29) for aceclofenac, to 24.74 (7.95-77.03) for ketorolac, and they were dose-dependent. There were few patients exposed to rofecoxib (OR = 7.22 [2.27-23.02]) and to celecoxib (OR = 0.32 [0.03-4.06]). There was no risk associated to topical NSAIDs. UGIB associated to NSAID's was significantly increased in patients with a history of peptic ulcer and in those under concomitant antiplatelet drugs; it was decreased among those under concomitant proton-pump inhibitors or nitrovasodilators.
Conclusions: NSAID-induced UGIB is a common cause of hospital admission. Its risk depends on the patient's age, sex, history of peptic ulcer, the particular drug, its dose and concomitant treatments.

28 June 2003 08:30 – 11:00

## Computer Surveillance of Adverse Drug Resctions in Hospital

Micha Levy
Hadassah University Hospital,Jerusalem,Israel

Objective: To develope and implement the use of information technology techniques as a detection support tool of adverse drug reactions (ADR) in hospital
Design: Retrospective and prospective observational studies of sequential medical admissions during a two months period. Setting: A 34- bed medical ward at the Hadassah University Hospital, Jerusalem, Israel. Measurements: Analysis of computerized laboratory data according to defined automated signals (AS) generated from the laboratory as potential indicators of ADR. Chart review for ADR and whether these were were recognized by the staff physicians.
Results: In one-quater to one-third of the admissions ADR were present. Duration of hospitalization increased by 50% in the ADR-positive admissions. About 60% of the ADR were identified by AS. AS were present in 49-58% of the ADR-negative admissions. Following application of AS the rate of AS-positive ADR not recognized by the attending physician decreased from 73% to 17%.
Conclusions: The routine implementation of computerized technique using the
hospitals' laboratory data base doubled the number of ADR recognized by the physicians while patients were hospitalized in the medical ward.. The use of the system appeared valid, simple amd potentially cost-effective. Further development of the system by including additional clinical information and drug safety profiles may provide early detection and prevent harm to patients.

28 June 2003 08:30 – 11:00

## How can one Assess the Effect of Teaching on the Competence of Prescribing by Health Professionals?

E. Sanz
Dept. Pharmacology. School of Medicine. Univ. La Laguna, Spain

Prescribing by health professionals is one of the most multivariate behaviours that physicians display in their daily routines. According with the mandates of medical ethics, the maximum benefit of the patients, at the lower risk should be the unique, or at least the most important, consideration before a prescription is finally written. But, there are many other, more or less subtle, conditionings of prescriptions. Among them, time and work settings considerations, the level of up-to-date knowledge on medicines and therapeutics, or the conflicts of interests, specially related to patient expectations or drug companies interests. How to evaluate prescription quality is also a difficult topic. Several "Quality indicators" have been used, with more or less acceptance by the scientific community. Nevertheless, the only evaluations that really can get to the core of the issue are therapeutic audits, provided that the clinical data of the patients and especially the outcomes can become a part of the analysis. To asses the competence of prescribing by health professionals is possible provided that competence of diagnosis and clinical care and workload and conditions are kept, or assumed to be, at the same level for the "sample". A pilot study with health professionals in Spain is exploring the possibility of using the criteria and structure of rationing of the WHO's "Guide to good prescribing" in Primary Care in a Public Health Service. The participating GPs, which will be compared with colleagues working in the same conditions, unaware of the study, will use the rationing of the guide with the help of the "P-Drugs 2.0" program to produce a list of their, up to 100, specialities to be used as primary, or secondary line, for the treatment of the most common conditions in Primary Care. Each GP will end with her or his "Personal Formulary" which will probably be similar, but never identical, to the rest of the participants. Compare and analyze the competence or quality of actual prescribing without stepping down to the real clinical data of each patient is always delicate, subject to numerous biases and highly ideological. Analyzing personal preferences after systematic and careful revision, and the degree of application or applicability of them, is a good tool to improve quality of prescription by pushing practitioners to do it by themselves.

28 June 2003 08:30 - 11:00

### The Development of Quality Measures for Therapeutics Reasoning

Ellen Vinge
Department of Clinical Pharmacology, University Hospital, Lund, Sweden

All students should be trained in defining the treatment objective(s) for each individual patient. All treatment indications and therapeutic goals should be clearly stated in the records. The student should define a method to assess the effect of the treatment, and indicate the criteria for a satisfactory response. The expected duration of the treatment should be noted, as well as a plan for how and when the effect should be evaluated. All treatment should be based on scientific evidence from clinical trials, as far as possible. Treatment guidelines may be useful if they are evidence-based and updated. When pharmacotherapy is the choice, drugs that are officially approved for the therapeutic indication(s) should be preferred. Lists of recommended drugs can give additional support for the choice of a particular drug.

The student should be trained in checking all contraindications, precautions and possible interactions with other ongoing therapy. If such information causes any action, such as reduced dosage, the reason for this should be noted in the records, and the patient should be informed. When the treatment is evaluated, the result of the effect measurement should be recorded in the files and assessed. Side effects should also be noted and assessed by severity. Any new actions should be recorded.

28 June 2003 11:30 - 12:15

### The Effects of Drugs on the Environment-Ecopharmacology

Klaus Kümmerer
Univeristy Hospital Freiburg

Pharmaceuticals are excreted into the aquatic environment via waste water. Unused medicaments and reminders are sometimes disposed of in drains. The drugs may enter the aquatic environment and eventually reach drinking water if they are not biodegraded or eliminated during sewage treatment. Additionally, antibiotics are supposed to disturb the waste water treatment process and the microbial ecology in surface waters. Furthermore, resistant bacteria may be selected in the aeration tanks of sewage treatment plants by the antibiotic substances present or other environmental compartments. An overview of the input and the concentrations of drugs in hospital effluents and municipal sewage and soil will be given. The biodegradability of some clinically important drugs and their effects against environmental bacteria will be reported. Only a few of the test compounds were biodegradable. The genotoxicity of some compounds was not eliminated in test systems. It can be concluded that the emission of drugs into the aquatic environment should be reduced. Reminders should therefore not disposed of via the drain. The environmental significance of drugs should be included into the curricula of doctors and pharmacists.

28 June 2003 Afternoon Course

### Clinical Pharmacological Principles in Therapeutic Drug Monitoring

Folke Sjöqvist
Department of Clinical Pharmacology, Huddinge University Hospital Stockholm, Sweden

TDM is perhaps the most sophisticated way to ascertain a drug treatment that is tailored towards the individual needs of the patient. Recent advances in pharmacogenetics clearly show that subpopulations of patients exist who need much higher or lower doses than those derived from controlled clinical trials, where usually a fixed dosage-schedule is used unless sharp pharmacological endpoints can be used for dose titration. TDM should be considered as part of a clinical pharmacological consultation aiming to explore the mechanisms involved in interindividual variability in drug response. The consultation should consider psychological (poor compliance) as well as pharmacological factors such as drug-drug interactions and pharmacogenetics. The combination of conventional TDM and pheno-genotyping of drug metabolic enzymes and transport mechanisms is particularly powerful in achieving sophisticated drug utilization (personalized medicine).

---

28 June 2003 Afternoon Course

**What Should a Clinical Pharmacologist Know About Drug Analytical Methods?**

Lennart Meurling
Dept. Clin. Pharm., Huddinge Univ. Hospital, Huddinge Sweden

Therapeutic drug monitoring ( TDM) aims at avoiding therapeutic failures due to, among other things, bad compliance, low dose of a given drug or adverse or toxic effects due to an excessive dose. Only by collaboration between scientists and clinicians meaningful TDM results may be obtained. Knowledge of clinical data, precise collection time, co-adminstered drugs and an idea of the therapeutic range of the drug, adapted to the population to which the patient belongs, are important parameters in this context.

However, scope and limitations of the analytical procedure used has also to be considered. During the last 30 years the world of laboratory medicine has experienced a period of enormous progress and development. Many new diagnostic techniques have been introduced in the clinical pharmacology laboratory. Two main development lines can be identified, namely in immunological and chromatographic techniques. An immunoassay can often be very rapidly performed, but often lacks adequate specificity. However, development of very specific immunoreagents has decreased this drawback. Chromatographic techniques, on the other side, are often very specific, but have sometimes been hampered by low sensitivity and relatively long turn around times. New chromatographic phases and the development of detection techniques such as LC-MS-MS has given chromatography a possibility to successfully compete with immunology as far as speed and logistics concern. Examples will be given in the presentation as well as a discussion of new trends in bioanalytical chemistry, like lab-on-a chip and analysis in a compact disc ( CD) format.

---

28 June 2003 Afternoon Course

**Recent Priorities in Therapeutic Drug Monitoring**

Lars Ståhle
Department of Clinical Pharmacology, Huddinge University Hospital, Stockholm, Sweden

Among the drugs recently added to the TDM arsenal in our laboratory are the immunomudulator sirolimus, a series of drugs against HIV, ribavirin, teicoplanin, busulphane and a range of antidepressants and antipsychotic agents. Analyses of drug metabolic genotypes are expanding but have not yet reached the position of routine methodology.

Bayesian methods to generate estimates of clearance and volume of distribution were introduced in the 80-ies and are becoming wide-spread with the availability of user friendly computer programs. However, the best estimates of population parameters are obtained with population methods such as the non-linear mixed-effect modelling of Sheiner and Beal. Here, there is a need for developing computer programmes based on modern user-interface design such that the parameters of more drugs can be obtained and implemented in the TDM-laboratories.

Concentration-effect studies of either epidemiological or controlled design are badly needed for many compounds. Much work has been done on drugs against HIV with efavirenz as the best example of a compound with an established therapeutic range.

It is important to point out that in many instances it is of value to analyse drug concentrations even in the absence of an established therapeutic range.

Finally, prospective studies of the value of TDM in terms of clinical efficacy and health economy are needed. The design of such studies is critical since average parameters are unlikely to guide decision makers as TDM is expected to affect the frequency of relatively unusual events. An obvious example is genotyping for TPMT where the frequency of homozygous mutated individuals is 0.3%. Their identification and subsequent dose adjustment of azathioprine is unlikely to influence average cost and effect but may never the less save lives.

---

28 June 2003 Afternoon Course

**The Practice of TDM - The Dialogue Between the Clinical Pharmacological Laboratory and the Prescriber**

Milan Grundmann
Department of Clinical Pharmacology, University Hospital and Medico Social Faculty, University of Ostrava, Ostrava, Czech Republic

In the 30 years TDM has moved from an abstract consideration to a routine intervention. The goal of TDM is to use drug concentrations to manage a patient´s medication regimen and optimise outcome. The TDM process involves the decision to request a drug level, the biological sample, the request, laboratory measurement, communication of results by the laboratory with clinical interpretation and therapeutic management. Clinical interpretation transforms drug concentration monitoring (DCM) into a TDM service and should be distributed to the requesting clinician as rapidly as possible. The ideal TDM team should consist of clinical pharmacologists, clinical pharmacists and analytical scientists. Pharmacokinetic interpretive services improve patient care. The dosage predictions, including a graph are ideally suited for incorporation into the report form issued by a TDM service. The clinician caring for a patient will modify a drug dosage regimen. If the members of the TDM team are well respected, many physicians will accept and implement their recommendations for dosage adjustment and seek their further advice.

---

28 June 2003 Afternoon Course

**TDM Data as a Source in Drug Utilization Research**

Blanka Koristkova
Department of Clinical Pharmacology, University Hospital and Medico Social Faculty University of Ostrava, Czech Republic

The TDM request form in its simplest version contains information about indication, prescribed daily dose, and basic characteristics about the patient (age, gender, and optionally body weight). More sophisticated request forms also specify co-administered drugs, other diseases, clinical outcome and sometimes the occurrence of adverse drug reactions.

The relation between prescribed daily dose (DDD) and drug concentration can be used to detect drug-interactions and poor compliance of the patient. It can also be used for pharmacoepidemiological purposes to assess the clinical relevance of the DDD (defined daily dose), which is widely used as a measure of drug utilization. TDM data can also be used to map out therapeutic patterns and drug combination used in different diseases. Examples will be given with antiepileptic drugs.

# Table of Abstracts

P -1 **Induction Of Apoptosis Of Human Nasopharyngeal Carcinoma Cell Line Cne-2 By Tubeimoside I Isolated From Bolbostemma Paniculatum**

XiYang Weng, RunDi Ma, LiJian Yu

*Issues in drug discovery and development*

P -2 **Effects of tubeimoside I on Cell Cycle and Apoptosis of Human Myeloblastic Leukemia Cells (HL-60)**

Zhang Hu, Rundi Ma, Lijian Yu

P -3 **Predominant Role For Nitric Oxyde In The Relaxation Induced By Acetylcholine In The Canine Uterine Artery**

Pesic S, Grbovic L, Radenkovic M, Stojic D, Cvetkovic Z.

*Cardiovascular pharmacology and therapeutics*

P -4 **Endothelium-Dependent Relaxation In The Human Facial Artery**

Pesic S, Grbovic L, Radenkovic M, Stojic D, Pesic Z.

*Cardiovascular pharmacology and therapeutics*

P -5 **Effects Induced By Cb-1 Receptor Agonists On Visual Evoked Responses And Oscillatory Potentials In The Mouse**

Capasso A., De Lovanna A., Giuliani G., Guarino I., Loizzo A.

*Miscellaneous*

P -6 **Hospital visits caused by adverse drug reactions (ADRs):a French study in primary care-emergency departments**

Queneau P.,Bannwarth B.,Carpentier F.,Guliana J.M.,Bouget J.,Trombert B.

*Quality indicators in drug use*

P -7 **Adenosine Induces Relaxation Of Isolated Rat Aorta And Caudal Mesenteric Artery: The Role Of Adenosine Receptors**

Grbovic L., Radenkovic M.

*Cardiovascular pharmacology and therapeutics*

P -8 **The Role Of Potassium Current In Adenosine-Induced Effect In The Peripheral Rat Arteries**

Radenkovic M., Grbovic L.

*Cardiovascular pharmacology and therapeutics*

P -9 **Digoxin Pharmacokinetics And MDR1 Genetic Polymorphisms**

Verstuyft C., Schwab M., Schaeffeler E., Kerb R., Brinkmann U., Jaillon P., Funck-Brentano C., Becquemont L.

*Pharmacogenetics and pharmacogenomics*

P -10 **Turkish And German Patients Of General Practitioners Diseases, Drug Expectations And Drug Presciptions**

Von Ferber L., Koester I., Erdogan N.

*Drug utilization*

P -11 **Bioavailability Of Arsenic From Arsenic Trioxide Solubalised For Oral Administration To Patients With Haemic Malignancies**

Kumana C.R., Au W.Y., Lee N.S., Kou M., Mak R.W.M., Lam C.W., Kwong Y.L.

*Therapeutic drug monitoring - Issues in drug discovery and development*

P -12 **Comparison Of The Efficacy Of Sclerotherapy Alone and a Therapeutic Combination of Octreotide and Sclerotherapy in the Control of Acute Bleeding in Patients with Portal Hypertensive Gastropathy: A Controlled Study**

González-Martin G., Urzúa L.D., Muñoz L., Rojas M.

*Gastrointestinal pharmacology and therapeutics*

P -13 **Bisoprolol Dose-Response Relationship in Patients With Congestive Heart Failure**

Simon T., Mary-Krause M., Funck-Brentano Ch., Lechat Ph., Jaillon P.(On behalf of the Cardiac Insufficiency Bisoprolol Study (CIBIS II) investigators)

*Cardiovascular pharmacology and therapeutics*

P -14 **Impact Of MDR1 (C3435T) Genetic Polymorphism In Patients Naïve Treated With Haart Including Indinavir (IDV)**

Verstuyft C., Marcellin F., Morand-Joubert L., Launay O., Peytavin G., Gerard L., Becquemont L., Aboulker Jp., for the ANRS 08 Study Group

*Pharmacogenetics and pharmacogenomics*

P -15 **Randomised Non-blinded Two-fold Cross-over Study to Assess the Relative Bioavailability of the ASA Dry Granules 500 mg Given with and without Water to 24 Healthy Male Subjects**

Latta G, Voith B, Nagelschmitz J

*Pharmacokinetics*

25. Jun 16:15-16:30

**The Role of CYP2C8 And CYP2C9 Genotypes In Acute Myocardial Infarction**

Yasar Ü., Bennet A., Eliasson E., Lundgren S., Wiman B., De Faire U., Rane A.

*Pharmacogenetics and pharmacogenomics*

P - 16 **Transdermal Penetration of Diclofenac After Multiple Epicutaneous Administration of a Novel Spray Gel Formulation**

Brunner M., Seigfried B., Dehghanyar P., Martin W., Piotrowiak R., Menke G., Müller M.

*NSAIDS*

P - 17 **Positron Emission Tomography for the Description of Target Tissue Pharmacokinetics of [18F] Fluorine-labelled Ciprofloxacin.**

Brunner M., Langer O., Dobrozemsky G., Müller U., Mitterhauser M., Wadsak W., Kletter K., Müller M.

*Pharmacokinetics*

P - 18 **Pattern of Prescription and Drug Use in Phthalmology in a Tertiary Hospital in Delhi**

Biswas N.R., Jindal S., Siddiquei M.M., Maini R.

*Drug utilization*

P - 19 **Can the Electophysiological Actions of Psychotrop Drugs Explain Their Cardiac Side Effects?**

Kecskeméti V., Magyar J., Bányász T., Pacher P., Nánási P.P.

*Cardiovascular pharmacology and therapeutics*

P - 20 **Indinavir-induced Nephrolithiasis in HIV-infected Patients**

Dragovic G., Jevtovic Dj.

*Antiviral pharmacotheraphy*

P - 21 **Influence of the HMG-CoA-Reductase Inhibitor Atorvastatin on Biochemical Bone Metabolism Parameters: A Randomized Controlled Trial in Postmenopausal Women**

Berthold H.K., Unverdorben S., Degenhardt R., Zittermann A., Gouni-Berthold I.

*Osteoporosis*

P - 22 **Dose Proportionality (7.5mg To 22.5mg) and Food Effect (22.5mg) of Meloxicam Oral Suspension. An Open 4-Way Crossover Trial in Healthy Volunteers**

Klüglich M., Scheuerer S., Wallenstein G.

*NSAIDS - Pharmacokinetics*

P - 23 **Influence Of Underlying Disease on Busulfan Disposition in Bone Marrow Transplant Children : A Non Parametric Population Pharmacokinetic Study**

Bonnet-Bertholle V., ,Bleyzac N., Magron P., Galambrun C., Bertrand Y., Souillet G., Maire P., Jelliffe R., ,Aulagner G.

*PKPD modelling*

P - 24 **The Effect of the Nitroanalog Tetrapeptidamid on the Syntheses of the b-Endorfin and Corticotropin**

Hazar H., Hazar A.

*Pharmacokinetics*

P - 25 **Evaluation of Markers for Glucuronidation and Sulfation Activities Following Acetaminophen Administration**

Yin O.Q.P., Tomlinson B., Chow M.S.S.

*Drug metabolism*

P - 26 **Cost Effectiveness of an Active Antibiotic Control Program**

Lustig A.

*Pharmacoeconomy - Drug utilization*

P - 27 **Effect Of Acetylic Salicyclic Acid (ASA) on the Pharmacokinetics and Pharmacodynamics Of XRP0673, a Direct Factor Xa Inhibitor.**

Hinder M., Frick A., Ozoux M.L., Scholz H., Gebauer A., Rosenburg R.

*Drug interactions*

P - 28 **The Role of Researchers and Physicians Chambers in Formulation of National Drug Policies**

Chrusciel T.L.

*Pharmacoeconomics*

P - 29 **A Study of Drug Prescribing Pattern in Gastroenterology in a Tertiary Teaching Hospital in India**

Sood P., Midha V., Sood A.

*Drug utilization*

P - 30 **Trends of Consumption of Antiasthmatic Preparations in Yaroslavl in 2001-2002 s**

Palyutin Sh.Ch., Yakusevitch V.V.

*Teaching and communication in clinical pharmacology*

P - 31 **Secondary Lusiotropic Efficiency of Riodipine and Nifedipine on the Right Heart Ventricle Diastolic Dysfunction**

Pukitis A., Skutelis A., Mikazans V.

*Cardiovascular pharmacology and therapeutics*

P - 32 **Influence of Menthol on Caffeine Disposition and Pharmacodynamics in Healthy Female Volunteers**

Gelal A., Guven H., Balkan D., Artok L, Benowitz N.L.

*Pharmacokinetics*

P - 33 **Toxicity of Lead Acetate on Rabbit Arteries: A Histological Evaluation**

Minaii B., Towfighi Z., Soltaninejad K., Abdollahi M.

*Cardiovascular pharmacology and therapeutics*

P - 34 **A Drug Utilization Study in 511 Patients Attending, Gynaecology and Obstetrics Out-door Department at a Tertiary Referral Centre of Industrial Town of Ludhiana, India**

Kaushal S., Chopra S.C., Kaushal K., Cheema T.S., Cheema R.

*Drug utilization*

P - 35 **Influence of Oral Placebo, Trapidil and Isosorbide Dinitrate on Norephinephrine-induced Hand Vein Constriction in Healthy Men**

Sziegoleit W., Dannenberg K., Konschak A., Presek P.

*Cardiovascular pharmacology and therapeutics*

P - 36 **Adenosine Receptor Mediated Cytotoxicity in the Breast Cancer Cell Lines: Focus on the A3 Receptor**

Panjehpour M., Karami-Tehrani F.

*Miscellaneous*

P - 37 **Different Patterns of Craving and Withdrawal Symptoms During Smoking Abstinence**

Teneggi V., Squassante L., Ziviani L., Milleri S., Bye A.

*Drug dependence*

P - 38 **Effects of Acetylsalicylate on Spinal Reflexes in Rats**

Genc O., Turgut S., Turgut G., Kortunay S.

*NSAIDS*

P - 39 **Effects of Metamizol (Dipyrone) on Spinal Reflexes in Rats**

Genc O., Turgut S., Turgut G., Kortunay S.

*NSAIDS*

P - 40 **The Effects of Zizyphus Jujuba Mill. Extractions On Heart Rates And Minute Respiratory Volume Of Rats**

Çelik A., Turgut G., Genç O., Turgut S., Altin R., Aydın M., Kortunay S.

*Miscellaneous*

P - 41 **A New, Rapid, Fully Automated Method for Determination of Fluconazole in Serum by Column-Switching Liquid Chromatography**

Kümmerer, K.

*Therapeutic drug monitoring*

P - 42 **Vasoconstrictor Hyporeactivity in Inflammation can be Corrected by Antioxidants**

Pleiner J.

*Cardiovascular pharmacology and therapeutics*

P - 43 **Effects of Sildenafil Citrate on Ejaculation Process**

Bilge S.S., Kesim Y., Kurt M., Aksoz E., Celik S.

*Miscellaneous*

P - 44 **Irrational Drug Use in Some Districts of Lithuania**

Maciulaitis R., Janusonis T.

*Ratinolpharmacotheraphy*

P - 45 **Efficacy of Myrrh in Comparison with Anticoccidial Drug Diclazuril ,on Performance of Broiler Chicks**

El -Ashmawy I.M., El- Lakany H.,,Salama O.M.

*Miscellaneous*

P - 46 **Role of Polyphorphic Human CYP2B6 in Cyclophosphamide Bioactivation**

Xie H., Yasar U., Lundgren S., Griskevicius L., Terelius Y., Hassan M., Rane A.

*Pharmacogenetics and pharmacogenomics*

P - 47 **Optimising the Treatment of Burned Patients by Usage of Tibetan Healing Techniques**

Fedorov V.M., Strakhov S.N., Philppov A.I., Kostyukova Z.I., Mikhailov A.G., Redkina V.Y.

*Miscellaneous*

P - 48 **Effects of Chronic Lead Acetate Intoxication on Blood Indices in Male Adult Rat**

Noori M.M.H.,Heidari Z., Mahmoudzadeh Sagheb H.R.

*Cardiovascular pharmacology and therapeutics*

P - 49 **Survival Following Severe Dapson Poisoning**

Vessal G., Moiensadat M., Shadnia S.

*Drug interactions*

P - 50 **Hange-koboku-to (Banxia-houpo-tang) Raises Neuropeptide Levels in Human Plasma and Saliva**

Naito T., Itoh H., Takeyama M.

*Gastrointestinal pharmacology and therapeutics*

P - 51 **Comparison Between the Analgesic Effect of Carum Copticum Extract and Morphine in Phasic Pain Modle in Mice**

Dashti M.H., Hejazian S.H. , Morshedi A.

*Pain*

P - 52 **The Analgesic Effect of Ethanolic Extract of Lactuca Sativa Seeds in Mice**

"Morshedi A.; Dashti M.H."

*Pain*

P - 53 **Commonly Prescribed Chemotherapeutics in Pregnancy in Trabzon, Turkey**

Kadioglu M., Yaris F., Ulku C., Kesim M., Yaris E., Kalyoncu N.

*Ratinolpharmacotheraphy*

P - 54 **Analgesics Prescribed in Pregnancy in Trabzon, Turkey**

Kadioglu M., Yaris F., Ulku C., Kesim M., Yaris E., Kalyoncu N.

*Ratinolpharmacotheraphy*

P - 55 **GABAergic Mechamisms in Nucleus Tractus Soliarius on Barareflex Sensitivitg in Acut Hypertension Rat**

Rafati A., Pourshanazari A.A., Ciriello J.

*Cardiovascular pharmacology and therapeutics*

P - 56 **Anti Nociceptive Effect of Carum Copticum in Mice**

Hejazian Yazdy S.H.

*Pain*

P - 57 **The Comparison between the Anti Nociceptive Effect of Chamomile Extract and Morphine in Mice**

Vahidi Mehrjardi,A.

*Pain*

P - 58 **Esrrogen Regulation of GABA Response in Nucleus Tractus Solitarii of Rats**

Pourshanazari A.A., Alaei H.A., Rafati A., Ciriello J.

*Cardiovascular pharmacology and therapeutics*

P - 59 **On GABAA Receptor to Increase Baroreflex Sensitivity in Rats**

*Alaei H.A., Pourshanazari A.A., Eslami H.R.*

P - 60 **Prescribing Pattern of Antipsycotic Drugs in Patients with Schizophrenia**

Chinellato A., Salvato C., Terrazzani G., Pullia G., Serraglia D., GiustiP., Lucioni C., Haycox A., Walley T.

*Pharmacoepidemiology*

P - 61 **Some Degradation Pathways Affecting the Biological Activity of IFN Alpha 2b, Interleukin 2 and Epidermal Growth Factor**

Ruiz L.

*Drug utilization*

P - 62 **The Influence of Some Formulation Factors on the Protein Stability**

Ruiz L.

*Drug utilization*

P - 63 **A Bioavaılability/Bioequivalence Study of Generic Fluoxetine Tablets**

Jovanovic D., Maksimovic M., Todorovic V., Srnic D., Stoj_ic D., Ciric B., Vehabovic M., Potogija N.

*Pharmacokinetics*

P - 64 **Development of Formulations of Interleukin 2 with a Long-Term Stability**

Reyes N.

*Drug utilization*

P - 65 **Development of New Albumin-Free Formulations of Interferon Alpha 2b for Clinical Purposes**

Hardy E.

*Drug utilization*

P - 66 **How Prevalent and How Rational is the Prescription of more han one Benzodiazepine to the Same Patient?**

De Las Cuevas C., Sanz E.

*Ratinolpharmacotheraphy-Quality indicators in drug use-Drug utilization-Pharmacoepidemiology*

P - 67 **Effect of Antıoxidant Vitamins on Serum Paraoxonase Activity and Lipid Peroxidation in Women With Type 2 Diabetes**

Gorshunska M., Karachenzev Y.

*Miscellaneous*

P - 68 **Loratadine Bioequivalence Study**

Jovanovic M., Vuksanovic J., Ivezic S., Segrt Z., Maksimovic M., Jovanovic D.

*Pharmacokinetics*

P - 69 **Comparative Bioavailability of Two Oral Formulations of Nitrazepam in Healthy Volunteers**

Jovanovic D., Jovanovic M., Maksimovic M., Kilibarda V., Vehabovic M., Potogija N.

*Pharmacokinetics*

**The Rational Use of Psychotherapeutic Agents in Primary Care**

Rihmer Z.

*Ratinolpharmacotheraphy*

P - 70 **6-Mercaptopurine Metabolites in Patients with Inflammatory Bowel Disease**

Derijks L.J.J., Gilissen L.P.L., Engels L.G.J.B., Lohman J.J.H.M., van Deventer S.J.H., Hommes D.W., Hooymans P.M.

*Pharmacokinetics*

P - 71 **High Serum Concentrations of the Acyclovir Main Metabolite 9-Carboxymethoxymethylguanine in Renal Failure Patients with Acyclovir-Related Neuropsychiatric Side Effects: An Observational Study**

Helldén A., Odar-Cederlöf I., Diener P., Barkholt L., Medin C., Svensson J.O., Säwe J., Ståhle L.

*Therapeutic drug monitoring*

P - 72 **The Effect of Chamomill Extract on Phasic Pain in Mice**

Mirvakili M., Dashti M.H., Vahidi A., Morshedi A.

*Pain*

P - 73 **Effects of Exposure to Selective Serotonin reuptake Inhibitors During Pregnancy on Infant Outcome**

Laine K., Heikkinen T., Ekblad U., Kero P.

*Pediatric clinical pharmacology*

P - 74 **Tauredon and Wobenzym Combination in Treatment of Rheumatoid Arthritis**

Shalamberidze L., Gongadze N., Kartvelishvili E., Chapichadze Z.

*Osteoporosis*

P - 75 **Treatment with Selective Cyclooxygenase 2 Inhibitor Rofecoxib in Mice Model of Parkinson's Disease.**

Przybylkowski A., Joniec I., Ciesielska A., Kurkowska-Jastrzebska I., Czlonkowski A., Czlonkowska A.

*NSAIDS*

P - 76 **Effects of Cimetidine on Male Reproductive System**

Takzaree A.R., Takzaree N., Rezayat M., Akbari M., Yarmohammady K.

*Drug metabolism*

P - 77 **OCP Intake During Pregnancy and Its Side Effects Leading to Anomalies**

Takzaree N., Yarmohammady K., Takzaree S., Rezayat S.M.

*Drug utilization*

P - 78 **Teratogenic Effects of Diazepam Intake During Pregnancy Leading to Visual System Anomalies**

Takzaree N., Yarmohammadi K., Takzaree A.R., Rezayat M., Akbari M.

*Drug utilization*

P - 79 **The Effect of Ginger on Hyperglycemia and Hyperlipidemia Induced by Cyclosporin a Drug in Male Rats**

Taghizadehafshari A.

*Drug utilization*

P - 80 **The Effect of Garlic On Cyclosporin a Induced Ldl Changes**

Shirpoor A.

*Drug utilization*

P - 81 **Dispensing Habits of The Community Pharmacists in Ümraniye Distiict Of Istanbul, Turkey**

Hale Toklu, Ahmet Akıcı, Sena Sezen, _anda Çalı, _ule Oktay, Meral Keyer-Uysal

*Pharmacoepidemiology*

P - 82 **Evaluation of Childhood Respiratory Tract Infections' Treatment**

"Akıcı A., Kalaça S.; U_urlu Ü., Oktay _."

*Pediatric clinical pharmacology*

P - 83 **The Effect of Rational Pharmacotherapy Training on Therapeutic Competence of Interns and General Practitioners**

Akıcı A., Kalaça S., U_urlu Ü., Akkan G., Karaalp A., Gören Z., Demir D.,Oktay _.

*Teaching and communication in clinical pharmacology*

P - 84 **Comparison of Osce and Unstructered Oral Examination to Assess Therapeutic Competence**

Akıcı A., Kalaça S., Kocaba_o_lu Y. E., Demir D., Oktay _.

*Teaching and communication in clinical pharmacology*

**25. Jun 10:15-10:30**

**Which Factors Affect Hypertension Management in Diabetic Patients?**

Denig P, Schaars CF, Kasje WN, Haaijer-Ruskamp FM.

*Ratinolpharmacotheraphy*

P - 85 **On the Pathophysiology of Schizophrenia**

Bjerkenstedt L., Farde L., Terenius L., Edman G., Venizelos N., Wiesel F. A.

P - 86 **Differential Effect of Cyclophosphamide on the Expression and Activity of Cytochromes P450**

Xie H., Mirghani R., Yasar Ü., Terelius Y., Lundgren S., Rane A., M Hassan M.

*Pharmacogenetics and pharmacogenomics*

P - 87 **Drug Treatment After Acute Myocardial Infarction in Estonia**

Marandi T, Thetloff M.

*Drug utilization*

P - 88 **Correlation Between Busulphan Concentration and Transplantation Related Toxicity in Patients Undergoing Stem Cell Transplantation**

Hassan M., Aschan J., Hassan Z., Ringden O., Winiarski J., Nilsson C., Öberg G.

*Pharmacokinetics*

**The Ethical Issues of Controlled Randomised Double Blind Clinical Trials**

Borvendég J.

*Miscellaneous*

**26. Jun 10:15-10:30**

**Early Exposure To Ciprofloxacin in A Bioequivalence Study**

Macedo T.R.A., Neta C., Martins F., Marques H., Silva J., Morgadinho M.T., Fontes Ribeiro C.A.

*Pharmacokinetics*

P - 89 **Accelerated Healing of Chronic Nonhealing Pressure Ulcer in a Patient Induced By the Lipid Calf Thymic Extract**

Majsimovic D., Pitic L., Beleslin D.B.

*Issues in drug discovery and development*

P - 90 **Comparison of the Rate and Extent of Absorption of Nimesulide Contained in Tablets and Granules**

Fontes Ribeiro C.A., Neta C., Martins F., Marques H., Silva J., Macedo T.R.A.

*Pharmacokinetics*

P - 91 **Analysis of Roscovitine Using Novel High Performance Liquid Chomatography and Uv-Detection Method: Pharmacokinetics and Tissue Distribution of Roscovitine and Its Major Metabolite in Rat**

Fernanda Vita M., Meurling L., Pettersson T., Cruz M., Sidén Å.,Hassan M.

*Pharmacokinetics*

P - 92 **Time Course of Platelet Aggregation and Inhibition of Thromboxane and Prostacyclin Biosynthesis after Administration of Different Single Oral Doses of Aspirin in 48 Male Healthy Subjects**

Becker A., Kornberger R., Völker M., Grossmann M.

*NSAIDS*

**P - 93** **Identification of a Novel G816A SNP in the Human MRP1 Gene Using a LightCycler Technique**

Oselin K., Mrozikiewicz P.M., Pähkla R., Roots I.

*Transporter systems*

**P - 94** **Euro-Med-Stat: Monitoring Expenditure and Utilisation of Medicinal Products in the European Union Countries. A Public Health Approach**

Van Ganse E., Pietri G.

*Pharmacoepidemiology*

**25. Jun 10:15-10:30**

**Tolerance of Antihypertensive Therapy : The Ota Study, Design and Overall Data**

Van Ganse E., Girerd X., Larguier J.S., Alamercery Y. , Laforest L., Mistretta F.

*Pharmacoepidemiology*

**25. Jun 10:30-10:45**

**Community Pharmacy Survey of Diabetes Patients**

Bauguil G., Catala O., Van Ganse E., Travier N., Chamba G.

*Pharmacoepidemiology*

**Identification of Cytochrome P4502C9 and 3A4 as the Major Catalysts of Phenprocoumon Hydroxylation**

Ufer M.

*"Pharmagenetics and pharmacogenomics; Drug metabolism"*

**P - 95** **Medicated Chewing-Gum : Formulation for Prevention of Dento- Periodontal Diseases**

Belgun - Florea S.

*Miscellaneous*

**P - 96** **Telomeres and Telomerase in Pediatric Patients with Acute Lymphoblastic Leukemia (T-All)**

Kleideiter E., Bangerter U., Schwab M., Niethammer D., Greil J., Klotz U.

*Miscellaneous*

**26. Jun 10:15-10:30**

**Eradication of Helicobacter Pylori (Hp) by Short-Term Lansoprazole Quadruple Therapy in Caucasians Depends on CYP2C19 Genotype**

Schwab M., Schäffeler E., Treiber G., Klotz U.

*Gastrointestinal pharmacology and therapeutics*

**P - 97** **Assessment of Drug-Induced Gastrointestinal Diseases in Sugery University Hospital**

Hippius J.M., Hegenbart U., Hoffmann A.

*Pharmacoepidemiology*

**P - 98** **Influence of Genetic Polymorphisms on Rifampicin-Mediated Induction of MRP2 (ABCC2) mRNA Expression**

Cascorbi I., Haenisch S., Gießmann T., Dazert P., Hecker U., Kroemer H.K., Siegmund W.

*Transporter systems*

**P - 99** **Embryotoxicitic Effects of Ranitidine**

Nassrollazadeh B., Lalaney M., Onsory D.

*Issues in drug discovery and development*

**P - 100** **Evaluation of Contraceptive Effects of Trimethoprim and 2,4-Diamino - 5 (3,4-Dichlorophenyl6-Isopropyloxmethyl Pyrimidine in Male Rats**

Sadeghipour Roudsari H.R.

*Issues in drug discovery and development*

**P - 101** **Efavirenz Plasma Concentrations in HIV-Infected Patients: Inter- and Intraindividual Variability and Clinical Effects**

Ståhle L., Moberg L., Svensson J.O., Sönnerborg A.,

*Antiviral pharmacotheraphy*

**P - 102** **Activity of CYP3A Determined by Quinine Hydroxylation in Pregnant and non Pregnant Women Infected with Plasmodium Falciparum**

Mirghani R.A., Elagib I., Hellgren U., Adam I., Elghazali G., Elbashir M.I., Gustafsson L.L.

*Drug metabolism*

**P - 103** **Pilot-Analysis of Pharmacogenetic Polymorphisms in Patients with Gastrointestinal Carcinoma**

Farker K., Merkel U., Wedding U., Höffken K., Hoffmann A.

*Miscellaneous*

**P - 104** **Autoimmune Thyroiditis in Patients with Chronic Hepatitis C during Treatment with Combination Therapy (Interferon Alfa Plus Ribavirin)**

Nesic Z., Delic D., Prostran M., Vuckovic S., Todorovic Z., Stojanovic R.

*Antiviral pharmacotheraphy*

**P - 105 The Priorities in Prescription of Ukrainian Cardiologists**

Sharayeva M.L., Victorov O.P., Khomenko Z.A.

*Ratinolpharmacotheraphy*

**P - 106 The Influence of Caffeine Preparations Intake on Pharmacodynamic Effects of Propranolole**

Brajovic T., Raskovic A. , Boljevic A., Jakovljevic V.

*Drug interactions*

**P - 107 Impaza - a New Promising Remedy for Erectile Dysfunction: Placebo-Controlled Trial**

Martyushev-Poklad A.V., Smolenov I.V., Petrov V.I., Dugina J.L.,.Sergeeva S.A, Epstein O.I.

*Clinicalpharmacologyofelderly*

**P - 108 Artrofoon in Treatment of Rheumatoid Arthritis Patients: A Pilot Randomized Clinical Study**

Petrov V.I., Babaeva A.R., Tcherevkova E.V., Martyushev-Poklad A.V., Sergeeva S.A., Epstein O.I.

*Pain*

**P - 109 Tissue Pharmacokinetics of Metronidazole**

Pähkla R., Karjagin J., Starkopf J.

*Pharmacokinetics*

**P - 110 Anaferon - A Novel Therapeutic For Influenza in Children: Clinical Efficacy and Immunomodulation**

Martyushev-Poklad A.V., Drinevskiy V.P., Osidak L.V., Dugina J.L., Kotelnikova M.P., Sergeeva S.A., Epstein O.I.

*Pediatric clinical pharmacology*

**P - 111 Anxiolytic and Antidepressant Action of Proproten: Experimental and Clinical Study**

Voronina T.A., Molodavkin G.M., Krylov E.N., Dugina J.L., Sergeeva S.A., Epstein O.I.

*Drug dependence*

**P - 112 Ketoconazole Increases Venlafaxine Plasma Concentrations Regardless of CYP2D6 Pheno/Genotype**

Lindh J., Annas A., Meurling L., Dahl M.L., AL-Shurbaji A.

*Drug interactions*

**P - 113 Population Kinetic Analysis of the Interactions Between Lamotrigin and Inducers and Inhibitors of Glucuronidation**

Böttiger Y., Ståhle L.

*Drug interactions*

**P - 114 Anar in the Treatment of Opiate Withdrawal Syndrome**

Bohan N.A., Abolonin A.F., Dugina J.L., Sergeeva S.A., Epstein O.I.

*Drug dependence*

**P - 115 Knowledge of Patients about Prescribed Drugs**

Akıcı A., Kalaça S., U_urlu Ü., Altunba_-Toklu H., _skender E., Oktay _.

*Pharmacoepidemiology*

**P - 116 Lack of Effect of Age, Weight and Body Mass Index on Trough and Peak Indinavir Plasma Concentrations in HIV-Infected Patients Treated with Different Indinavir Boosted Regimens**

*Zouai O., Poirier J.M., Meynard J.L., Lacombe K., Guiard-Schmid J.B., Girard P.M., Jaillon P.*

**P - 117 Identification and Characterisation of Novel SNPs in the 5'-Flanking Region of the CYP2C9 Gene**

Sandberg M., Bloethner S., Malmebo S., Rane A., Johansson I., Eliasson E.

*Pharmacogenetics and pharmacogenomics*

**P - 118 Bufrenorphine Treatment in Heroin Addicts**

Guglielmino L., Vigezzi P., Silenzio R., De Chiara M., Corrado F., Marzorati P., Cocchi L., Cozzolino E.

*Drug dependence*

**27. Jun 10:15-10:30**

**Lowering of LDL and Raising of HDL by High-Dosage Itraconazole in Men**

Lütjohann D., Gerdsen R., Lindenthal B., Locatelli S., Diczfalusy U., Björkhem I., Neuvonen P., Bieber T., Von Bergmann K.

*Cardiovascular pharmacology and therapeutics*

**P - 119 Ezetimibe Effectively Reduces Serum Plant Sterols in Patients with Sitosterolemia**

Lütjohann D., Von Bergmann K., Salen G., The Multicenter Sitosterolemia Study Group

*Cardiovascular pharmacology and therapeutics*

P - 120 **Use of Non-specific Intravenous Human Inmunoglobulins, Need for a Hospital Protocol.**

Cabrera García L., Ruiz A.S., Antorán B.R., Valderas M.S., Torralba A., Solá C.A.

*Drug utilization*

P - 121 **Lead and Cadmium Content of Korbal Rice in Northern Iran**

Bakhtiarian A., Gholipour M., Ghazi-Khansari M.

*Miscellaneous*

P - 122 **Replacement Therapy With L?Thyroxine Plus Triiodothyronine (14:1) Is Not Superior to Thyroxine Alone with Respect to the Psychical and Physical Wellbeing of Patients with Hypothyroidism**

Siegmund W., Spieker K., Giessmann T., Jasmann D., Modess C., Engel G., Kirsch G., Hamm A., Meng W.

*Miscellaneous*

P - 123 **Disposition of Oral Carvedilol Is Inducible by Rifampicin Mainly Dependent on Up-Regulation of Intestinal P-Glycoprotein and MRP2**

Siegmund W., Giessmann T., Zschiesche M., Hecker U., Kunert-Keil C., Warzok R., Engel G.,, Dazert P., Cascorbi I., Kroemer H.K.

*Transporter systems*

**27. Jun 10:15-10:30**

**COX-2 Selective Inhibitors Rofecoxib and Celecoxib Protect Against Colorectal Adenomas Occurrence and Recurrence. A Nested Case-Control Study.**

Rahme E., Barkun A.N., Toubouti Y., LeLorier J., Bardou M.

*Pharmacoepidemiology*

P - 124 **Postoperative Analgesia After Traumatic and Orthopaedic Surgery: a Methodological Qualitative Systematic Review**

Montané E, Vallano A, Aguilera C, Laporte JR.

*Pain*

**26. Jun 10:30-10:45**

**Proton Pump Inhibitors Used as High Dose Intravenous Infusion Decrease Both Re-Bleeding and Mortality in High-Risk Patients with Acute Peptic Ulcer Bleeding: a Series of Meta-Analyses.**

Bardou M., Toubouti Y., Benhaberou-Brun D., Rahme E., Barkun A.

*Gastrointestinal pharmacology and therapeutics*

P - 125 **Intra- and Inter-Individual Variability in Losartan Metabolic Ratio, a Specific Marker of CYP2C9 Activity in Vivo.**

Eliasson E., Sandberg M., Christensen M., Dahl M.L., Yasar Ü.

*Drug metabolism*

P - 126 **Real Time RT-PCR: A method for the Assessment of Immun-Response on mRNA Level. A case study on fosfomycin.**

Joukhadar C., Jilma B., Müller M., Wagner O., Marsik C.

*Antimicrobial theraphy*

**25. Jun 16:30-16:45**

**Microdialysis: An Innovative Method for the Assessment of Penetration Properties of Antimicrobial Agents into Target Tissues in Humans**

Joukhadar C., Zeitlinger M., Müller M.

*Pharmacokinetics*

P - 127 **Are We Participants or Bystanders?**

Milan Stanulovic, Vid Stanulovic, Dusan Duric

*Issues in drug discovery and development*

P - 128 **Assessment of Opiates and Cocaine Consumption During Pregnancy by Self-Reported Questionnaire and Meconium Analysis**

Pichini S., Zuccaro P., Marchei E., Pellegrini M., , Perez-Alarcón E., Puig C., Vall O., Pacifici R., Ordobas L., García-Algar Ó.

*Pediatric clinical pharmacology*

**The Emerging Problem of Therapy Resistant Tuberculosis.**

Kiivet R.

*Antimicrobial theraphy*

P - 129 **Resistance on Ceftriaxone in two Periods: First of Restricted Usage and Second of Unrestricted Usage**

Knezevic A.,Dobrovic K., Morovic M.

*Ratinolpharmacotheraphy*

P - 130 **Effects of the Administration Schedule of Oral Salmon Calcitonin on Bone Resorption Markers**

Bucher M., Buclin T., Cosma M., Azrıa M., Attinger M., Mcleod J., Biollaz J., Burckhardt P.

*Osteoporosis*

**P - 131** **Nociceptin Levels During the Cluster Headache Period**

Ertsey Cs., Hantos M., Bozsik Gy., Tekes K.

*Clinical Pharmacologyinneurology*

**P - 132** **Efficacy and Safety of Cizolirtine Citrate in the Treatment of Acute Pain Caused by an Attack of Renal Colic.**

Abadías M., Suchı J., Sust M., Toufarová P., Villoria J., Bartlett A.

*Pain*

**P - 133** **Heavy Users of NSAIDs in Finland. A Prescription Database Study**

Huupponen R., Helin-Salmivaara A., Klaukka T.

*NSAIDS*

25. Jun 10:30-10:45

**Initial Drug Therapy of Hypertension in Estonia**

Irs A., Thetloff M.

*Pharmacoepidemiology*

**Contribution of a Poison Information Centre (PIC) in the Evaluation of Adverse Drug Effects (ADEs) to the German National Pharmacovigilance System**

Mey C., Hentschel H., Hippius M., Tiaden J.D., Müller-Oerlinghausen B., Balogh A.

*Pharmacoepidemiology*

**P - 134** **Chronic Ethanol Consumptıon and Papillary Muscle Responses to Nifedipine**

Rasic A., M.Prostran, Stevanovic H.L., Todorovic Z., Vuckovic S., Stojanovic R., Nesic Z.

*Drug interactions*

**P - 135** **Investigatıon of the Pharmacokinetics and Metabolism of Promegestone in Healthy Female Volunteers Following Single Oral Administration of 1 Mg Promegestone**

Gualano V., Geneteau A., Chassard D., Fordham P., Schatz B.

*Drug metabolism*

27. Jun 16:30-16:45

**Considerations When Investigating Association between Drug Exposure and Hepatic Function.**

Ghahramani P., Lennon S.M.

*Pharmacokinetics*

**P - 136** **Chemotherapy for Lung Cancer: Rationalization of Costs**

Cervellino J.C., Araujo C.E., Fligman M.D., Pires E.A.

*Pharmacoeconomy*

**P - 137** **Pentoxifylline: Pharmacokinetics of an Acqueous Oral Solution and _nfluence on PTH Secretion in Healthy Volunteers.**

Rochat M.C., Buclin T., Decosterd L.A., Sanderson P., Biollaz J.

*Osteoporosis*

**P - 138** **Effects of Paracetamol on Antioxidant Enzymes in Erythrocytes in Febrile Children**

Bajcetic M., Mitrovic J., Divac N., Samardzic R.

*Pediatric clinical pharmacology*

**P - 139** **Newer Hypnotic Drugs for Short-Term Pharmacotherapy for Insomnia: a Systematic Review**

Dundar Y., Boland A., Dickson R., Haycox A., Strobl J., Walley T.

*Clinical Pharmacologyinneurology*

**P - 140** **Sustained Hemodynamic Effects of Intravenous Levosimendan**

Lehtonen L.A., Kivikko M., Colucci W.S.

*Cardiovascular pharmacology and therapeutics*

**P - 141** **The three-arm Trial: Report of a Practical Case Illustrating the Utility of This Approach to Assess the Assay Sensitivity**

Videla S., Sust M., Villoria J., Abadías M., Fresquet A., Costa A., Bartlett A.

*Issues in drug discovery and development*

**P - 142** **Food Effect on the Double Peak Phenomenon Occurrence in Famotidine Bioequivalence Studies**

Kopecky J., Zoulova J., Filipova K., Pastera J., Chladek J., Svoboda D., Macek K., Kvetina J.

*Pharmacokinetics*

**P - 143** **The Relationship of in Vitro Dissolution and Human Bioavailability on the Model of Two Oral Isosorbide-5-Mononitrate (Is-5-Mn) Formulations**

Vyslouzil L., KopeckyJ., Pastera J., Macek K., Chládek J., Rezanka V., Kvetina J.

*Pharmacokinetics*

**P - 144 The Effect of Food on Bioavailability of Propafenone**

Zoulová J., Kopecky J., Perlík F., Anzenbacherová E., Svoboda D., Chládek J., Kvetina J.

*Pharmacokinetics*

**P - 145 CYP1A2 Activity in Caucasians - Relationship to Smoking Habits, Use of Oral Contraceptives and 3 SNPs in Intron 1 of the CYP1A2 Gene.**

Christensen M., Nordmark A., Aklillu E., Schrey S., Ingelman-Sundberg M., Bertilsson L.

*Pharmacogenetics and pharmacogenomics*

**P - 146 Paraoxon Induces Apoptosis in EL4 Cells via Activation of Mitochondrial Pathways.**

Saleh A.

*Miscellaneous*

**P - 147 Fluconazole in Anuric Patients Undergoing Continuous-Veno-Venous- Hemodialysis (CVVHD): Pharmacokinetics and Dosage Simulation**

Mueller S.C., Majcher-Peszynska J., Mundkowski R.G., Hickstein H., Drewelow B.

*Antimicrobial theraphy*

**P - 148 The Effect of Caffeine-Containing Coffee Versus Decaffeinated Coffee on Serum Clozapine Concentrations in Hospitalised Patients**

Raaska K., Raitasuo V., Laitila J., Neuvonen P.J.

*Drug interactions*

**27. Jun 10:30-10:45**

**The Management of Hyperlipidaemia in CAPD Patients**

Velickovich- Radovanovich R., Avramovich M., Raicevich R., Mitich B., Kostich S., Djordjevich V.

*Cardiovascular pharmacology and therapeutics*

**P - 149 Efficacy and Safety Fluvastatın Compared to Simvastatin in Capd Patients**

Raicevic R., Velickovic- Radovanovic R., Avramovic M., Kostic S.

*Cardiovascular pharmacology and therapeutics*

**P - 150 HLA Class II Molecules and Drug-Induced Idiosyncratic Liver Disease. A Multicenter Study**

Lucena M.I., Andrade R.J., Alonso A., Fernández M.C., Durán J.A., Torres E.L., Seoane J., Verge C., De la Cuesta F.S.

*Miscellaneous*

**P - 151 Consumption Trend of Anticonvulsant Agents in Sarajevo Svjetlana**

Loga S., Loga S., Mulabegovic N., Skaljic A., Kusturica J., Rakanovic M., Becic F.

*Drug utilization*

**P - 152 Application Dossier for Marketing Authorization in the European Union and Federation of Bosnia and Herzegovina**

Todic M., Becic F., Loga-Zec S., Kusturica J.

*Miscellaneous*

**P - 153 Diclofenac Systemic Exposure is not Increased When Topical Diclofenac is Applied on Uv-Induced Erythema**

Magnette J.L., Kienzler J.L., Sallin D., Ménart C., Nollevaux F., Knops A.

*Pharmacokinetics*

**P - 154 Information about Drugs Available for our Medical Staff**

Beèiæ F., Mulabegoviæ N., Kapiæ E., Kusturica J., Loga-Zec S., Todiæ-Rakanoviæ M.

*Ratinolpharmacotheraphy*

**P - 155 Drugs Available for Treatment of Asthma Bronchale**

Beèiæ F., Mulabegoviæ N., Kapiæ E., Kusturica J., Rakanoviæ-Todiæ M., Zec S.L.

*Miscellaneous*

**P - 156 Incorporating Pharmacology Education into an Intergrated Medical Curriculum.**

Franson K.

*Teaching and communication in clinical pharmacology*

**P - 157 Attitudes to Feed-Back with Prescribing Profiles among Prescribers in Rijeka, Croatia and Stockholm, Sweden**

Palcevski V.V., Wettermark B., Prpic I., Bergman U.

*Quality indicators in drug use*

**P - 158 Pharmaco-economic Comparison of Switch and Intravenous Antibiotic Therapy for Lower Respiratory Tract Infections in Elderly Patients**

Wawruch M.,Bozekova L.,Krcmery S.,Slobodova Z.,Kozlikova K.,Lassan S.,Kriska M.

*Pharmacoeconomy*

**P - 159 Hepatic Toxicity of Benzarone and Benzbromarone**

Kaufmann P. , Hänni A., Gasser R., Török M., Krähenbühl S.T.

*Drug metabolism*

**P - 160 Onset of Action of Alfuzosin Once-Daily in Men with Symptomatiic Benigin Prostatic Hyperplasia**

"Jacobs S., Leonard S.M., City C., CA; Roehrborn C., Gittelman M., Forrest J. "

*Therapeutic drug monitoring*

**P - 161 Veno-Occlusive Disease (VOD) in a Patient Treated with Cyclophosphamide (CPA) and Roxithromycin (ROX)**

Kaufmann P., Beltinger J., Wenk M., Bogman K., Török M., Krähenbühl St.

*Drug interactions*

**P - 162 'Selective' Switching from Non-Selective to Selective Non-Steroidal Anti-Inflammatory Drugs (NSAIDs).**

Bennett K., Teeling M., Feely J.

*Pharmacoepidemiology*

**The Effect of Gemfibrozil on the Pharmacokinetics of Rosuvastatin**

Schneck D.W., Birmingham B.K., Zalikowski J.A., Mitchell P.D., Lasseter K.C., Raza A.

*Drug interactions*

**P - 163 A Role for Aldosterone in Essential Hypertension**

Mahmud A.

*Cardiovascular pharmacology and therapeutics*

**P - 164 Chronopharmacologic Study of the Local Anaesthetic Activity of Mepivacaïne in Children Dental Care**

Boughattas N.A., Amor S.H., Attia M.B., Letaief M., Maatoug F., Bouzouita K..

*Clinical Pharmacologyinneurology*

**P - 165 The Improvement of Digoxin Therapy after Implementation of Pharmacokinetic Interpretation**

Grundmann M., Kacirova I., Koristkova B., Brozmanova H.

*Therapeutic drug monitoring*

**P - 166 A Novel in-vivo PK/ in-vitro PD Model for the Combined Simulation of Bacterial Killing of Two Antimicrobial Agents: A case Study on Fosfomycin and Cefpirome**

Zeitlinger M., Müller M., Joukhadar C.

*PKPD modelling*

**P - 167 An Exploration of the Therapeutic Arsenals of Antibiotics in European Countries Using the Drug Utilisation 90% Method**

Ferech M., Stichele R.V., Elseviers M., Goossens H.

*Drug utilization*

**P - 168 Pattern of Use of Benzodiazepines (BDZ) in Hypertensive Patients in General Practice (GP) in Serbia**

Divac N., Veljkovic S., Bajcetic M., Samardzic R.

*Pharmacoepidemiology*

**P - 169 Pharmacoeconomical Evaluation of Antimicrobial Treatment Patients with Antibiotic-Resistant Pseudomonas Aeruginosa Pneumonia in Intensive Care Units**

Kadusevicius E., Zmuidaite V., Stankeviciene I., Zaliaduonyte D.

*Pharmacoeconomy*

**P - 170 26. Jun 14:40-15:05**

**Effect of St. Johns Wort (Hypericum Perforatum, SJW) on Human CYPs**

Wenk M., Todesco L., Krähenbühl S.

*Drug interactions*

**P - 171 Interactions Between Herbal Drugs and Warfarin**

Dobric S., Dragojevic-Simic V., Kilibarda V., Bokonjic D.

*Drug interactions*

**P - 172 Influence of Glyceryl Trinitrate on Anti-Inflammatory and Ulcerogenic Actions of Indomethacin in Rats**

Dobric S., Velev R., Cupic V., Milovanovic Z., Jacevic V., Bokonjic D.

*NSAIDS*

**P - 173 The Organization and Teaching of Clinical Pharmacology in Serbia and Montenegro Army**

Dragojevic-Simic V., Dobric S., Jandric D., Stojiljkovic M.P., Jovanovic D., Bokonjic D.

*Teaching and communication in clinical pharmacology*

P - 174 **Dose Selection of Cytoprotector Amifostine for Chronic Rat Study of Doxorubicin Toxicity**

Dragojevic-Simic V., Dobric S., Bokonjic D.

*Issues in drug discovery and development*

P - 175 **Retrospective Prospective Analysis of Pilot Study of Pharmaco-Economy at the Model of Application of Antibiotics in Surgical and Internal Medicine Department Through the Analysis of ATC/DDD and ABC.**

Begovic B., Zulic I., Hadzovic S.

*Pharmacoeconomy*

P - 176 **Clinical Research of Efficiency, Tolerability and Safety Using Repaglinide in Treatment of Patients with Diabetes Mellitus Type 2**

Begovic B., Zulic I., Grujic M., Stevanovic D., Babic D., Ler Z., E.S. Waltonand, Kanc K.

*Miscellaneous*

25. Jun 16:15-16:30

**Population Pharmacokinetics of Rac-, (R)- and (S)-Methadone in Methadone Maintenance Subjects**

Somogyi A.A., Foster D.J.R, Bochner F., White J.

*Pharmacokinetics*

P - 177 **Grapefruit Juice even in Small Amounts Increases Considerably Plasma Concentrations of Simvastatin and Simvastatin Acid**

Lilja J.J., Neuvonen M., Neuvonen P.J.

*Drug interactions*

P - 178 **Input and Elimination of Resistant Bacteria in Sewage Treatment Plants**

Kümmerer K., Unger J., Wiethan J., Tietze A.B.

*Antimicrobial theraphy*

**Orange Juice Greatly Reduces Plasma Concentrations of Celiprolol**

Lilja J.J., Juntti-Patinen L., Neuvonen P.J.

*Drug interactions*

P - 179 **Patterns of Systemic Antibiotic Use in a Tertiary Hospital in Israel in the Years 1998-2000**

Kitzes-Cohen R., Coos D., Levy M.

*Drug Utilization*

27. Jun 10:15-10:30

**Chemotherapy for Lung Cancer: Rationalization of Costs**

*Cervellino J.C., Araujo C.E., Fligman M.D., Pires E.A.*

P - 180 **Association Angiotensin Converting Enzyme Inhibitor-Antagonists of Angiotensin II Receptors to Reduce Renal Risk in Diabetic Patients Study Among 25 Patients**

*Ory J.P., Combes J.*

P - 181 **Investigation of the Functional Responses of Corpus Cavernosum Smooth Muscle in Secondhand Smoked Rabbits**

Göçmez S.S., Utkan T., Duman C., Yıldız F., Gacar M.N., Ulak G., Erden F.

*Miscellaneous*

P - 182 **Risk Factors for Extrapyramidal Symptoms (EPS) During Treatment with Selective Serotonin Reuptake Inhibitors (SSRI's)**

Hedenmalm K., Yue Q.Y., Dahl M.L., Spigset O.

*Pharmacokinetics*

P - 183 **Concentrations of Ciprofloxacin and Ceftazidime in Surface Waters**

Wiethan J., Al-Ahmad A., Henninger A., Kümmerer K.

*Antimicrobial theraphy*

P - 184 **Effects of Combined Hypolipemic Diet on Serum Lipids**

Krehic J., Cabaravdic A., Begovic B., Veletovac-Causevic V.

*Cardiovascular pharmacology and therapeutics*

P - 185 **Pharmacokinetics of Ciprofloxacin and Levofloxacin in Patients with Liver Cirrhosis: Influence of Albumin Dialysis**

Majcher-Peszynska J., Klammt S., Mundkowski .R, Berg A., Mueller S.C., Peszynski P., Mitzner S.R., Drewelow B.

*Antimicrobial theraphy*

**Incidence of Drug-Related Visits in a Hospital Emergency Room**

Juntti-Patinen L., Kuitunen T., Pere P., Neuvonen P.J.

*Pharmacoepidemiology*

**ADR's leading to Hospital Admission**

Ibáñez L., Laporte J.R., Leone R., Vendrell L., Vidal X.

*Gastrointestinal pharmacology and therapeutics*

**P - 186 Adverse Events in Healthy Volunteers: a Phase I 5-years Survey**

Lutfullin A., Kuhlmann J., Wensing G.

*Miscellaneous*

**P - 187 Monitoring Digoxin Serum Concentrations**

Donado E., García M., Tato F., Tarragó J., Velasco M., Durán C.

*Drug utilization*

**P - 188 Dynamics of a Level of Endothelin-1 and Parameters of an Immunological Homeostasis in Patients with Myocardial Infarction Under Influence of Thrombolytic Therapy**

Pivovar S., Rudyk Y., Gorb Y.

*Cardiovascular pharmacology and therapeutics*

**P - 189 Lack of Influence of Glutathione S-transferase (GSTM1) and (GSTT1) Null Genotypes and T-allele Frequency at the MDR-1 Gene on Susceptibility to Parkinson's Disease**

Bernal L.

*Pharmacogenetics and pharmacogenomics*

**P - 190 GH Deficiency and rhGH Treatment Alter CYP3A Activity in Children: Influence of: Gender and Pubertal Status**

Sinues B.

*Growthhormone*

**P - 191 Polypharmacy and Adverse Drug Reactions in Patients of Different Age**

Dakovic-_vajcer K., Vujisic A.

*Pharmacoepidemiology*

**P - 192 Experience with Transdermal Fentanyl in Hospitalised Chronic Pain Patients**

Girardin F., Piguet V., Desmeules J., Escher M., Vernaz N., Offner J.M., Dayer P.

*Pain*

**P - 193 Lumiracoxib does not Affect the Pharmacokinetics of Methotrexate in Patients with Stable Rheumatoid Arthritis**

Hartmann S., Scott G., Rordorf C., Milosavljev S., Branson J., Chales G., Juvin R., Lafforgue P., Le Parc J.M., 8Tavernier C., 9Meyer O.

*Drug interactions*

**P - 194 Fluconazole does not Affect Lumiracoxib Pharmacokinetics in Healthy Subjects: a two-stage, open-label, randomized, crossover study**

Yih L., Scott G., Yeh C.M., Milosavljev S., Laurent A., Rordorf C.

*Drug interactions*

**P - 195 Pharmacokinetics of Lumiracoxib in Synovial Fluid and Plasma of Patients with Rheumatoid Arthritis**

Reynolds C., Scott G., Looby M., Milosavljev S., Huff J.P., Ruff D.A., Rordorf C.

*Pharmacokinetics*

**P - 196 Lumiracoxib Shows Similar Bioavailability at Different Sites in the Gastrointestinal Tract**

Wilding I.R., Connor A.L., Carpenter P., Rordorf C., Branson J., Milosavljev S., Scott G.

*Pharmacokinetics*

**P - 197 Multiple-dose Lumiracoxib Shows Rapid Absorption and COX-2 Selectivity without Accumulation in Patients with Rheumatoid Arthritis**

Scott G., Rordorf C., Milosavljev S., Chase W., Fleischmann R., Kivitz A.

*Pharmacokinetics*

**P - 198 Lumiracoxib does not Alter the Pharmacokinetic Profile or Efficacy of the Triphasic Oral Contraceptive Triphasil®-28**

Kalbag J., Rordorf C., Wang Y., Caldwell J., Leese P., Scott G.

*Drug interactions*

**P - 199 Lumiracoxib Demonstrates High Absolute Bioavailability in Healthy Subjects**

Hartmann S., Scott G., Rordorf C., Campestrini J., Branson J., Keller U.

*Pharmacokinetics*

P - 200 **Co-administration of Lumiracoxib and Warfarin does not Alter the Pharmacokinetic Profile of R- or S-Warfarin**

Bonner J., Scott G., Branson J., Milosavljev S., Rordorf C.

*Drug interactions*

P - 201 **Omeprazole and Maalox® Antacid do not Affect Lumiracoxib Pharmacokinetics in Healthy Subjects: an open-label, randomized crossover study**

Reynolds C.V., Scott G., Milosavljev S., Langholff W., Shenouda M., Rordorf C.

*Drug interactions*

**25. Jun 16:15-16:30**

**Light Evoked Pupillography - a Sensitive Clinical Biomarker for 5-HT1A Compounds**

Boettcher M., Heinig R., Wensing G., Kuhlmann J.

*Clinical Pharmacologyinneurology*

P - 202 **Safety of Neuroleptics in Schizophrenic Patients in Correlation with the Total Oxidative Hepatic Capacity.**

Ziganshina L.E., Kuchaeva A.V., Vedernikova O.O., Yakhin K. K., Gatin F.F.

*Drug metabolism*

P - 203 **Pharmacokinetics (PK) of Melagatran, the Active Form of the Oral Direct Thrombin Inhibitor Ximelagatran, and the Relationship to Clinical Response in Extended Secondary Prevention of Venous Thromboembolism**

Cullberg M., Clason S.M., Eriksson H., Karlsson M.O., Lundström T., Nyström P., Schulman S., Wåhlander K.

*Pharmacokinetics*

P - 204 **Subdosing of Parenteral Antibiotics in General Practice (GP) in Serbia**

Samardzic R., Divac N., Bajcetic M., Vujnovic M.

*Drug utilization*

P - 205 **Clinical and Pharmacoeconomical Outcomes of Posternotomy Mediastinitis due to Staphylococcus Aureus Methicillin-Resistant and Methicillin-Susceptible Infection**

Kadusevicius E., Zaliaduonyte D., Zmuidaite V., Stankevicienë I., Benetis R.

*Pharmacoeconomy*

P - 206 **Dermal Absorption of Permethrin Following Administration to the Haired Area of the Head**

Lazar A., Tomalik-Scharte D., Bastian B., Meins J., Ihrig M., Wachall B., Jetter A., Fuhr U.

*Pharmacokinetics*

P - 207 **Increased Concentrations of the Acyclovir Main Metabolite 9-Carboxymethoxymethylguanine (CMMG) in CSF in patients with Neuropsychiatric Side Effects**

Helldén A., Lycke J., Ståhle L.

*Transporter systems*

P - 208 **Flavonoids Modulate Endothelial Function and Have Protective Role on Cardiovascular System**

Ilic K., Kuntic V.

*Cardiovascular pharmacology and therapeutics*

P - 209 **New and rapid LC-MS Method to Determine Piperacillin and Tazobactam in Sputum of Patients with Cystic Fibrosis**

Trittler R., König A., Frank U., Kümmerer K.

*Therapeutic drug monitoring*

P - 210 **Impact of the Directive 2001/20/EC on Clinical Trial Regulation and Process in Hungary**

Eggenhofer J., Borvendég J.

*Miscellaneous*

P - 211 **Cystic Fibrosis: Pharmacoeconomic Analysis in Hospitalized Patients in the University Paediatric Hospital**

Vitezic D., Rosovic-Bazijanac V., Rozmanic V., Ahel V.

*Pediatric clinical pharmacology*

P - 212 **Regional Clusters in Antibiotic Consumption in Europe Monique**

Elseviers M., Robert H., Stichele V., Ferech M., Goossens H.

*Pharmacoepidemiology*

P - 213 **A Tolerability and Pharmacokinetic Study of a New Formulation of Disodium Clodronate in Comparison with Two Marketed Formulations in Healthy Female Volunteers**

Mariotti F., Corrado M.E., Acerbi D.

*Osteoporosis*

P - 214 **Nonparametric Expectation Maximization (NPEM) population pharmacokinetic analysis of caffeine disposition from sparse data in adult**

Terziivanov D., Bozhinova K., Dimitrova V., Atanasova I.

*Pharmacokinetics*

P - 215 **Randomised Trial of Candesartan and Enalapril (RACE) in the Treatment of Hypertension**

Cheung B.M.Y., Law C.Y, Fung P.C.W., Sang K.W.T.T., Tan K.C.B., Kumana C.R., Lau C.P.

*Cardiovascular pharmacology and therapeutics*

P - 216 **Effect of Renal and Hepatic Function on Oxaliplatin Pharmacokinetics: a Pilot-Analysis in Patients with Gastrointestinal Carcinoma**

Merkel U., Zimmer M., Wedding U., Roskos M., Höffken K., Hoffmann A.

*Pharmacokinetics*

P - 217 **Drug Committee Work: To Recommend Or Not To Recommend Activated Protein C (Apc) In The Treatment Of Severe Sepsis**

Victor J., Christophersen A.B., Christensen H.R.

*Miscellaneous*

P - 218 **Cobalamin Prescribing: Increase in Overall Use and Regional Differences in Prescription Pattern**

Christophersen A.B., Andersen S.E., Christensen H.R.

*Cobalamin Prescribing*

P - 219 **"Cobalamin Prescribing in a Geriatric Outpatient Clinic; Old Drug, New Indication"**

Andersen S.E., Christophersen A.B., Christensen H.R.

*Cobalamin Prescribing*

P - 220 **Correlation of Tramadol Pharmacokinetics in Relation to CYP2D6 Activity in Healthy Volunteers**

Perlík F., Nobilis M., Slanar O., Kvetina J.

P - 221 **Bioequivalence Study With Two Preparations Containing Selegiline**

Skreblin M., Staresinic-Sernhorst I., Saric-Kuzina S.

28. Jun **Documentation Grading - a Signalling and Quality Assurance Tool for International Adverse Reaction Data**

Lindquist M., Kiuru A., Pettersson M., Meyboom R., Edwards R.

P - 222 **Succinate Treatment in Children with Lactic Acidosis**

Globa O.V., Jourkova N.V., Kondakova O.B., Bacanov M.I., Maslova O.I., Balkanskaya S.V., Andreenko N.V., Basargina E.N.

P - 223 **"On the Classification of Sets of Experimental Points and Curves in Biopharmacy. Dissolution And Bioequivalence ""Metrics"" ."**

Mircioiu C.

*Pharmacokinetics*

P - 224 **On Pharmacokinetic of Orally Administered Glyburide**

Mircioiu C., Miron D.S. , Taranu B., Mircioiu I.

*Pharmacokinetics*

P - 225 **Comparative Bioavailability of Two Metoprolol Formulations in Healthy Volunteers**

Voicu V.A., Mircioiu C., Miron D.S. , Lovin I.

*Pharmacokinetics*

P - 226 **Enterohepatic Circulation and Bioequivalence Evaluation**

Voicu V.A., Mircioiu C.

*Pharmacokinetics*

P - 227 **Purinergic Modulation of Voltage-Dependent Calcium Channels in Rat Dorsal Root Ganglion Neurons**

Borvendeg S.J., Gerevich Z., Gillen C., Illes P.

P - 228 **The Influence of Drug Bulletins on Prescribing**

Ksenija M.A., Igor F., Bozidar V.

*Teaching and communication in clinical pharmacology*

P - 229 **Randomised Controlled Trial of Low Salt Diet in the Treatment of Hypertension**

Cheung B.M.Y., Law C.Y., Ho G.Y.Y., Ng P.P.Y., Kumana C.R., Lau C.P.

*Cardiovascular pharmacology and therapeutics*

26. Jun 15:40-15:55

**Survey on Prescribing of Antimicrobial Agents (AA) in University Hospital in Two Consecutive Years**

Francetic I., Bilusic M., Macolic-Sarinic V., Huic M., Mercep I., Erdeljic V., Makar-Ausperger K., Katalinic R., Likic R.

*Antimicrobial theraphy*

P - 230 **Nasal Sumatriptan Effectively Relieves Migraine Attacks in Children**

Ahonen K., Hämäläinen M.L., Rantala H., Hoppu K.

*Pediatric clinical pharmacology*

P - 231 **Orange Juice Greatly Reduces Plasma Concentrations of Celiprolol**

Lilja J.J., Juntti-Patinen L., Neuvonen P.J.

*Drug interactions*

P - 232 **Bioequivalence Study of Two Enalapril Formulations (20 mg) in Healthy Volunteers**

Portolés A., García-Arenillas M., Terleira A., Almeida S., Vargas E.

*Pharmacokinetics*

P - 233 **Incidence of Drug-Related Visits in a Hospital Emergency Room**

Juntti-Patinen L., Kuitunen T., Pere P., Neuvonen P.J.

*Pharmacoepidemiology*

28. Jun **Do Medical Students Copy the Drug Treatment Choice of Their Teachers or Do They Think for Themselves ?**

Richir M.C.

*Ratinolpharmacotheraphy*

**Drug Interactions with New Psychotropic Drugs**

Spina E.

*The rational use of psychotherapeutic drugs*

P - 234 **NSAIDs Sensitive to Radiant Tail Flick Test When Given Peripherally**

Dogrul A., Ossipov M.H., Porreca F., Tulunay F.C.

*NSAIDS*

P - 235 **The Effect of Gemfibrozil on the Pharmacokinetics of Rosuvastatin**

Schneck D.W., Birmingham B.K., Wang Y., Zalikowski J.A., Mitchell P.D., Lasseter K.C., Raza A.

*Drug interactions*

P - 236 **The Influence of Senna\'S Leaves Water Extract on Rat Liver Enzymes Activity**

Samajlik I., Djakovic-Svajcer K., Popovic M.

*Gastrointestinal pharmacology and therapeutics*

P - 237 **Consumption of Medicines in Southwestern Russian Medical or Social Disabled Person Population: The Most Reimbursed vs. Most Utilized Drugs**

Tatarkin A., Kalinichenko V., Mamontov A., Kalinichenko D., Gorokhov S., Shevchenko N.

*Pharmacoepidemiology*

P - 238 **The Infuence of Hormone Replacement Therapy on Bone Mineral Density and Risk Factors for Occurence of Osteoporosis**

Knezevic N., Dragovic G., Beljic T.

*Osteoporosis*

P - 239 **Influence of CYP2C9, 2C19 and 2D6 Genetic Polymorphisms on Plasma Levels of Fluoxetine and Norfluoxetine Enantiomers**

Scordo M.G., Spina E., Dahl M.L., Gatti G., Perucca E.

*Pharmacogenetics and pharmacogenomics*

P - 240 **Rosuvastatin Pharmacokinetics in Heart-Transplant Recipients Administered Cyclosporin**

Simonson S.G., Schneck D.W., Martin P.D, Mitchell P.D., Jarcho J.A., Raza A.

*Drug interactions*

P - 241 **Calcitonin Gene-Related Peptide-Induced Vasodilation in the Human Forearm is Inhibited by CGRP8-37**

De Hoon J.N.J.M., Vanmolkot F.H.M.

*Clinical Pharmacology in neurology*

P - 242 **A Placebo-Controlled Study of the Inhibition of Pentagastrin-Induced Gastric Acid Secretion by Single Oral Doses of Pantoprazole**

Paul J., McKeand W., Abell M., Baird S., Mako B., Smout A., Patat A.,

*Gastrointestinal pharmacology and therapeutics*

27. Jun 16:15-16:30

**Quality Assured Sources in Knowledge Databases for Computerised Drug Prescribing**

Eiermann B., Julander M., Gustafsson L.L.

*Ratinolpharmacotheraphy*

27. Jun 16:15-16:30

**Operational Problems of a Pilot Study in Usual Clinical Practice: Reasons for a Failure**

Durán M., Morralla C. Vidal X. Laporte J.R.

*Miscellaneous*

P - 243 **Novel Antioxidant L-2264 Prevents Insulin Resistance Development In Rats**

Ivanova O., Poltorak V., Gorbenko N., Lipson V., Leshchenko Z.

*Drug discovery and development*

P - 244 **Effect of Glipizide on Nephropathy Development in Streptozotocin-Diabetic Rats**

Poltorack V., Gorbenko N., Gladkih A.

*Clinical pharmacology of elderly*

P - 245 **Antiatherogenic Effect of Novel Antioxidant Phensuccinal in Diabetic Rabbits**

Gorbenko N., Poltorak V., Gladkich A., Ivanova O.

*Cardiovascular Pharmacology And Therapeutics*

**Jurilab Ltd, a high-tech R&D Bioscience Company, with an Extensive Experience in the Fields of Cardiovascular Diseases, Diabetes and Hypercholesterolemia.**

Jukka T.S.

*Drug metabolism*

P - 246 **Determination Of Ciprofloxacin In Gingival Crevicular Fluid And Plasma By High-Performance Liquid Chromatography**

Dincel A., Yildirim A., Caglayan F., Bozkurt A.

*Pharmacokinetics*

P - 247 **Contribution of a Poison Information Centre (PIC) in the Evaluation of Adverse Drug Effects (ADEs) to the German National Pharmacovigilance System**

Mey C., Hentschel H., Hippius M., Tiaden J.D., Oerlinghausen B.M., Balogh A.

*Pharmacoepidemiology*

P - 248 **Alfentanil-Induced Miosis in Patients**

,Slanar O., Urban M., Roots I., Perlík F.

*Drug metabolism*

P - 249 **Prevalence of MRSA Infections in a Clinical Hospital Centre in Croatia**

Bilusic M., Mercep I., Kalinic S., Francetic I., Macolic-Sarinic V., Huic M., Mimica S.

*Antimicrobial theraphy*

**The Effects of Drugs on the Environment-Ecopharmacology**

Kümmerer K.

*Miscellaneous*

P - 250 **Teratogenic Effects of Diazepam Intake During Pregnancy to cleft palate & cleft lip**

Takzaree N., Yarmohammadi K., Takzaree A.R., Semiyari H.

*Drug utilization*

P - 251 **Study of Antiviral Activity of Cyclocitidin-monophosphate**

Novikova I.V., Kevra M.K., Trukhacheva T.V., Boreko E.L.

*Antiviral pharmacotheraphy*

P - 252 **Synergism of NSAIDs with Pentoxiphylline in rheumatoid Arthritis Treatment**

Kevra M.K., Dubovic B.V., Keura V.M.

*NSAIDS*

P - 253 **Pentoxiphylline in Combination with Methylprednisolone in Treatment of Sepsis**

Kevra M.K., Dubovic B.V., Leonovich S.I., Keura Zh.S.

*Ratinolpharmacotheraphy*

P - 254 **Rationalization of Expenses for Lung Cancer Chemotherapy**

Cervellino J.C., Araujo C.E., Fligman M.D., Pires E.A.

*Issues in drug discovery and development*

P - 255 **The Efficacy of Adsorbent's Mixture in Protection of Animals Poisoned with Bromadiolone**

Cupic V., Dobric S., Milovanovic Z., Bokonjic D.

*Gastrointestinal pharmacology and therapeutics*

P - 256 **Comparison of Serious Adverse Drug Reactions (ADRs) Associated with Non-Selective and Selective COX2-Inhibitors**

Haase G., Kohlen K., Riethling A.-K., Drewelow B.

*NSAIDS*

P - 257 **Serious Adverse Drug Reactions (ADR) Associated with Herbal Drugs**

Haase G., Riethling A.-K., Drewelow B.

*Pharmacoepidemiology*

P - 258 **Pharmacokinetics of Gapapentin in Neonates and During Lactation**

Öhman I., Vitols S., Tomson T.

*Ratinolpharmacotheraphy*

P - 259 **CYP3A5*3 Polymorphism as Risk Factor for Prostate Cancer**

Karypidis H., Söderström T., Lundgren S., Rane A.

*Pharmacogenetics and pharmacogenomics*

P - 260 **Computer Simulations of the Regional Manufestation of Asthma**

Apiou G.S., Lemaire M., Katz I., Conway J., Floming J., Martonen T.

*Issues in drug discovery and development*

P - 261 **Psychologic Profile of Patients wiih History of Drug Hypersensitivity**

Sarinic V.M., Herceg M., Bilusic M., Francetic I., Huic M., Mercep I.

*Miscellaneous*

P - 262 **New Applications of Nebulizers in the Treatment of Asthma**

Martonen T., Apiou G.S., Lemaire M., Katz I., Conway J., Floming J.,

*Issues in drug discovery and development*

P - 263 **Inhibitory Effect of 5-Fluorouracil in CYP2C9 Activity**

Güne_ A., Co_kun U., Börüban C., Günel N., Sencan O., Bozkurt A., Rane A., Hassan M., Zengil H., ,Ya_ar Ü.

*Drug interactions*

P - 264 **Role of Cytochrome P450 2C9 in the Metabolism of Ketobemidone**

Annas A., Yasar Ü., Svensson J.O., AL-Shurbaji A.

*Drug Metabolism and Pharmacogenetics*

P - 265 **Caffeine as a Probe for the Assessment of CYP1A2, CYP2A6, NAT2 and Xanthine Oxidase Activities in Turkish Subjects**

Dincel A., Ya_ar Ü., Babaoglu M.O., Bozkurt A., Basci N., Kayaalp S.O.

*Drug metabolism ve Pharmacokinetics*

P - 266 **Effect of Ketoconazole on the Pharmacokinetics of Erlotinib (TarcevaTM) in Healthy Adult Male Subjects**

Abbas R., Fettner S., Riek M., Davis S., Hamilton M., Frohna P., Rakhit A.

*Drug Interactions*

P - 267 **Academic Fluoroquinolone Prescribing, Resistance and Impact of Guidelines**

Mol P.G.M., Panday P.V.N., Degener J.E., Van Der Werf T.S., Haaijer-Ruskamp F.M., Gans R.O.B.

*Antimicrobial theraphy*

P - 268 **When are Antimicrobial Treatment Guidelines Not Followed?**

Mol P.G.M., Denig P., Panday P.V.N., Gans R.O.B., Degener J.E., Laseur M., Haaijer-Ruskamp F.M.

*Antimicrobial theraphy*

P - 269 **The Patient Administration System Registry Contained Several Severe Adverse Drug Reactions Never Reported to the Regulatory Authorities. Shame or Opportunity?**

Grundmark B., Göransson V., Söderström T.

*Quality indicators in drug use*

P - 270 **Impaired Gastric Motility in the Gastroesophageal Reflux Rat Model: An in Vitro Study**

Yıldız F., Tugay M., Utkan T., Gacar N.

*Gastrointestinal pharmacology and therapeutics*

P - 271 **Chronic Unilateral Cavernous Nerve Denervation-Related Changes in Neurogenic- and Endothelium-Dependent Relaxant Responses of Rabbit Corporal Smooth Muscle**

Sarıo_lu Y., Utkan T., Yıldırım S., Yıldız F.

*Miscellaneous*

P - 272 **Ambiguous Diagnoses in the ICD-10 Classification System Make it an Unsatisfactory Tool in the Development of Quality Indicators of Drug Use**

Göransson V., Grundmark B., Söderström T.

*Quality indicators in drug use*

**P - 273 Renal Impairment and Dose Adjustment**

Lafay C., Raylet D., Barrière M., Favrelière S., Perault M.C.

*Drug utilization*

**P - 274 Effect of Losartan on the Cardiovascular Response to Cold Pressor Test in Healthy Volunteers**

Israel A., Zavala L.E.

*Cardiovascular pharmacology and therapeutics*

**28. Jun "Use of the "Pharmapac" Tool in a Regular Course in Clinical Pharmacology for Medical Students"**

Törnqvist E., Böttiger Y., Lars L.

*Teaching and communication in clinical pharmacology*

**P - 275 Lack of a Pharmacokinetıc (PK) Interaction Between Sirolimus (SRL) And Cyclosporıne (CsA) When SRL is Administered 2 Hours Before CsA**

Parks V., Patat A., Zimmerman J.J., Richards J.

*Pharmacokinetics*

**P - 276 Absolute/Relative Bioavailability of Bazedoxifene Acetate in Healthy Postmenopausal Women**

Bellaire S.B., McKeand W., Patat A., Ermer J., Le Coz F.

*Pharmacokinetics*

**P - 277 Esophagıtıs Impairs Esophageal Smooth Muscle Reactivity in the Rat Model: An in Vitro Study**

Yıldız F., Tugay M., Utkan T.

*Gastrointestinal pharmacology and therapeutics*

**P - 278 Esophageal Smooth Muscle (Tunica Muscularis Mucosae) Reactivity in Diabetic Rats**

Yıldız F., Utkan T., Ulak G., Gacar N., Goçmez S.

*Gastrointestinal pharmacology and therapeutics*

**P - 279 Effects of Various Agonists on Lower Esophageal Sphincter Strips Isolated from Diabetic Rats**

Yıldız F., Utkan T., Ulak G., Gacar N.

*Gastrointestinal pharmacology and therapeutics*

**P - 280 Chronic Ethanol Consumption Impairs Cholinoreceptor-Mediated Contractions and Nanc-Mediated Relaxations of Isolated Rat Lower Esophageal Sphincter and Tunica Muscularis Mucosae**

Yıldız F., Utkan T., Tugay M.

*Gastrointestinal pharmacology and therapeutics*

**P - 281 Ecstasy (MDMA) is a Mechanism-Based Inhibitor of CYP2D6**

Heydari A., Rowland Yeo K., Rostami-Hodjegan A., Lennard M.S., Tucker G.T.

*Drug metabolism*

**P - 282 The Effects of Age and Gender on Fluvoxamine Caffeine Interaction in Rats**

Eminoglu O., Kalkan S., Guven H., Benker T., Gelal A., Gidener S.

*Drug interactions*

**P - 283 The Effects of Gender and Menopause on Serum Lidocaine Levels in Smokers**

Oztekin S., Kalkan S., Mavioglu O., Elmas T., Elar Z., Guven H.

*Pharmacokinetics*

**P - 284 Dextromethorphan Test and Enzyme Inhibition - Comparative Results with Urine and Serum Analysis**

Kuhn U.D., Kirsch M., Merkel U., Eberhardt A.M., Beier T., Maurer I., Härtter S., Hiemke C., Volz H.P., Balogh A.

*Pharmacogenetics and pharmacogenomics*

**P - 285 Adrenomedullin Suppresses Migration Inhibitory Factor Production and Cytokine Response of Rat Macrophages to Lipopolysaccharide**

Cheung B.M.Y., Wong L.Y.F., Li Y.Y., Tang F., Lan H.Y.

*Cardiovascular pharmacology and therapeutics*

**P - 286 The Interaction of the Diltiazem with Oral and Intravenous Cyclosporıne in Rats**

Kalkan S., Gumustekin M. , Aygoren O., Tuncok Y., Gelal A., Guven H.,

*Drug interactions*

**P - 287 Relation of Caffeinated Beverage Consumption With Serum Liver Enzymes, Serum Lipids and Caffeine Levels: A Preliminary Study.**

Güven H., Gumustekin M., Balkan D., Benker T., Eminoglu E., Arslan S., Musal B., Tunca M.

*Miscellaneous*

**The Influence of Hemp on CNS Depression Induced by Pentobarbital**

Horvat O., Jakovljevic V., Sabo A., Berenji J., Stanojevic Z.

*Drug interactions*

P - 288 **The Comparison of Pharmacotherapy of Epilepsy in the Czech Republic and in Sweden**

Koristkova B., Grundmann M., Bergman U., Sjöqvist F.

*Pharmacoepidemiology*

P - 289 **Antibiotic Prescribing in Pediatric Hospitalized Patients**

Radosevic N., Bajcic P., Palcevski G., Ahel V., Francetic I., Vlahovic-Palcevski V.

*Drug utilization*

**The Role of Circadian Rhythm in the Pharmacokinetic of Methotrexate in Sidm Rats**

Gumustekin M., Kalkan _., Murat N., Gur Ö., Hocaoglu N., Gıdener S.

*Miscellaneous*

P - 290 **Identification of Cytochrome P4503A4 and 2C9 as the Major Catalysts of Phenprocoumon Hydroxylation**

Ufer M., Tybring G., Svensson J.O., Rane A.

*Drug metabolism*

P - 291 **Essential Drug Lists a Way Towards a Rational Use of Medicines. A Venezuelan Model.**

Landaeta L., Valdivieso L.H., Briceño E.

*Drug utilization*

P - 292 **The Effects of Age and Gender on Fluvoxamine Caffeine Interaction in Rats**

Emınoglu O., Kalkan S., Guven H., Benker T., Gelal A., Gıdener S.

*Drug interactions*

**26. Jun 17:55-18:10**

**Validation of a Predictive Model for Individualizing Clozapine Dose**

Rostami-Hodjegan A., Ros J.E., Van Der Weide J., Flanagan R.J., Lennard M., Tucker G.T.

*Therapeutic drug monitoring*

P - 293 **Tropical Climatic Conditions Affect Bioavailability of Diclofenac Formulations**

Van Bortel L., Risha P.G., Van den Abeele W.M., Vergote G., Vervaet C., Remon J.P.

*Miscellaneous*

**27. Jun 16:30-16:45**

**Comparison of Quality of Life with Nebivolol and Losartan**

Van Bortel L., Mäkel W., Fici F.

*Cardiovascular pharmacology and therapeutics*

P - 294 **Utilization of Fluoroquinolones and the Development of Bacterial Resistance**

*Urbanek K., **Kolar M.

*Drug utilization*

P - 295 **The Role of Endothelin in Rat Gastric Mucosal Injury by Nonsteroidal Antiinflammatory Drugs**

Murat N., Gidener S., Koyuncuo_lu M.

*NSAIDS*

**27. Jun 16:15-16:30**

**Multidisciplinary Medication Review among Nursing Home Residents - What are the Most Significant Drug-Related Problems? The Bergen District Nursing Home (BEDNURS) Study**

Ruths S., Straand J., Nygaard H. A.

*Pharmacoepidemiology*

P - 296 **Detection of Sulbactam Ampicilin Susceptibilty with Microdilution Method in Proteus, Citrobacter and same Gram Negative Bacteria**

Uraz G., Öncül Ö.

*Drug interactions*

P - 297 **Pharmacokinetics and Pharmacodynamics of Subcutaneous Interferon Alpha-2b**

Kinzig-Schippers M., Jetter A., Tomalik-Scharte D., Szymanski J., Fuhr, Illauer M., Skott A., Sörgel F.

*Antiviral pharmacotheraphy*

P - 298 **Role of Amoxicillin Prophyilactic Therapy in Third Molar Surgery**

Sillet M., Orellana A., Mathison Y.

*Antimicrobial theraphy*

**P - 299 Predicting Drug Clearance Allowing For The Influence Of P-Glycoprotein Activity Using SIMCYP™**

Howgate E.M., Proctor N.J., Rostami-Hodjegan A., Tucker G.T.

*Drug metabolism*

**Assessing the Prevalence of Adverse Drug Reactions in a French University Hospital: A Capture-Recapture Study Using Data From PMSI And The French Pharmacovigilance Database**

Lugardon S., Desboeuf K., Fernet P., Montastruc Jl., Lapeyre-Mestre M.

*Pharmacoepidemiology*

**P - 300 Comparative Study of Initial and Acquired Drug Resistance in Pulmonary Tuberculosis in National Research Institute of Tuberculosis and Pulmonary Disease**

Arami S., Mansoori D., Mirabolhasani Z., Farnia P.

*Antimicrobial theraphy*

**P - 301 Influence of Long-term Anticonvulsant Drug Therapy on Bone Mass Status in Childrens: A Quantitative Ultrasound Study**

Pedrera J.D., López-Lafuente A., López-Rodríguez M.J., Borrella S., Rodríguez T., Canal M.L.

*Osteoporosis*

**P - 302 Ultrasound Bone Mass in Patient Treated with Long-Term Oral Anti-Coagulants**

Pedrera JD, Canal ML, Bote JL, Morales ML, Retortillo C, Lavado JM

*Osteoporosis*

**P - 303 Ultrasound Bone Mass in Schizophrenic Patients on Long-Term Neuroleptic Therapy**

Rey P., Lavado J.M., Morales M.L., Rodríguez T., Borrella S., Pedrera J.D.

*Osteoporosis*

**P - 304 The Influence of Sibutramine on the Therapy of Obese Patients Representing Different Behaviour Patterns**

Bogdanski P., Szulinska M., Pupek-Musialik D.

*Miscellaneous*

**P - 305 Evaluation of Blood Pressure Values in 3-Month Obesity Treatment with Use of Sibutramine**

Bogdanski P., Pupek-Musialik D., Bryl W., Luczak M., Jabecka A.

*Cardiovascular pharmacology and therapeutics*

**P - 306 Evaluation of Influence of Angiotensin Converting Enzyme Inhibitor Treatment on Blood Pressure and Serum Endothelin-1 Concentration in Young Hypetensives During 6-Month Therapy.**

Bryl W., Miczke A., Bogdanski P., Luczak M., Cymerys M., Pupek-Musialik D.

*Cardiovascular pharmacology and therapeutics*

**P - 307 Prescribing and Health Care Utilisation - Is it Possible to Analyse the Effects of Interventions Using Aggregate Data?**

Wettermark B., Krakau I.,Bergman U.

*Drug utilization*

**P - 308 Paracetamol Poisoning and N-Acetylcysteine Treatment in Patients without Liver Damage. Which one Modifies the Prothrombin Time?**

Lopez-Torres E., Seoane J., Verge C., Martinez A.,Andrade R.J., Sánchez de la Cuesta F., Lucena M.I.

*Drug interactions*

**P - 309 Reproducibility of Prostaglandin D2 Induced Nasal Obstruction Using Active Anterior Rhinomanometry in Healthy Subjects**

Van Hecken A., de Hoon J.N., Depré M., Ragab A., De Lepeleire I., Laethem T., Deutsch P., Mazina K., Thach C., Hartford A., Clement P.

*Miscellaneous*

**P - 310 Effect of Aprepitant on the Pharmacokinetics and Pharmacodynamics of Warfarin**

Depré M., Van Hecken A., Oeyen M., De Lepeleire I., Laethem T., Rothenberg P., Petty K., Majumdar A., Crumley T., Panebianco D., Bergman A., de Hoon J.N.

*Drug interactions*

**P - 311 Therapeutic Drug Monitoring in North Eastern Greece: Focus on Digoxin and Cyclosporin**

Manolopoulos E.G.

*Pharmacoepidemiology*

**28. Jun Smart Choice List : A New Concept to Reach the Prescribers with Evidensbased Recommendations**

Sjoberg S., Bahr C., Bergman U., Granberg-Stange M., Jagre I., Persson P., Tryselius R., Thornwall G., Gustafsson L.L.

**P - 312 Circadian Change in Ondansetron (Zophren®) and in Oxaliplatin Toxicities in Mice**

Khedhaier A., Ben Attia M., Sani M., Gadacha W., Chouchane L., Boughattas N.A., Bouzouita K.

*Drug utilization*

**P - 313 Antibiotic Resistance in Catheter-Associated Urinary Infections at the Clinical Center of Banja Luka - Bosnia and Herzegovina**

Verhaz A., Skrbic R., Stojisavljevic-Satara S., Babic-Djuric D., Stojakovic N., Nezic L.

*Antimicrobial theraphy*

**P - 314 Drug Utilization Analyses in Banja Luka region (North-West Bosnia)**

Stojakovic N., Skrbic R., Stoisavljevic-Satara S., Babic-Djuric D., Nezic L., Sabo A.

*Drug utilization*

**P - 315 "Therapeutic Approach to the Patients with Coronary Heart Disease; The results of Coronary Prevention Study in Republic of Srpska (ROSCOPS) - Bosnia and Herzegovina"**

Skrbic R., Vulic D., Lazarevic A., Keric L., Krneta M.

*Cardiovascular pharmacology and therapeutics*

**P - 316 Antibiotic Utilization in Banja Luka Region (North-West Bosnia) During the Past Decade**

Stoisavljevic-Satara S., Babic-Djuric D., Vucen M., Skrbic R., Stojakovic N., Nezic L.

*Drug utilization*

**P - 317 Protective Role of Glutathione S-transferase P1 (GSTP1) Val105Val Genotype in Patients with Bronchial Asthma**

Aynacioglu A._., Nacak M., Filiz A., Ekinci E., Roots I.

**P - 318 Cytochrome P450 2C19 Genotype-Phenotype Correlation Using Omeprazole as a Probe Drug**

Aynacioglu A._., Öngen H.Z., Bauer S., Roots I., ,Brockmöller J.

**P - 319 Length Of Gambling History as a Predictor Of Treatment Participation**

Brands B., Toneatto T., Selby P., Selhi Z., Gorthy L.

*Drug dependence*

**P - 320 The Permeability of Haemofilter, Haemodialyzer and Plasma Separator Membranes for Amphotericin B: Implications for Plasma Pharmacokinetics during Haemofiltration and for investigation of Target Site Pharmacokinetics by Microdialysis**

Bellmann R., Joukhadar C., Dehghanyar P., Egger P., Müller M., Wiedermann CJ.

*Pharmacokinetics*

**P - 321 The Influence Of Hemp On Cns Depression Induced By Pentobarbital**

"Horvat O., Jakovljevi&# V, Sabo A., Stanojevi&#; Z."

*Drug interactions*

**Does Problem-Based Learing (PBL) Improve Rational Drug Prescribing?**

Vollebregt J., Richir M., Vries de ThPGM.

*Ratinolpharmacotheraphy*

**P - 322 Treatment of Schizophrenic Out-patients with Depot Haloperidol: Impact of CYP2D6 Polymorphism on Pharmacokinetic Parameters and Clinical Outcome.**

Holger W. A., Panagiotidis G., Dahl M.L., Sjöqvist F.

*Pharmacogenetics and pharmacogenomics*

**P - 323 Influence of genetic polymorphisms on rifampicin-mediated induction of MRP2 (ABCC2) mRNA expression**

Cascorbi I., Haenisch S., Gießmann T., Dazert P., Hecker U., Kroemer HK., Siegmund W.

*Transporter systems*

**P - 324 Mutations in the drug transporter genes MDR1 and MRP2 and pharmakokinetics in patients treated with saquinavir/lopinavir**

Cascorbi I., Breske A., Moecklinghoff C., Stocker H., Kruse G., Sawyer A., Staszewski S., Kurowski M.

*Transporter systems*

**28. Jun Assessıng the Prevalence Of Adverse Drug Reactıons In a French University Hospital : A Capture-Recapture Study Usıng Data From Pmsi And the French Pharmacovigilance Database**

Lugardon S., Desboeuf K., Fernet P., Montastruc JL., Lapeyre-Mestre M.

*Pharmacoepidemiology*

**P - 325 Perception of The Risk Of Gastro-Intestinal Adrs With Non Steroidal Antiinflammatory Drugs (Including Coxibs) : Differences Between General Practitioners, Gastro-Enterologists and Rheumatologists**

Montastruc J.L., Bongard V., Lapeyre-Mestre M.

*Pharmacoepidemiology*

**25. Jun 10:30-10:45**

**Pediatric counselling in community pharmacies : knowledge of pharmacists and pharmacy technicians about drug utilisation in children**

Pin M., Lapeyre-Mestre M.

*Pharmacoepidemiology*

**P - 326 Effect of rifampin on pravastatin pharmacokinetics**

Kyrklund C., Backman JT., Neuvonen M., Neuvonen PJ.

*Pharmacokinetics*

**P - 327 Giving feedback on prescribing at a primary health care center - important element in quality control of drug prescribing in Stockholm, Sweden**

Nyman K., Wettermark B., Bergman U.

*Teaching and communication in clinical pharmacology*

**P - 328 On an Open, One-centre, Comparative, Randomized, Clinical Trial on Efficacy and Safety of Topical Application of Stomatidin (Hexetidine) in Treating Patients Having Catarrhal Pharyngitis and Tonsilopharyngitis**

Kapidzic A., Baksic D. D., Cabaravdic A., Resic M.

*Antimicrobial theraphy*

**P - 329 The Role Of Circadian Rhythm in the Pharmacokinetıc of Methotrexate in Sidm Rats**

Gümü_tekin M., Kalkan _., Murat N., Gur Ö., Hocaoglu N., S. Gidener

*Pharmacokinetics*

**P - 330 Effect of short-term ibuprofen treatment on gastroduodenal mucosa**

Tomalik-Scharte D., Goeser T., Sörgel F., Lehmacher W., Jetter A., Szymanski J., Töx U., Fuhr U., Kinzig-Schippers M.

*Transporter systems*

**P - 331 A pilot study addressing the role of renal function in phenotyping for intestinal transporter activity using oral marker substrates**

Jabrane W., Kinzig-SchippersM., Malchau G., Tönnes E., Jetter A., Lück H., Hering U., SörgelF., Fuhr U.

*Transporter systems*

**P - 332 Losartan as a Probe for Phenotyping of Cyp2c9 in a Turkish Population**

Babaoglu M.O., Yasar Ü., Dincel A., Eliasson E., Dahl M.-L., Bozkurt Atila

*Drug Metabolism and Pharmacogenetics*

**27. Jun 10:30-10:45**

**Cytochrome P450 2d6 Polymorphism in Patients with Cancer**

Babaoglu M.O., Bayar B., Aynacioglu A. S., Abali H., Kerb R., Celik I., Bozkurt A.

*Drug Metabolism and Pharmacogenetics*

**P - 333 Relationship Between Neonatal Hyperbilirubinemia and Bilirubin UDP-Glucuronosyl Transferase 1A1 Gene Polymorphism**

Babaoglu M. O., Yigit S., Aynacioglu A.S., Kerb R., Bayar B., Yurdakok M., Bozkurt A.

*Drug Metabolism and Pharmacogenetics*

**P - 334 Annual Rhythm of the Acute Neurotoxicity of Sodium Nitroprruside in Mice**

Attia M. B., Tchacondo T., Reinberg A. & Boughattas N.A.

*Drug utilization*

**26. Jun 10:15-10:30**

**The Anti Doping Hot-Line, A Means to Detect and Prevent the Abuse of Doping Agents in The Swedish Society And a new Service Function in Clinical Pharmacology**

Sjöqvist F., Eklöf A.C., Thurelius A.M., Garle M., Rane A.

*Teaching and communication in clinical pharmacology*

**P - 335 The comparison of the Treatment of Epilepsy in Czech Republic and Sweden**

Koristkova B., Grundmann M., Bergman U., Sjöqvist F.

*Therapeutic drug monitoring*

P - 336 **Melatonin Protects Against Oxidative Organ Injury in a Rat Model of Sepsis**

Toklu H., _ener G., Kapucu C., Kaçmaz A., Tilki M., Ye_en B.Ç.

*Cardiovascular pharmacology and therapeutics*

P - 337 **Sistemic Apsorption of 2% Lidocaine Hydrochloride Gel after Colonoscopically Examined Patients**

Siuc Valkovic D., Vitezic D., Oguic R., Stimac D., Niksic M.

*Pharmacokinetics*

P - 338 **Influence of CYP2D6 And CYP2C9 Genotypes on Fluoxetine Plasma Concentrations in Psychiatric Patients**

, Llerena A., Dorado P., Berecz R., González A.P., Cáceres M.C.

*Drug Metabolism and Pharmacogenetics*

P - 339 **QTc Interval Lengthening and CYP2D6 in Patients Treated with Risperidone**

, Llerena A., Berecz R., Dorado P., de-la-Rubia A., Sanz-de-la-Garza C.

*Drug Metabolism and Pharmacogenetics*

P - 340 **Influence of CYP2D6 ON Haloperidol Plasma Concentration and QTc Interval**

Berecz R., de la Rubia A., Dorado P., González I.,,Llerena A.

*Drug Metabolism and Pharmacogenetics*

P - 341 **Thioridazine Plasma Concentrations, CYP2D6 and QTc Interval Lengthening**

de la Rubia A., Berecz R., Dorado P., Fernández-Salguero P., ,Llerena A.

*Drug Metabolism and Pharmacogenetics*

P - 342 **Reproducibility Over Time of the Diclofenac/4'-OH Diclofenac Urinary Ratio Among Different CYP2C9 Genotypes**

Dorado P., Berecz R., Cáceres M.C., González I., Llerena A.

*Drug MetabolismPharmacogenetics,NSAIDS*

P - 343 **Analysis of Debrisoquine and 4-Hidroxydebrisoquine in Human Urine by High-Performance Liquid Chromatography**

Llerena A., González I., Dorado P., Berecz R., Cáceres M.C.

*Pharmacogenetics*

P - 344 **Frequencies of CYP2C9 Allelic Variants Among Cubans and Spaniards**

González I., Dorado P., Calzadilla L.R., Pérez B., Llerena A.

*Pharmacogenetics*

P - 345 **Drug Treatment of Schizophrenia First Episode in Hungary, Spain And Cuba**

Llerena A., González I., Berecz R., Cáceres M.C., de la Rubia A., Calzadilla L.

*Drug utilization*

P - 346 **Anticancer Effects of Aspirin on A549, HeLa, HT-29, MCF-7 Cancer Cells : A Comparative Study with NIH3T3 Fibroblast Cells**

Korkmaz S., Öztürk Y.

*NSAIDS*

P - 347 **Attenuation of Ischemia-Reperfusion-Induced Myocardial Infarct Size in Rats by Aminoguanidine**

Parlakpinar H., Ozer M.K., Sahna E., Acet A.

*Cardiovascular pharmacology and therapeutics*

P - 348 **Protective Effect of Aminoguanidine Against Cardiotoxicity Induced by Doxorubicin In Rats**

Parlakpinar H., Ozer M.K., Sahna E., Ci_remi_ Y., Acet A.

*Cardiovascular pharmacology and therapeutics*

P - 349 **Reduction of Amikacin-Induced Nephrotoxicity in Rats by Caffeic Acid Phenethyl Ester (CAPE)**

Parlakpinar H., Ozer M.K., Sahna E., Gaffaroglu M., Acet A.

*Antimicrobial theraphy*

P - 350 **Effects of Captopril and Losartan on Ischemia-Reperfusion-Induced Myocardial Infarct Size in Rats**

Parlakpinar H., Ozer M.K., Acet A.

*Cardiovascular pharmacology and therapeutics*

P - 351 **Psychopharmacological Issues in Latin America**

Pacheco Hernandez A.

*Drug utilization*

P - 352 **Higher Methadone Maintenance Doses are Associated with a Longer Stay in Methadone Maintenance Therapy**

Dickinson G.L., Rostami-Hodjegan A., Pratt P., Lennard M.S.

*Drug dependence*

P - 353 **Reversal of the Oxidative Organ Damages and Dysfunction Due to Chronic Nicotine Administration by Melatonin in the Rat**

_ener G., Kapucu C., Paskalo_lu K., Ayano_lu-Dülger G., Alican _.

*Cardiovascular pharmacology and therapeutics*

P - 354 **Studies Concerning the Gastric Damage Induced by Alendronate Sodium and Protective Effects of Melatonin and Omeprazole Against This Damage**

_ener G., Gören F., Ayano_lu-Dülger G.

*Osteoporosis*

P - 355 **Investigation of the Effects of Melatonin Treatment on Streptozotocin (STZ)-Induced Diabetic Rat Corpus Cavernosum in Vitro**

Paskaloglu K., _ener G., Ayano_lu-Dülger G.

*Cardiovascular pharmacology and therapeutics*

P - 356 **A Population Model of Dexecadotril and Racecadotril Pharmacokinetics in Healthy Adults and Children with Diarrhoea.**

Dartois C., Ben Becher S., Pons G., Thebault J.J., Denis E., Robert P., de Paillette L., Tod M.

*Pharmacokinetics*

P - 357 **A Pharmacokinetic-Pharmacodynamic (PK-PD) Study of Racecadotril and Dexecadotril in Healthy Adults**

Dartois C., Pons G., Denis E., Thebault J.J., de Paillette L., Tod M.

*Gastrointestinal pharmacology and therapeutics*

27. Jun 16:15-16:30

**Lamivudine Combined with Corticosteroids in Prolonged Acute Hepatitis**

Kosseva B.O., Jelev D., Spasova Z., Avramova B., Krastev Z.

*Gastrointestinal pharmacology and therapeutics*

P - 358 **The Effect of Methadone on Mood State is Shorter Than its Effect on Subjective Opiate Withdrawal Score in Patients Undergoing Methadone Maintenance Therapy (MMT)**

Shiran M.R., Rostami-Hodjegan A., Lennard M.S., Iqbal M.Z., Lagundoye O., Seivewright N., Tucker G.T.

*Drug dependence*

25. Jun 10:15-10:30

**The Impact of Unlicensed and Off-Labeled Drug Use on Adverse Drug Reactions in Pediatric Patients**

Neubert A.

*Pharmacoepidemiology*

P - 359 **The Economic Impact of Adverse Drug Reactions and Readmissions in Medical Gastroenterology**

Dormann,Harald

*Gastrointestinal pharmacology and therapeutics*

P - 360 **Pharmacokinetics of Gapapentin in Neonates and During Lactation**

Öhman I., Vitols S., Tomson T.

*Pediatric clinical pharmacology*

P - 361 **Allele and Genotype Frequencies of Polymorphic CYP2C9 and CYP2C19 in the Beninese and Belgian Populations**

Allabi A.C., Gala J.L., Desager J.P., Heusterspreute M., Horsmans Y.

*Pharmacogenetics and pharmacogenomics*

27. Jun 16:30-16:45

**Incidence of Cytochrome-P450-polymorphisms in Geriatric Patients and Their Association with Adverse Drug Reactions**

Egger T.

*Pharmacogenetics and pharmacogenomics*

P - 362 **The Relative Sensitivity of the Metabolic Ratios of CYP2D6 Probes (Debrisoquine (DB), Dextromethorphan (DM) And Metoprolol (MP)) to Urine pH.**

Özdemir M., Aktan Y., Rostami-Hodjegan A., Crewe K.H., Tucker G.T.

*Drug metabolism*

**P - 363 The Role of Nitric Oxide in Iron-Induced Rat Renal Injury**

Kadkhodaee M., Gol A., Keshavarz M., Shams S., Aryamanesh S.

Miscellaneous

*Updated today*

**P - 364 A Randomized Comparison of Venlafaxine and Fluoxetine For Anxiety Side Effect in the Early Stage of Antidepressant Therapy**

Sa_lam E., Mırsal H., Beyazyürek M., Sur H.

*Clinical Pharmacology in neurology*

**P - 365 Application of a Modified Two-Portion Absorption Model to Famotidine Plasma Concentrations with Double Peaks or Irregular Shaped Single Peaks**

Yin O.Q.P., Tomlinson B., Chow A.H.L., Chow M.S.S.

*Pharmacokinetics*

**P - 366 Antibiotics Consumption in Hungarian Hospitals 1996-2002**

Matuz M., Nagy G., Soos Gy.

*Drug utilization*

**P - 367 Phenytoin Metabolic Ratio (PMR) Correlates with Formation Clearance of (S)-7-OH-Warfarin**

Adar L., Bialer M., Blotnick S., Caraco Y.

*Pharmacogenetics and pharmacogenomics*

**P - 368 Use of Antibiotics in Estonian Children Under 4 Years of Age**

Rootslane L., Kiivet R.A., Irs A.

*Pharmacoepidemiology*

**P - 369 Safety of Propiverine Hydrochloride in Patients with Glaucoma**

Gatchev E., Petkova N., Rankova C., Vlahov V., Braeter M., de Mey C.

*Ratinolpharmacotheraphy*

**P - 370 A New Ontology for Computerized Detection of Adverse Drug Reactions**

Dormann N.

*Miscellaneous*

**P - 371 Epitestosterone Crucial in Doping Tests. Genetic Cause of Large Variation?**

Jakobsson J., Ekström L., Garle M., Björkhem I., Rane A.

*Pharmacogenetics and pharmacogenomics*

**P - 372 Nonesterified Fatty Acids Induce Alterations of Haemodynamics in Humans**

Stojiljkovic M.P., Mitchell J.M., Zhang D., ,Lopes H.F., Lee C.G., Goodfriend T.L., Egan B.M.

*Cardiovascular pharmacology and therapeutics*

**P - 373 Comparison the Effects of Steroidal Therapy by Measuring Exhaled Carbon Monoxide in Bronchial Asthma and COPD.**

Bicak M., Gul H., Ozkan M., Yildiz O., Ekiz K., Saygı _., Demirci N.

*Miscellaneous*

**P - 374 A New Role for Application of Botulinum Toxin Injection in Patients with Idiopathic Chalasia:A Case-Control Study**

Mikaeli J., Yaghoobi M., Montazeri G., Nouri N., Malekzadeh R.

*Gastrointestinal pharmacology and therapeutics*

**26. Jun 10:30-10:45**

**Inequivalence Between 2 Reference Drugs**

Bakracheva N., Koytchev R., Vlahov V.

*Ratinolpharmacotheraphy*

**P - 375 Adverse Events after 24 Month Treatment with Betaferon in Patients with Multiple Sclerosis**

Kostadinova I., Manova M., Vasileva T., Trenova A.

*Ratinolpharmacotheraphy*

**P - 376 Effect of Vitamin C on Body Lead Levels in Children**

Gilani A.H., Tariq S.A., Shah A.J., Zaidi S.A.H., Butt S.A.H., Ghayur M.N.

**P - 377 Population Pharmacokinetic Modeling in Evaluating Comparative Average Bioavailability of Two Oral Preparations of Ampicillin**

Terziivanov D., Christov E., Bozhinova K., Atanasova I.

*Pharmacokinetics*

25. Jun 16:30-16:45

**C3435T Polymorphism of the MDR1 Gene is Correlated with Endometrial Cancer**

Seremak-Mrozikiewicz A., Drews K., Semczuk A., Mrozikiewicz P.M.

*Transporter systems*

P - 378 **Polymorphisms of CYP1A1 Gene: Susceptibility for Uro-Genital Cancers**

Seremak-Mrozikiewicz A., Drews K., Semczuk A., Mrozikiewicz P.M.

*Transporter systems*

P - 379 **Vitamin D Receptor Polymorphism in Women with Low Bone Mineral Density**

Seremak-Mrozikiewicz A., Drews K., Mielcarek S., Kopyra P., Mrozikiewicz P.M.

*Transporter systems*

P - 380 **Rapid Detection of MDR 1 Mutations Using Fluorogenic Hybridization Probes in the Sample from Polish Population**

Mrozikiewicz P.M., Niewinski P., Nowakowski-Gashaw I., Roots I.

*Transporter systems*

P - 381 **A Study on the Rational Use of Antibacterial Means Under Special Regime of Prescription and Usage at St Anna University Hospital, Varna**

Georgieva M., Eliseev V.

27. Jun 10:30-10:45

**NSAIDs, Inflammatory Mediators and on Cartilage Changes in Osteoarthritis**

K.D. Rainsford, P.A. Revell, S. Rashad, F.S. Walker (deceased), R. Seabrook, R.A.D.

P - 382 **Goitrogenic Effects of P-Coumaric Acid in Rats**

Taha R.A., Touhami F.K., Badary O.A., Lezzar A., Hamada F.M.

28. Jun **The Waste of Drugs Among Families Living in Ankara**

Gulmez S. E., Tulunay F. C., Ergun H.

P - 383 **Prescription Knowledge of Turkish Medical Doctors**

Ergun H., Tulunay F. C., Gulmez S. E.

P - 384 **Effects of Armagnac or Vodka on Platelet Aggregation in Healthy Volunteers: A Randomized Clinical Trial.**

Umar A., Depont F., Jacquet A., Lignot S., Bégaud B., Segur M.C., Boisseau M., Moore N.

P - 385 **The Efficacy and Safety of Dipyrone (NovalginÒ) Tablets in the Treatment of Acute Migrane Attacks: A Double-Blind, Cross Over, Randomized, Placebo-Controlled Multi-Center Pilot Study**

Tulunay F. C., Ergun H., Gulmez S. E. , Ozbenli T., Ozmenoglu M. , Boz C. , Erdemoglu A. K., Varlikbas A., Goksan B, Inan L.

P - 386 **The Pre-emptive Analgesic Efficacy of Dipyron (Novalgin®) During Removal of Nasal Packings After Septal Surgery**

Tulunay E. O., Tulunay F. C, Gulmez S. E. , Ergun H., Demireller A.

P - 387 **Drug Use in Pharmacies in Novi Sad, Serbia And Monte Negro. Comparison Between State and Private Pharmacies**

Sabo A., Vukmirovic A., Jakovljevic V., Papuga M.

# Abstracts

## P - 1

Induction Of Apoptosis Of Human Nasopharyngeal Carcinoma Cell Line Cne-2 By Tubeimoside I Isolated From Bolbostemma Paniculatum

XiYang W., RunDi M., LiJian Y.
Guangdong Provincial Key Laboratory of Marine Materia Medical-Zhanjiang Ocean University, Zhanjiang, China

The aim of this study is to examine whether tubeimoside I induce apoptosis of CNE-2. Growth inhibition by tubeimoside I was measured using MTT assay. The effect of tubeimoside I on apoptotic induction of CNE-2 cell line was studied by the fluorescent microscopy, electronic microscopy, DNA agarose gel electrophoresis, flow cytometry analysis. Western blotting was performed for detecting the apoptosis-related genes. The growth of CNE-2 cells was inhibited obviously by tubeimoside I. CNE-2 cells showed typical apoptotic features observed by fluorescent microscopy, electronic microscopy. DNA fragmentation into multiples of low molecular weight DNA(¡«200bp) was detected by agarose gel electrophoresis of DNA; Sub-G1 peak was found by flow cytometry analysis, and the apoptosis index was 72.8%. The low expression of p53, the phosphorylation of bcl-2, an inhibitor of apoptosis, was apparently detected at 1h after the addition of tubeimoside I. In contrast, the levels of bax appeared to be significantly elevated at 1, 3, 5 h after the addition of tubeimoside I. In conclusion, tubeimoside I can induce the apoptosis of CNE-2 cells, and the induction of apoptotsis by tubeimoside I is closely associated with p53 inhibition, bcl-2 phosphorylation and bax activation.

## P - 2

Effects of Tubeimoside I on Cell Cycle and Apoptosis of Human Myeloblastic Leukemia Cells (HL-60)

Zhang H., Rundi M., Lijian Y.
Guangdong Provincial Key Laboratory of Marine Materia Medical Zhanjiang Ocean University

Objective: To study the effects of tubeimoside I on cell cycle and apoptosis of human myeloblastic leukemia cells (HL-60). Methods: The growth inhibitory activity of tubeimoside I was evaluated in HL-60 cells with MTT assay. Cell cycle and the induction of apoptosis were evaluated by flow cytometry, fluorescent microscopy, electron microscopy and agarose gel electrophoresis. Western blot analysis was used to determine bcl-2 and CyclinB1 expression. Results: Tubeimoside I displayed growth inhibitory activity against HL-60 cells with IC50 values ranging from 13.0 ~30.7ılmol¡€L-1. HL-60 cells underwent G2/M arrest within 24 hours of exposure to tubeimoside I, and had morphologic and biochemical evidences of apoptosis after 72 hours. Western blot analysis of tubeimoside I-treated cells revealed low CyclinB1 expressing level consistent with G2/M arrest. Conclusion: Tubeimoside I has in vitro activity against HL-60 cells, and this activity is associated with G2/M arrest, the induction of apoptosis, and low CyclinB1 expressing level. These findings suggest that further evaluation of the activity of tubeimoside I in HL-60 cells is reasonable and that the pharmacologic modulation of cell cycle arrest and apoptosis pathways deserves further study as a potential anticancer strategy.

## P - 3

Predominant Role For Nitric Oxyde In The Relaxation Induced By Acetylcholine In The Canine Uterine Artery

Pesic S, Grbovic L, Radenkovic M, Stojic D, Cvetkovic Z.
Department of Pharmacology, Medical School, University of Nis, YU

The effect of acetylcholine on the isolated canine uterine artery rings was investigated. Acetylcholine ($10^{-10}$-$3x10^{-3}$M) induced concentration- and endothelium- dependent relaxation ($pEC_{50}$=6.59±0.03; Emax=90.67% relaxation of contraction induced by phenylephrine ($10^{-5}$M) of the pre-contracted arterial segments. Indomethacin, 4-aminopyridine ($10^{-5}$M) and precontraction with $K^+$-rich Krebs-Ringer-bicarbonate solution had no effect on acetylcholine induced relaxation ($pEC_{50}$=6.65±0.02, Emax=92.50%; $pEC_{50}$=6.67±0.01, Emax=87.00%; $pEC_{50}$=6.48±0.02, Emax=91.20%; respectively). $N^G$-monomethyl-L-arginine (L-NMMA) ($10^{-5}$M) antagonized relaxation induced by acetylcholine (Emax=52.9%). It is concluded that in the canine uterine artery acetylcholine induces endothelium-dependent relaxation. It is suggested that the acetylcholine-induced relaxation of isolated canine uterine artery is probably mediated via endothelial nitric oxide formation.

## P - 4

Endothelium-Dependent Relaxation In The Human Facial Artery

Pesic S, Grbovic L, Radenkovic M, Stojic D, Pesic Z.
Department of Pharmacology, Medical School, University of Nis, YU

The purpose of the present study was to examine the effect of acetylcholine on the human facial artery. Acetylcholine ($10^{-10}$-$3x10^{-3}$M) induced concentration- and endothelium- dependent relaxation ($pEC_{50}$=6.35±0.02. Emax=89.74 relaxation of contraction induced by phenylephrine $10^{-5}$M) of the pre-contracted arterial segments. 4-aminopyridine ($10^{-5}$M) had no effect on acetylcholine induced relaxation ($pEC_{50}$=6.67±0.01, Emax=87.00%). $N^G$-monomethyl-L-arginine (L-NMMA) ($10^{-5}$M) and indomethacin ($10^{-5}$M) antagonized, only partially, relaxation induced by acetylcholine (Emax=62.23%; Emax=68.43 respectively). Indomethacin applied together with L-NMMA provoked further inhibition of acetylcholine-induced relaxation (Emax=38.55%). 4-aminopyridine, in the presence of indomethacin, L-NMMA or both of them had no provoked further inhibition of relaxation (Emax=65.9%; Emax=60.9%; Emax=37.25%, respectively). It is concluded that in the human facial artery probably exists secretion of both nitric oxide and prostacyclin in response to acetylcholine. There is no further activation of some alternative pathway of endothelium-dependent relaxation, when NO- and cyclooxigenase products sythesis are inhibited.

## P - 5

Effects Induced By CB-1 Receptor Agonists On Visual Evoked Responses And Oscillatory Potentials In The Mouse

Capasso A., De Iovanna A., Giuliani G., Guarino I., [1]Loizzo A.
Departement of Pharmaceutical Sciences University of Salerno and [1]Istituto Superiore di Sanità, viale Regina Elena 299, Roma Italy

The aim of this study was to describe a method to reliaby record Visual Evoked Potentials (VEPs) and then extract oscillatory potentials (Ops) in freely moving, unanaesthetized mice and evaluate them in the frequency and time domains to describe their variation according to changes in frequency and intensity of the flash stimulus. The preparatory work of this study consists in a logic course : •Valuation of Visual Evoked Potentials in smart mice •Valuation of mice responses after administration with anandamide (CB-1 agonist). Oscillatory potentials (OPs) consist of short lasting (15-30 ms) low voltage (5-30 microV) bursts of sinusoidal waves, which are embedded inside traditional visual evoked response waveforms, and can be extracted through off-line high-pass filtering. We started studies in order to verify: whether CB-1 agonists induce excitatory (or vice-versa depressant) effects on visual evoked responses induced by flash stimuli (F-VER) and on OP in the free-moving, unanesthetized mouse. Preliminary results show that anandamide at lower dose (5 mg/Kg i.p.) induces a decrease of amplitude (from an average of 75 microV ES 9, to 52, ES 8) and of latency (from 31 ms, ES 4 to 26.5, ES 4) of F-VEPs, with quite analogous changes of OPs, while higher doses (15 and 45 mg/kg) induce dose-dipendent decrease of amplitude and increase of latency. These data suggest that some CB-1 agonists induce an exitatory effect on the visual pathways, without influencing general brain excitability. Further studies are in progress to compare anandamide effects with methanandamide, with WIN 55,212-2 and with $\Delta^9$ THC .

## P - 6

Hospital visits caused by adverse drug reactions (ADRs):a French study in primary care-emergency departments.

Queneau P.,Bannwarth B.,Carpentier F.,Guliana J.M.,Bouget J., [1]Trombert B.
Hôpital Bellevue,Saint-Etienne,France, APNET[1]

Objective: To assess the incidence and preventability of ADRs leading to hospital visits. Design:The study was conducted over 2 periods of one week, the first in June, the second in December, 1999.All patients aged 15 and over and consulting for a medical reason in primary care-emergency departments of 5 university hospitals and 5 general hospitals were included.Each patient was assessed by 2 clinicians to determine whether the visit was the result of an ADR.
Results:Out of a total of 1937 patients consulting, 1562 were taking at least one drug during the previous week, so they were included in the analysis according to the protocol.Altogether, 328 patients (21%; 95% CI:19%-23%)receiving at least one drug consulted because of an ADR.On average,these patients were older and took more drugs than those without ADR(63.5 vs 54.8 years, and 5.2 vs 3.8 drugs, respectively,P<0.001). Furthermore, 37.9% of ADRs were considered as being preventable because a contra-indication or a warning about drug use had not been respected.
Conclusions:In spite of its limitations (possible sampling bias,short study period),our study suggests that ADRs leading to hospital visits are frequent,with a great proportion of them appearing to be preventable

## P - 7

Adenosine Induces Relaxation Of Isolated Rat Aorta And Caudal Mesenteric Artery: The Role Of Adenosine Receptors

Grbovic L., Radenkovic M.
Department of Clinical Pharmacology, Pharmacology and Toxicology, Medical Faculty, Belgrade, Yugoslavia

Adenosine predominantly induces endothelium-independent vasodilatation. This paracrine effect is generally consequence of the vascular smooth muscle adenosine receptors activation. Nevertheless, many experimental results suggest the important role of the endothelial adenosine receptors in this process. Therefore, the present experiments were undertaken in order to establish the type and location of adenosine receptors involved in adenosine-produced effect on the isolated rat aorta (RA) and caudal mesenteric artery (CMA). Adenosine (0.1 - 300 microM) induced concentration-dependent relaxation in both examined arteries. After mechanical removal of endothelium adenosine-elicited effect in RA and CMA remained unaltered. DPCPX (10 nanoM), an A1-antagonist, did not affect adenosine-produced relaxation in the examined vessels. On the other hand, CSC (0.3 - 3 microM), an A2A-antagonist, significantly reduced adenosine-evoked dilation in the concentration-dependent manner in both RA and CMA. The obtained results showed that adenosine-induced relaxation in the studied arteries is most probably initiated after direct activation of A2A receptors located on smooth muscle cells. Moreover, in isolated rings of RA and CMA adenosine-elicited dilation doesn't depend upon functional integrity of endothelium.

## P - 8

The Role Of Potassium Current In Adenosine-Induced Effect In The Peripheral Rat Arteries

Radenkovic M., Grbovic L.
Department of Clinical Pharmacology, Pharmacology and Toxicology, Medical Faculty, Belgrade, Yugoslavia

The effect of adenosine (Ado) in isolated rat aorta (AO), caudal mesenteric artery (CMA) and renal artery (RA) was examined, as well as possible involvement of potassium current in this process. Ado (0.1 - 300 microM) induced endothelium-independent relaxation in AO and CMA, but endothelium-dependent one in RA. In the presence of KCl (100 mM) or ouabain (100 microM), an inhibitor of $Na^+/K^+$ -ATPase, Ado-induced relaxations in denuded AO and CMA were strongly inhibited. Glibenclamide (1 microM), an ATP-sensitive $K^+$ channel (KATP) blocker, reduced denuded AO response to Ado. In denuded CMA inhibition of Ado-induced relaxation was obtained with concomitant incubation of glibenclamide and TEA (an $Ca^{++}$ - activated $K^+$ channel blocker). In intact RA glibenclamide and KCl produced comparable inhibition of Ado-evoked vasodilation. The obtained reduction in the presence of KCl or glibenclamide was similar to that one induced by denudation. Ouabain didn't alter RA response to Ado. These results indicate significant role of potassium current in Ado-induced action in examined arteries. It may be proposed that in AO and CMA adenosine increases potassium current and subsequently produces relaxation via predominant activation of $Na^+/K^+$ -ATPase on smooth muscles, while in RA by indirect opening of smooth muscle KATP with released endothelium-derived hyperpolarizing factor.

## P - 9

Digoxin Pharmacokinetics And MDR1 Genetic Polymorphisms

Verstuyft C., Schwab M., Schaeffeler E., Kerb R., Brinkmann U., Jaillon P., Funck-Brentano C., Becquemont L.
Saint-Antoine University, Medical School of Pharmacology, Paris, France

Background : The influence of MDR1 C3435T single nucleotide polymorphism (SNP) in exon 26 on digoxin pharmacokinetics has been recently challenged.

Objective : To clarify the relations between MDR1 genetic polymorphisms in exon 26 (C3435T) and 21 (G2677T/A) and digoxin pharmacokinetics.

Material and methods : MDR1 genotypes for C3435T and 2677T/A SNPs were determined in 32 healthy subjects whose single oral dose digoxin pharmacokinetics had been measured over 48 h.

Results : A significant relation was observed between C3435T SNP and digoxin AUCs ($p<0.05$). Homozygous TT subjects had 20% higher digoxin plasma concentrations compared to CT and CT subjects and a trend for higher 48 h digoxin urinary recoveries (TT > CT > CC). Similar results, although not statistically significant, could be observed from the MDR1 G2677T/A SNP.

Conclusion : Our results confirm that the MDR1 C3435T SNP significantly influences digoxin disposition kinetics, homozygous TT subjects presenting the highest plasma concentrations. G2677T/A genetic polymorphism does not bring additional informations.

## P - 10

Turkish and German Patients of General Practitioners. Diseases, Drug Expectations and Drug Presciptions

von Ferber L., Koester I., Erdogan N.
Clinik for Child and Adolescent Psychiatry University Koeln, Germany

Aim of the study: to assess the diseases and complaints for treatment of patients relative to their ethnic origin: Turkish immigrants (T) or German citizens (D).

Methods: Questionnaire survey of patients of general practioners before and after consultation. The survey was conducted separately for Turkish and German patients, involving nine GP`s practices for each group.

Sample: sizes were 216 Turkish and 357 German patients respectively. Only responses of patients younger than 60 years of age were evaluated (T: 216; G: 357).

Results: The two most frequent reasons for a visit to the doctor by Turkish migrants were pains of varied origin (T: 44%; G: 20%; p>0,001) and colds or diseases of the respiratory tract (T: 43%; G: 25%; p>0,001). Turkish and German patients differ significantly with respect to their mentioning of pains and colds.

The physicians' prescribing frequency on the other hand conforms primarily to the disease of the patients and not to their ethnic group. To confirm this, we compared the share of drug recipients per disease group: Respiratory tract: T: 79% / D: 84%, alimentary system: T: 58% / D: 60% and locomotive system: T: 49%/ D: 39%. Medicaments. Significantly more Turkish than German patients (T: 23%/ D: 9%; p<0,001) received pain killing drugs.

Consequences: The treatment concept of Turkish patients is more directed to drugs. They request a drug more intensively and are more convinced of the medicaments' effectiveness than German patients are.

## P - 11

Bioavailability Of Arsenic From Arsenic Trioxide Solubalised For Oral Administration To Patients With Haemic Malignancies

Kumana C.R., Au W.Y., Lee N.S., Kou M., [1]Mak R.W.M., [2]Lam C.W., Kwong Y.L.
Department of Medicine, The University of Hong Kong; [1]Department of Pharmacy, Queen Mary Hospital; [2]Department of Chemical Pathology, The Chinese University of Hong Kong.

Arsenic trioxide ($As_2O_3$) is used increasingly to treat refractory haemic malignancies. Typically such treatment entails daily intravenous (IV) dosing for 1 or 2 months with its attendant drawbacks. We therefore set out to develop and administer a formulation by the oral route to suitable patients and compare the ensuing systemic availability of arsenic to that of IV dosing. With ethics committee approval, 9 patients with relapsed acute leukaemia were recruited with their informed consent. On day 1, each received 10 mg of $As_2O_3$ by IV infusion over 1 hour and on day 2 (24 hours after starting the infusion) swallowed 10 ml of our clear $As_2O_3$ solution for oral use. Prior to and up to 48 hours after starting IV infusion, timed venous samples were drawn and plasma and whole blood arsenic concentrations assayed by atomic absorption spectroscopy. The area under the curve (AUC) of each concentration versus time plot was determined by the trapezoidal rule and used as a measure of systemic bioavailability of arsenic. The day 2 AUC attributable to oral dosing was calculated as the difference in AUCs between the day 2 AUC and the day 2 AUC extrapolated from the day 1 AUC post IV dosing. From these AUCs for plasma and for whole blood, the mean day 2 AUCs attributable to oral dosing were estimated to be equivalent to 99% and 87% respectively of the day 1 (post IV dose) bioavailability. Thus, apart from being more convenient and cost-effective, our oral $As_2O_3$ formulation appeared to have similar bioavailability for arsenic as IV dosing.

Kumana CR et al, 2002. Eur J Clin Pharmacol 58 521-6

## P - 12

Comparison Of The Efficacy Of Sclerotherapy Alone and a Therapeutic Combination of Octreotide and Sclerotherapy in the Control of Acute Bleeding in Patients with Portal Hypertensive Gastropathy: A Controlled Study

[1]González-Martin G., [1]Urzúa L.D., [2]Muñoz L., [2]Rojas M.
Department of Pharmacy, Faculty of Chemistry, Pontifical Catholic University of Chile[1], and Pharmacy Service, Clinical Hospital of University of Chile[2]. Santiago, Chile

Background: Portal hypertensive gastropathy is an important complication of liver cirrhosis and it contributes to acute gastric bleeding. Effective management of this condition remains a clinical challenge. We assessed and compared the efficacy of sclerotherapy alone with a therapeutic combination of octreotide and sclerotherapy in the treatment of acute bleeding in patients with portal hypertensive gastropathy.

Methods: Seventy patients with portal hypertensive gastropathy were randomized into sclerotherapy, and a combination of sclerotherapy and octreotide groups. Bleeding was monitored by observing the contents of the nasogastric tube. Blood transfusion requirements, days of hospitalization and mortality rate were recorded. Repeat endoscopies were scheduled 2 weeks after treatment.

Results: Complete bleeding control after 48 h of drug infusion was achieved in 31/35 patients receiving the combination of octreotide and sclerotherapy (88.6%), and 24/35 patients with sclerotherapy alone (68.6%) (x2=3.9; d.f=1; p<0.049). The combination octreotide and sclero therapy group required much less time and significantly fewer blood transfusions to control bleeding (2.2±1.4 vs. 3.5±2.4) (t=2.8;p=0.007). There was not statistically significant difference between the days of hospitalization in both groups (11.4±6.7 and 15.5±7.4 days respectively) (t=0.6; p=0.5). Four patients (11.0%) died due to bleeding in the groups of sclerotherapy only, and none in the group who received octreotide in combination with sclerotherapy.

Conclusions: Octreotide appeared to be more effective in controlling acute bleeding in patients with hypertensive gastropathy, with significantly rapid action, smaller transfusion requirements, and minor mortality.

## P - 13

Bisoprolol Dose-Response Relationship in Patients With Congestive Heart Failure

Simon T., Mary-Krause M., Funck-Brentano Ch., Lechat Ph., Jaillon P.(On behalf of the Cardiac Insufficiency Bisoprolol Study (CIBIS II) investigators)
Department of Pharmacology, Saint Antoine University, Paris, France

Several betablockers have demonstrated a reduction of mortality in congestive heart failure (CHF). We examined whether survival was dose-related by classifying the patients into groups according to the last tolerated dose before event: low dose (LD : 1.25, 2.5 or 3.75 mg/day, n= 434), moderate dose (MD : 5 or 7 mg/day, n= 328) and high dose (HD : 10 mg/day, n = 565) of bisoprolol or placebo (LD=234, MD=278, HD=808). After adjustment, mortality in bisoprolol group was reduced in HD (RR = 0.38, 95%CI = 0.25-0.59, p = 0.0001), and MD groups (RR = 0.56, 95%CI = 0.37-0.86, p = 0.009) compared to LD group. Compared to placebo, all cause mortality was significantly reduced in the bisoprolol group regardless of the dose level considered : LD (HR=0.64, 95%CI = 0.46-0.88), MD (RR = 0.34, 95%CI = 0.22-0.52) or HD (RR = 0.63, 95%CI = 0.426-0.938). PTW was associated with a significant increase of mortality in the bisoprolol group (RR=2.15, 95%CI = 1.45-3.20, p=0.002). These results indicate that bisoprolol reduces mortality in CHF patients in all tolerated dose levels and its withdrawal increases the risk of mortality. The goal for a given patient should be to maintain the individual tolerated dose.

## P - 14

Impact Of MDR1 (C3435T) Genetic Polymorphism In Patients Naïve Treated With Haart Including Indinavir (IDV)

[1]Verstuyft C., [2]Marcellin F., [3]Morand-Joubert L., [4]Launay O., [5]Peytavin G., [2]Gerard L., [1]Becquemont L., [2]Aboulker Jp., for the ANRS 081 Study Group
[1]Pharmacology Department, Faculty of Medicine, Saint-Antoine Hospital, Paris. [2]INSERM SC10, Villejuif, [3]Laboratory of Virology, Saint-Antoine Hospital, Paris. [5] Pharmacie, hôpital Bichat-Claude Bernard, Paris, France.

Background: Bioavailability of IDV is mainly dependent on the activity of a liver and intestinal enzyme, cytochrome P450 3A4. However it has been recently shown that the P-glycoprotein, encoded by the MDR1 gene, limits IDV intestinal absorption. Moreover, MDR1 genetic polymorphism located in exon 26 (C3435T) has been shown to regulate P-gp expression in intestine and circulating lymphocytes. The aim of this study was to assess whether MDR1 (C3435T) genetic polymorphism in exon 26 predicted not only plasma drug concentration but also response to treatment, as expressed by CD4 T cell counts, plasma HIV-1 RNA level and, proviral HIV-1 DNA level. IDV plasma concentrations (peak and trough) were assessed after 8 and 24 W of therapy. The subsequent analysis was performed on the 76 HIV-1 infected patients who were naïve. Subjects were genotyped for the MDR1 genetic polymorphism (C3435T) in exon 26 by TaqMan allelic discrimination. Results: The frequencies of MDR1 exon 26 genotypes CC, CT and TT in the population studied were 35%, 40.8% and 23.7%, respectively. We did not identify a relation between peak and trough plasma levels of IDV and the 3 MDR1 genotypes. Conclusions: The MDR1 (C3435T) genetic polymorphism did not predict IDV concentrations, although we observed a trend to a higher immune recovery after initiation of antiretroviral treatment in patients with the CC genotype.

## P - 15

Randomised Non-blinded Two-fold Cross-over Study to Assess the Relative Bioavailability of the ASA Dry Granules 500 mg Given with and without Water to 24 Healthy Male Subjects

[1]Latta G, [2]Voith B, [2]Nagelschmitz J
[1]R&D Medical Department, Consumer Care Europe, Bayer AG, 51368 Leverkusen, Germany, [2]Institute of Clinical Pharmacology, Pharma Research Center, 42096 Wuppertal, Germany

The Aspirin® dry granules are a new powder formulation of acetylsalicylic acid (ASA) The pharmacokinetic characteristics of this new galenic formulation of ASA and its safety and tolerability were assessed after single administrations without and with water. After approval by an independent ethics committee, a randomised, non-blinded 2-way cross-over study in 24 healthy male volunteers assessed safety, tolerability and pharmacokinetics for ASA and salicylic acid (SA) after a dose of 500 mg ASA given as ASA dry granules with and without water in the fasted state. The concentration of SA after acid hydrolysis was measured in urine as Aeur. The treatments were safe and well tolerated, no serious or drug related adverse events occurred. Absorption rate of ASA was similar compared after administration without and with water resulting in a similar Cmax (4.02 mg/L vs. 4.68 mg/L) and similar median time to peak (0.667 h vs. 0.5 h). No changes in pharmacokinetic behaviour were detected with regard to the administration with or without water. The observed Cmax and AUC values for ASA and SA of the 500 mg doses of ASA dry granules were in the same range as seen in a previous study.1 In conclusion, the Aspirin® dry granules are safe and show pharmacokinetic characteristics which allow an effective treatment of pain, administrating this new formulation with or without water.

## ORAL

The Role of *CYP2C8* And *CYP2C9* Genotypes In Acute Myocardial Infarction

[1]Yasar Ü., [2]Bennet A., [1]Eliasson E., [1]Lundgren S., [3]Wiman B., [2]De Faire U., [1]Rane A.
[1]Division of Clinical Pharmacology, Karolinska Institutet, Huddinge University Hospital, Sweden, [2] Division of Cardiovascular Epidemiology, Karolinska Institute, Sweden. [3] Division of Blood Coagulation Research, Karolinska Hospital, Sweden

Cytochrome P450 (CYP) 2C8 and 2C9 are polymorphic enzymes and responsible for the biosynthesis of some vasoactive substances; arachidonic acid metabolites, i.e. epoxy-eicosatrienoic acids and endothelium-derived hyperpolarizing factors. These substances are important in the regulation of vascular tone that might be a contributory factor in the pathogenesis of acute myocardial infarction and hypertension. In the present study, 1172 acute myocardial infarction patients and 1503 control subjects that participated in the Stockholm Heart Epidemiology Program were genotyped by allelic discrimination using a 5'-nuclease assay. The frequencies of *CYP 2C8*1, 2C8*3, 2C9*1, 2C9*2* and *2C9*3* variants in the control group were 0.91, 0.095, 0.83, 0.11 and 0.065, respectively. Those of *CYP2C8*1* and *CYP2C9*1* were significantly lower in the acute myocardial infarction group. The risk of acute myocardial infarction in the female individuals carrying the **2* or **3* variant alleles of *CYP2C9* and that of individuals carrying **3* variant of *CYP2C8* were significantly higher (OR (95% CI): 1.3 (1.0-1.9); 1.5 (1.0-2.2) and 1.2 (1.0-1.5), respectively). The frequency of genotypes with *2C8*1*3/2C9*1*1* (but not *2C8*1*1/ 2C9*1*2*) was significantly higher in the acute myocardial infarction group compared to the control (95% CI for the difference was 0.02-0.11). Polymorphisms of *CYP2C8* and *CYP2C9* may be a contributing factor in the pathogenesis of acute myocardial infarction. Further studies including different subgroups of acute myocardial infarction are warranted.

## P - 16

Transdermal Penetration of Diclofenac After Multiple Epicutaneous Administration of a Novel Spray Gel Formulation

[1]Brunner M., [2]Seigfried B., [1]Dehghanyar P., [3]Martin W., [2]Piotrowiak R., [4]Menke G., [1]Müller M.
Department of Clinical Pharmacology, Division of Clinical Pharmacokinetics[1], Vienna University Medical School, Vienna, Austria; MIKA Pharma GmbH[2], Limburgerhof, Germany; and Pharmakin GmbH[3], Ulm, Germany; Biostatician[4], Frankfurt/Main, Germany.

Background: Transdermal application of diclofenac should combine the advantage of achieving a therapeutic effect at the target site without risking potentially severe systemic side effects. Recently, a novel topical Spray Gel formulation (MIKA Diclofenac Spray Gel 4%) with enhanced penetration characteristics has been developed. Aims: To evaluate the relative diclofenac bioavailability in plasma, subcutaneous adipose and skeletal muscle tissue after repeated topical (MIKA Diclofenac Spray Gel 4%) and oral (VOLTAREN® 50mg enteric coated tablet) administration of comparable daily doses. To assess safety and local tolerability of the new formulation. Methods: 48 mg diclofenac were topically administered t.i.d. for 3 days onto a defined area on the thigh of 12 male healthy volunteers. After a 14 days wash out period, volunteers were orally treated with 50 mg diclofenac t.i.d. In vivo microdialysis in target tissues was performed after both treatments immediately after a final dose on day 4 and 48 hours later. Plasma samples were simultaneous taken. Results: Diclofenac bioavailability in subcutaneous adipose and skeletal muscle tissue was substantially higher after topical compared to oral dosing, i.e. 324% and 209%, respectively, whereas relative plasma bioavailability was 500fold lower. Both treatments were well tolerated. Conclusion: Due to its favorable penetration characteristics and low systemic availability MIKA Diclofenac Spray Gel 4% qualifies as rational alternative to oral diclofenac formulations for the treatment of conditions affecting soft tissues.

## P - 17

Positron Emission Tomography for the Description of Target Tissue Pharmacokinetics of [18F] Fluorine-labelled Ciprofloxacin

[1]Brunner M., [1]Langer O., [2]Dobrozemsky G., [1]Müller U., [2]Mitterhauser M., [2]Wadsak W., [2]Kletter K., [1]Müller M.
Department of Clinical Pharmacology, Division of Clinical Pharmacokinetics[1], and the Department of Nuclear Medicine[2], Vienna University Medical School, Vienna, Austria

Background: Effective antimicrobial therapy is dependent upon the delivery of sufficiently high drug concentrations to the target site of infection, which is located in peripheral tissues rather than in serum for most antibiotics. A detailed description of target site pharmacokinetics (PK) of antibiotics, has so far often been prevented by a lack of appropriate methodology. Recent advances in non-invasive imaging techniques, such as positron emission tomography (PET), however, have greatly expanded the scope of PK measurements that can be performed in humans. Aims: To characterize the distribution of [18F]Fluorine-labelled ciprofloxacin to relevant target tissues including the central nervous system (CNS) employing PET. Methods: 4 healthy male volunteers orally received unlabelled ciprofloxacin (Ciproxin 250mg-Filmtabletten, Bayer Austria, Vienna, Austria) twice daily for 5 days plus a final oral dose on day 6. After the final dose, an intravenous bolus of approximately 740 MBq of [18F]ciprofloxacin was administered. Serial PET imaging was performed for 6 hours for specific groups of organs. Venous blood samples were taken simultaneously. Results: A first descriptive analysis indicated a very low CNS distribution of ciprofloxacin. Tissue concentrations could be quantified in lung, heart, skeletal muscle and liver for up to 6 hours. Conclusion: PET allows to obtain quantitative information about drug PK in various tissues including the central nervous system for several hours and might thus be useful for the evaluation of standard or new drug therapies.

## P - 18

Pattern of Prescription and Drug Use in Phthalmology in a Tertiary Hospital in Delhi

Biswas N.R., Jindal S., Siddiquei M.M., Maini R.
Dr. Rajendra Prasad Centre for Ophthalmic Sciences, All India Institute of Medical Sciences, New Delhi - 110 029 and College of Pharmacy, Pushp Vihar, Sec-III, New Delhi - 110 017, India

Aims: The present study was carried out to describe the patterns of prescription and drug use in Ophthalmology in out-patients at Dr. Rajendra Prasad (R.P.) Centre for Ophthalmic Sciences of All India Institute of Medical Sciences (A.I.I.M.S.), New Delhi. Methods: Prescriptions of 1017 outpatients were audited through a specially designed form and analysed for the following: average number of drugs per prescription, duration of treatment (recorded or not), dosage forms prescribed, frequency of administration (recorded or not),number of encounters with antibiotics and percentage of drugs prescribed by generic name. Results: Prescription analysis showed that the average number of drugs per prescription was 3.03. Duration of treatment was recorded for only 26.4% of the drugs prescribed. The maximum number of drugs prescribed were in the form of eye drops (76%), followed by tablets (10.9%), ointments (6.4%), syrups (1%), capsules (0.7%), lotions (0.3%) and injections (0.1%). No dosage form was recorded for 4.6% of the drugs prescribed. The frequency of administration was recorded for only 77.9% of the drugs prescribed. The number of antibiotics prescribed was 1059 which constitutes 34.2% of the total number of drugs prescribed. The percentage of drugs prescribed by generic name was only 35%. Conclusions: The results obtained in this study indicated an awareness of polypharmacy but a high incidence of common prescription writing errors such as not recording the duration of therapy, frequency of administration and dosage form. Moreover prescribing by generic name was also low.

## P - 19

Can the Electophysiological Actions of Psychotrop Drugs Explain Their Cardiac Side Effects?

Kecskeméti V., [1]Magyar J., [1]Bányász T., Pacher P., [1]Nánási P.P.
Department of Pharmacology and Pharmacotherapy, Semmelweis University, Budapest, [1]Department of Physiology, University Medical School of Debrecen, Hungary

The most frequent cardiac side effects of psychotrop (antidepressant , antipsychotic) drugs are brady- or, tachycardia, ECG alterations (prolongation of QRS, QT interval), AV-block, ventricular arrhythmias (tachycardia, torsade de pointe). The actions of antidepressant and antipsychotic drugs on cardiac ion channels (Na+, K+ Ca2+) may underlie their different cardiac effects. Aim: in this study the actions of fluoxetine (F), the well-known selective serotonin reuptake inhibitor antidepressant and risperidone (R), an atypical (DA2/5-HT2 antagonist) antipsychotic drug on isolated canine ventricular myocytes and guinea-pig papillary muscles were analysed using conventional microelectrode and whole cell clamp techniques. Results: at concentrations of 0.5-50 μM, F exhibited depressant effects on force of contraction on Ca2+ and Na+- dependent electrophysiological parameters of cardiac preparations and on cardiac Ca2+ current with EC50 of 5.4 ± 0.94 μM. F had no effect on the amplitude of K+ currents (IK1 and Ito). R (0.1-10 μM) caused a concentration-dependent lengthening of action potential duration (APD) in both preparations (EC50 = 0.29±0.02 and 0.48±0.14 μM). R caused concentration-dependent block of the rapid component of the delayed rectifier K+ current (IKr), with EC50 of 0.92±0.26 μM. Conclusion: the inhibition of cardiac Ca2+ and Na+ currents by F and the depression of IKr current by R may explain the cardiac side-effects observed occasionally with these drugs. Our results suggest that both fluoxetine and risperidone may have antiarrhythmic (class I + IV and III type, respectively), as well as proarrhythmic properties.Supported by grants OTKA T 037334, FKFP 0243/2000, ETT 52/2000, 155/2000, 244/2000.

## P - 20

Indinavir-induced Nephrolithiasis in HIV-infected Patients

[1]Dragovic G., [2]Jevtovic Dj.
[1]Institute of Clinical Pharmacology, School of Medicine, University of Belgrade, Belgrade, Yugoslavia; [2]Institute of Infective and Tropical Desease, School of Medicine, University of Belgrade, Belgrade, Yugoslavia

Background: Nephrolithiasis is known adverse effect of indinavir therapy. The objective of this study was to examine the association with indinavir use and the risk of incidence nephrolithiasis. We performed prospective cohort study in HIV-infected and AIDS patients on antiretroviral therapy and their association with indinavir-containing (IDN+) and non-containing (IDN-) regimens. Methods: Data were obtained from patients continuously monitored for incident cases of nephrolithiasis at the HIV/AIDS Unit, a university teaching hospital, Belgrade, Yugoslavia. The prevalence of nephrolithiasis between groups of patients on IDN+ and IDN- regimens were compared using the chi-square test. The probability of developing nephrolithiasis was estimated by the Univariate logistic regression. Results: In a cohort of 112 HIV-infected 64 patients were on IDN+ and 48 patients were on IDN- regimens, respectively. Average follow-up was 4.6 years. During this period nephrolithiasis developed in 14 (12.5%) patients. It's prevalence was 9.8% among patients on IDN+ regimens vs. 2.71% on IDN- regimens ($p<0.005$; df=1). Univariate logistic regression shown that the risk of nephrolithiasis is almost 6-fold grater when indinavir was used (RR=5.8; 95%CI 1.5-22.1). Conclusion: This study suggest that indinavir use increase the risk of developing nephrolithiasis and suggest the importance of managing this side effect.

## P - 21

Influence of the HMG-CoA-Reductase Inhibitor Atorvastatin on Biochemical Bone Metabolism Parameters: A Randomized Controlled Trial in Postmenopausal Women

[1]Berthold H.K., Unverdorben S., Degenhardt R., Zittermann A., Gouni-Berthold I.
[1]Drug Commission of the German Medical Association; from the Institute for Clinical Research, Center for Cardiovascular Diseases Rotenburg an der Fulda; Medical Policlinic, Univer- sity of Bonn; and Dept. of Medicine II, University of Cologne, Germany.

In vitro findings suggest that statins may stimulate bone for- mation. There is evidence from epidemiological studies that statins reduce the risk of bone fractures, but prospective studies investigating their effects on bone metabolism are missing. We investigated in a double-blind randomized placebo- controlled trial the effects of atorvastatin (20 mg per day, N = 24) or placebo (N = 25) on bone metabolism in postmenopausal women (age 61 ± 5 yrs). Treatment duration was 8 weeks. The bone formation marker, osteocalcin, increased by 9.0 ± 23 % (P = 0.02) in the placebo group and changed by +6.7 ± 22.7 % (n.s.) in the atorvastatin group. The bone resorption marker, C-telopeptide, was unchanged (+10.0 ± 25.7 %, n.s., under placebo and +2.6 ± 25.9 %, n.s., under atorvastatin). The C-telopeptide/osteocalcin-ratio (an indicator of bone remodel- ing) also remained unchanged (-3.1 ± 24.3 %, n.s., under pla- cebo and -1.9 ± 27.0 %, n.s., under atorvastatin). Compliance was assessed by measuring blood lipid concentrations. LDL cholesterol decreased under atorvastatin (-49 ± 12 %, P < 0.0001), while it remained unchanged under placebo (+0.9 ± 15 %, n.s.). We conclude that short-term treatment with atorva- statin has no effect on bone metabolism in postmenopausal women. Conflicts of interest: none.

## P - 22

Dose Proportionality (7.5mg To 22.5mg) and Food Effect (22.5mg) of Meloxicam Oral Suspension. An Open 4-Way Crossover Trial in Healthy Volunteers

Klüglich M., Scheuerer S., Wallenstein G.
Boehringer Ingelheim GmbH & Co. KG Human Pharmacology Centre, Ingelheim, Germany

Introduction : Clinically relevant characteristics such as dose proportionality and food effect were assessed for a newly developed meloxicam oral suspension.
Method : 24 healthy subjects received 7.5mg (fasted), 15mg (fasted) and 22.5mg (fed and fasted) single doses of the meloxicam oral suspension in an open-label, randomised, four-way crossover design. Influence of food was studied following a standard high fat, high caloric meal. Meloxicam plasma concentrations were measured by a validated HPLC assay until 96h p.a..
Results/Discussion : Treatments were safe and well tolerated. Mean $C_{max}$ was 0.601, 1.09, 1.57 and 1.60mcg/mL; mean $AUC_{0-\infty}$($AUC_{0-tf}$) was 16.9(15.8), 34.1(32.4), 49.3(46.8) and 48.5(46.1) mcg·h/mL in the fasted (7.5/15/22.5mg) and fed (22.5mg) groups, respectively. Application of the regression model y=a·dose$^b$ demonstrated that $C_{max}$, $AUC_{0-\infty}$ and $AUC_{0-tf}$ increased dose-proportionally. Point estimators of the slope (ideally:unity) were: 0.8848 for $C_{max}$ (CI: 0.8060-0.9637), 0.9740 for $AUC_{0-\infty}$ (CI:0.9218-1.0262), and 0.9963 for $AUC_{0-tf}$ (CI:0.9437-1.0490). No food effect (22.5mg) was found: 90% CIs for both $C_{max}$ and AUCs were contained within the range of 0.8-1.25 ($C_{max}$: 0.94-1.10, $AUC_{0-\infty}$: 0.93-1.04, $AUC_{0-tf}$: 0.94-1.04).
Conclusion : Dose proportionality was confirmed for meloxicam oral suspension over the dose range from 7.5mg to 22.5mg (fasted). Food had no effect on both, peak and total exposure, of meloxicam.

## P - 23

Influence Of Underlying Disease on Busulfan Disposition in Bone Marrow Transplant Children : A Non Parametric Population Pharmacokinetic Study

[1]Bonnet-Bertholle V., [1,3]Bleyzac N., [1]Magron P., [2]Galambrun C., [2]Bertrand Y., [2]Souillet G., [3]Maire P., [4]Jelliffe R., [1,5]Aulagner G.
[1]Pharmacy department, [2]Paediatric Haematology Department, Debrousse Hospital,29 Rue Sœur Bouvier, 69005 Lyon, France, [3]ADCAPT, A. Charial Hospital, 40 Avenue de la Table de Pierre, 69340 Francheville, France, [4]Laboratory of Applied Pharmacokinetics, USC, Los Angeles, USA, [5]Henry Poincarré University, rue Lebrun, 54000 Nancy, France.

Busulfan is an alkylating agent characterised by a narrow therapeutic index with major liver toxicity (veno-oclusive disease). Furthermore, previous studies pointed out the wide inter-patient and intra-patient pharmacokinetic variability. The aim of this study is to present the results of a population pharmacokinetic analysis where we tested different models based on pathology classes justifying the bone marrow transplantation. Fifty five children (5,9  5,1 years old) received bone marrow transplantation after busulfan-based conditioning regimen (1mg/kg theorically every 6 hours over 4 days) between March 1998 and February 2002. In a first step, a population pharmacokinetic model based on the overall population's data has been selected using NPEM program. The models differed from each other by the errror pattern assay included in the NPEM algorithm. With this selected model, pharmacokinetic parameter estimates of the patients (Ka, Kel and Vs) were studied. Patients were divided into four groups according to their initial diagnosis : metabolic storage disease, non malignant hematological disease (thalassemia or sickle cell anemia), malignant disease and immune deficiency. Ka and Kel were significantly different in the four groups and several differences in the pharmacokinetic parameter estimates were observed in each sub-population. The results confirmed the wide inter-patient variability. Furthermore, the relevance of a non parametric method was confirmed by the non gaussian distribution of the parameters. The predictive performances of these different models were better for models based on population classified according to the type of pathology than for the « overall population » model, excepted for the « malignant diseases » population model.

## P - 24

**The Effect of the Nitroanalogue Tetrapeptidamid on the Syntheses of the β-Endorfin and Corticotropin**

Hazar H., Hazar A.
Department Pharmacology of Medical School, Yuzuncu Yıl University, Van, Turkey

Objectives: In recent studies, the importance of the opioids has been shown in the regulation of the blood circulation. In this study, the purpose is to study the effect of the nitroanalog terapeptidamid on the levels of β-endorfin and corticotropin in blood plazma and spino-cerebellar fluid.
Methods: The studies were performed on cats under general anesthesia with sodium pentobarbital (Nembutal, 40 mg/kg, intravenously)The blood taken from jugular vein and from spinal fluids were withdrawn from a part of the thoraxic region of the vertebral column by steriotaxis devices. Nitroanalog tetrapeptidamid was injected iv at a dose of 1 mg/kg. Blood and spinal fluid were withdrawed at the 3 and 20 minutes before and after the application of the tested substance.
The level of the β-corticotropin were assessed by the radioimmunological methods (Tracor Europa, France).
Results: 20 minutes after the application of tetrapeptidamid, the blood level of
β-endorfin decreased significantly to a mean value of 39±9.5 pkmol/l. The intensity of the β-endorfin were 33±9.5 and 11±2.9 at 3 and 20 minutes after the application of the tested substance. Similar changes were seen in the spinal fluid. Nitroanalog tetrapeptidamid did not effect on the intensity of the plasma corticotropin at 3 and 20 minutes after the application of the tested substance in plasma and spinal fluid.
Conclusions: The decrease in plasma and spinal fluid β-endorfin can be explained by the effect of the nitroanalog tetrapeptidamid onthe opioids synthesis in the brain. We can say that nitroanalog tetrapeptidamid inhibited the synthesis of the β-endorfin by the negative feedback as a result of the stimulation of the opioid receptors.

## P - 25

**Evaluation of Markers for Glucuronidation and Sulfation Activities Following Acetaminophen Administration**

[1]Yin O.Q.P., [2]Tomlinson B., [1]Chow M.S.S.
[1]School of Pharmacy and [2]Dept. of Medicine & Therapeutics, The Chinese University of Hong Kong, Shatin N. T., Hong Kong

PURPOSE: Acetaminophen has been extensively used as a probe for the study of phase II metabolism. This study is to evaluate potential markers in plasma and urine for assessing glucuronidation and sulfation activities following acetaminophen administration in humans.
METHODS: A 500mg acetaminophen was administered to 14 healthy subjects in a crossover manner. Multiple blood and urine samples were collected over 24 h. Concentrations of acetaminophen (A), acetaminophen glucuronide (AG) and acetaminophen sulfate (AS) were determined by an HPLC method. Metabolite formation clearance, determined as the ratio of urinary metabolite to acetaminophen plasma AUC, was used as the reference marker of glucuronidation and sulfation activities.
RESULTS: Formation clearance of AG and AS accounted for 59.8 ± 8.6% and 30.8 ± 7.8% of an apparent total clearance. Urinary metabolic ratios of AG to A at 0-8, 0-12 and 0-24h interval correlated significantly with AG formation clearance (r=0.60, 0.62, 0.62, all p<0.05). AUC ratio of AG to A correlated significantly to AG formation clearance, so are plasma ratios of AG to A obtained 2 to 6h after dosing. Similar results were observed with AS. Plasma ratios of AG to A and AS to A, both at 3h, showed the highest correlations with AG and AS formation clearance (r=0.92 and r=0.79, both p<0.001).
CONCLUSION: Based on our data of different urinary and plasma markers, a single plasma ratio of AG/A or AS/A at 3h appears to be most attractive and convenient. However, further work is warranted to determine its utility in large population.

## P - 26

**Cost Effectiveness of an Active Antibiotic Control Program**

Lustig A.
Pharmacy Department, Barzilai Medical Center, Ashkelon, affiliated with the Faculty of Health Sciences, Ben-Gurion University of the Negev, Israel

Analysis of antibiotic drug expenditures as part of an assessment of various forms of management interventions is rarely reported. The objective of this study was to compare the expenditure and usage of antimicrobials in an Israeli general hospital before and after implementation of an active antibiotic management program. Information for all antimicrobial drugs used was collected during a three-year period-2000 to 2002. Antibiotic usage was standardized by defined daily doses (DDDs) and inflation- adjusted cost was expressed in dollars. All data was adjusted to 100 patient- days. Paired samples test was used and significance was defined as P<0.05 by use of a two- tailed test. For the years 2000 to 2001, a passive antimicrobial program was used based on limited drug formulary, standardized antimicrobial order form, and usage of restricted drugs according to ID physician approval. In 2002, an additional active antibiotic program was implemented based on changes in the classification of some drugs from non- restricted to restricted ones and of guidelines regarding specific restricted drugs. After the active management program was implemented, usage of all antibiotics increased by 0.8%, compared to 2000 (68.28 to 67.73DDD/100patient-days). Expenditure decreased by 44.4%(from $467.56/100 patient days in 2000 to $260.22 /100 patient days in 2002, p=0.015). This standardized method for conducting and reporting an antibiotic control program can help to analyze and compare antibiotic use in an individual institution among other hospitals.

## P - 27

**Effect Of Acetylic Salicyclic Acid (ASA) on the Pharmacokinetics and Pharmacodynamics Of XRP0673, a Direct Factor Xa Inhibitor.**

[1]Hinder M., [2]Frick A., [3]Ozoux M.L., [4]Scholz H., [1]Gebauer A., [1]Rosenburg R.
Aventis Pharma, Depts. of: [1]Clinical Discovery & Human Pharmacology, Frankfurt, Germany; [2]DMPK, Frankfurt, Germany; [3]Bioanalytics Pharmacodynamics, Antony, France and [4]Farmovs-Parexel, Bloemfontein, South Africa

Combination therapy with anticoagulants and platelet aggregation inhibitors is common medical practice in the treatment of acute coronary syndromes. In this double-blind, 3-way crossover design, the effects of coadministration of ASA (300 mg po) on the pharmacokinetics (PK) and pharmacodynamics (PD) of 2 different doses of XRP0673 (0.3, 0.5 mg/kg continuous iv infusion over 6h) in healthy male volunteers. PK was determined as Cmax, Tmax, AUC. PD was determined as (a) coagulation tests, (b) platelet function tests and (c) skin bleeding time. Interaction analysis was performed by calculation of the ratio of geometric means and 90% confidence intervals for the 3 different treatments, respectively. PK-parameters (Cmax, Tmax, AUC) of XRP0673 remained constant in the presence and absence of ASA. XRP0673 and ASA alone did not prolong significantly the skin bleeding time Although the combination of the two compounds prolonged the skin bleeding time, no clinically relevant bleeding was observed. For all other PD-parameters (coagulation- and platelet function- parameters) no interaction between ASA and XRP0673 was detected. No serious adverse event and no drug-related drop-out occurred. This study demonstrates the lack of interaction on PK and PD parameters (coagulation-& platelet-function-tests) after concomitant administration of ASA with XRP0673. The clinical relevance of prolongation of skin bleeding time will be assessed in future studies.

## P - 28

The Role of Researchers and Physicians Chambers in Formulation of National Drug Policies

Chruściel T.L.
National Council of the Physicians Chamber,Warsaw, Poland

There is a constant need for changes in the drug (medicaments) policy. It depends heavily on the governmental system of National Health Service; particularly on the financial system of provision of health services to the population; however it is also related sometimes, in some countries, to the activities of self-governing bodies and local authorities. A complete information on many aspects of drug utilization, drug epidemiology, tradition of drug use and local habits, financial aspects of drug use by the population, and policy of drug manufacturers is a skeleton of such data. Local drug policies may differ in some aspects from national policy, although, obviously the governmental regulations must be followed.
In Poland a fundamental change in financing the health services is taking place since the beginning of the year 2003. The changes in organization of system of provision of health services will follow shortly. In this change the appreciation of the progress of pharmacotherapy calls for participation of learned medical societies in drafting a new drug policy, while the chambers will react to practical aspects of its implementation. The governmental regulations already indicate the right and obligation of medical societies of presenting the candidates for the newly created Drug Advisory Council. The Physicians Chambers by their representatives participate in drafting and continuous revisions of hospital medicaments formularies, as well as in educating pharmacoeconomics. The National Physicians Chamber created a body to prepare drug policy that will enable the discussion with government and may, by the Deputies to the Parliament, be proposed for the national discussion. Draft drug policy will be presented.

## P - 29

A Study of Drug Prescribing Pattern in Gastroenterology in a Tertiary Teaching Hospital in India

Sood P., Midha V., Sood A.
Dayanand Medical College &Hospital, Ludhiana, India

This study was conducted to define the drug prescribing pattern at gastroenterology speciality out- patient clinic of Dayanand Medical College & Hospital ,Ludhiana, from April-July 2002.
Six hundered & thirty six prescriptions were audited with average number of drugs per prescription as 3.03. The majority (n=249) of these contained 3 drugs while 18 were for 1 drug, 68 for 2, 168 for 4 and 135 containing >4 drugs. In 3 (0.47%) prescriptions only investigations were ordered . Brand prescribing was in 92%. The prescribing frequency of proton pump inhibitors (PPIs) was maximum (16.13%) followed by H2 blockers (12.9%). In PPI's maximum prescriptions were for Omeperazole (70.7%) followed by Lansoprazole (19.1%), Pantoprazole (6%), Rabeprazole & Esomeprazole (4.1%). Famotidine was prescribed in 164. Amongst prokinetics (10.9%) maximum prescription was for Domperidone (61.4%) followed by Mosapride (22.9%) & Cisapride (15.7%). Anti spasmodics accounted for 7.9% , Drotaverine being the commonest (77.6%).The prescribing frequencies of other therapeutic classes were:laxatives in 7.9%., antihelminthics 5.1%, antibiotics 5.8%,multivitamins 19.8% & miscellaenous 9%. The least frequently prescribed drugs were NSAIDs (5.1%), the most common were Nimesulide (79.5%), Celecoxib & Rofecoxib (15.3%).. This study indicates the general trend in the prescribing habits of gastroenterologists in a tertiary teaching hospital.

## P - 30

Trends of Consumption of Antiasthmatic Preparations in Yaroslavl in 2001-2002 Palyutin S.C., Yakusevitch V.V.
Yaroslavl State Medical Academy, Department of Clinical Pharmacology, Yaroslavl, Russia

Purpose: analysis of consumption of preparations for the treatment of bronchial asthma in Yaroslavl in 2001-2002 through analysis of recipes from the drug stores.
Results and discussion: treatment of bronchial asthma must be made 0n the principles, stated in GINA. Main base preparations are inhaled glucocorticoids but the medical program for the patients' asthma not always is identical. In the first half 2001 the patients have received 3060 packs of beclometasone 50 mcg (Bec), 1239 - budesonide 200 mcg (Bud), 8637 - β2-agonists short action (salbutamol, fenoterol - SalFen), 2193 - prolonged theophylline (Theo), 2191 - perorales glucocorthicoids (prednisolone, triamcinolone - PreTri). On one patients was come to average near 0,6 packing an Bec, 0,25 Bud, 1,7 SalFen, 0,4 Theo, 0,4 PreTri. Noted essential prevalence in using the patients preparations β2- agonists short action, but base drugs are used insufficiently actively. In the same time near 20% patients bronchial asthma constantly got perorale steroids. Educational programs amongst physicians have brought about that in the first half 2002 a spectrum of drawing recipes on antiasthmatic preparations several is changed in the best side. In particular, is enlarged amount inhalations steroids: Bec - 3165, Bud - 3828. With provision for greater dose Bud possible value a given speaker positively. Amount of drawing recipes on Bud is enlarged in 3 times, but β2-agonists the whole on 30%.
Conclusion: in the structure of consumption of antiasthmatic preparations are saved more essential defect, which do not correspond principles of permanent and identical pharmacotherapia, stated in GINA. Correction to situations possible under active educational functioning with physicians.

## P - 31

Secondary Lusiotropic Efficiency of Riodipine and Nifedipine on the Right Heart Ventricle Diastolic Dysfunction

Pukitis A., Skutelis A., Mikazans V.
Laboratory of Pharmacology and Toxicology, Latvia Institute of Cardiology, Riga, Latvia

Objective: It has been suggested that, calcium channel blockers showed diastolic effects. The diastolic changes are known as early signs of the arterial hypertension (AH) induced heart ischaemic cascade, where diastolic dysfunction is observed as early symptom of the myocardium contractility insufficiency.
Design and Methods: Comparison of the lowest effective doses of nifedipine (40mg/daily) and riodipine (40mg/daily) was made in 15 pts. groups each (54 to 68 years age) with arterial hypertension (grade II) and diastolic dysfunction (grade II according the RKCG) to 15 pts. control in a ten days treatment course. Radiokinetocardiography (RKCG) was used for the right ventricle function and heart wall mechanical movement studies combined with (ECG) and impedance cardiography (IC).
Results: Riodipine increased diastolic relaxation period (RP) of 12,5±3,1% (p<0,01,), nifedipine decreased RP for 8,3±1,6, p<0,05). Hemodynamic studies showed riodipine reduced minute volume, middle arterial pressure (-9.3±1.5%) which correlates with systemic vascular resistance (-8.4±0.9%, p<0.05) and diastolic dysfunction decrease (from grade II to I).
Conclusions: Riodipine data will extend new indications for the early and effective diastole modulating therapy, based on hemodynamic and local diastolic effect. Riodipine showed more expressed antihypertensive and lusiotropic effect in comparison to nifedipine.

## P - 32

Influence of Menthol on Caffeine Disposition and Pharmacodynamics in Healthy Female Volunteers

[1]Gelal A., [1]Guven H., [1]Balkan D., [2]Artok L, [3]Benowitz N.L.
DEU Medical Faculty, Dept. of Pharmacology[1], IIT, Faculty of Science, Dept. of Chemistry[2], UCSF, Div Clin Pharmacol, CA[3].

The present study was undertaken to determine whether menthol affects the *in vivo* metabolism of caffeine and pharmacological responses to caffeine in people.

This was a randomized, double-blind, 2-phase crossover study. Eleven female subjects took 200 mg caffeine within coffee with 100 mg menthol or placebo capsules. Serum concentrations, cardiovascular and subjective parameters of caffeine were measured.

During the menthol and placebo phase, the $(AUC)_{0-24}$ and $(AUC)_{0-\infty}$ values of caffeine were not significantly different. Caffeine $t_{max}$ values were 76.4 min (95%CI, 57.5 to 95.2) and 43.6 min (95%CI, 29.8 to 57.5) in menthol and placebo phase, respectively (p<.05). The $C_{max}$ values of caffeine were slightly lower in menthol phase than in placebo phase (p=0.0653). Maximum values for heart rate (HR) change in menthol and placebo phases were -8.9 (95%CI, -5.9 to -11.9); -13.1 (95%CI, -11.5 to -14.7); respectively (p<.05). Systolic and diastolic blood pressures were slightly higher in the menthol phase than in the placebo phase (p>.05).

We conclude that pure menthol delays caffeine absorption and blunts the HR slowing effect of caffeine, but does not affect caffeine metabolism. The possibility that menthol slows the absorption of other drugs should be considered.

## P - 33

Toxicity of Lead Acetate on Rabbit Arteries: A Histological Evaluation

[1]Minaii B., [1]Towfighi Z., [2]Soltaninejad K., [2]Abdollahi M.

Lead is a toxic environmental contaminant that induces many biochemical and structural changes in biological systems. Lead has toxic effects on cardiovascular system and could induce hypertension. It is well known that one element in pathogenesis of hypertension is vascular damage. Therefore, we were studied the toxic effects of lead acetate on rabbit arteries. Ten male albino rabbits, chosen by simple randomized sampling and were divided into two groups. Treated animals received lead acetate solution (0.1% w/v) for 2 month (group B). Controls received tap water for the same period (group A). After termination of exposure period, aorta and subclavian arteries were removed by surgery and stained with H&E for microscopic analysis. Results showed marked histopathological changes in treated animals. Endothelial cells damage in intima, acidiophilic changes of connective layer, thrombosis in lumen of arteries, fibrosis and dystrophic calcification in media were the most important alterations on arteries. It is concluded that chronic lead acetate exposure and resulted alterations in arteries might be a cause of hypertension reported in previous studies.

## P - 34

A Drug Utilization Study in 511 Patients Attending, Gynaecology and Obstetrics Out-door Department at a Tertiary Referral Centre of Industrial Town of Ludhiana, India

[1]Kaushal S., [1]Chopra S.C., [2]Kaushal K., [2]Cheema T.S., [2]Cheema R.
[2]Department of Gynaecology and Obstetrics, Dr. B. L. Kapoor Memorial Hospital, Ludhiana, [1]Department of Pharmacology, Dayanand Medical College and Hospital, Ludhiana Punjab, India

This prospective study was conducted at the Gynaecology and Obstetrics Out-door Patient Department; of a tertiary care hospital of Ludhiana, Punjab, India to the study drug utilization in this speciality. The study was conducted over three consecutive calendar months and 511 prescriptions were evaluated. The percentages of prescriptions containing no drug, one, two, three, four and five or more drugs were 22.11%, 8.42%, 20.94%, 20.94%, 17.61% and 9.98% respectively, with mean number of drugs being 2.52/ prescription. The commonly prescribed drugs were haematinics (17.81%), multivitamins and anti-oxidant preparations (14.54%), calcium supplements (13.76%), antimicrobial agents (including antibiotics, anti-fungal and probiotics) (8.63%), folic acid supplements (7.08%), analgesics (6.22%), styptytics (5.5%), tocolytics (4.59%), hormonal preparations (4.28%), protein supplements (3.89%), anti-emetics (2.18%) and anti-spasmodic (1.17%). The drugs not included in the above groups were prescribed in 13.45% of prescriptions. Only 2.41% of patients received Injectable preparations, which were mostly tetanus toxoid and hormonal preparations. Most commonly prescribed drugs were haematinics, calcium supplements and multivitamin preparations as majority of patients evaluated had come for antenatal check up. No patient called for procedures was prescribed any drug indicating that the drugs were prescribed only when thought fit by the prescriber.

## P - 35

Influence of Oral Placebo, Trapidil and Isosorbide Dinitrate on Norephinephrine-induced Hand Vein Constriction in Healthy Men

Sziegoleit W., Dannenberg K., Konschak A., Presek P.
Sektion Klinische Pharmakologie, Martin-Luther-Universität Halle-Wittenberg, Halle, Germany

In three studies the influence of an oral dose of the vasodilators trapidil (200 mg, study T) and isosorbide dinitrate (20 mg, study I) and of placebo (study P) on norepinephrine-induced venoconstriction has been investigated in healthy male volunteers, using the dorsal hand vein compliance technique. Study P and study T were done in 10 subjects aged 20 to 30 years in a cross-over design, 8 subjects aged 22 to 29 years took part in study I. In each study dose-response curves for venoconstriction by locally infused norepinephrine were established before and 1 h, 2 h and 3 h after oral medication. The mean ED50- values of norepinephrine were 12.1a/32.4d/21.3e/ 31.7a,b,f ng/min in study P (a p < 0.02), 9.6/20.6/13.5/ 12.6b ng/min in study T (b p < 0.05) and 9.4c/7.3d/3.3c,e/ 6.0f ng/min in study I (c p < 0.05, d p < 0.01, e p < 0.01, f p < 0.01). They show that the norepinephrine effect weakened in the course of study P and that oral administration in contrast to local intravenous administration of vasodilators did not diminish a peripheral venoconstriction but increases it slightly (study T, study I), perhaps reflectory to dilatation of large vessels.

## P - 36

Adenosine Receptor Mediated Cytotoxicity in the Breast Cancer Cell Lines: Focus on the A3 Receptor

Panjehpour M., Karami-Tehrani F.
Cancer Research Lab, Clin. Biochem. Dept., School of Medical Sci., Tarbiat Modarres University, Tehran, Iran

Objective: The nucleoside adenosine is present in all cells and body fluids of all living organisms. The physiological effects of adenosine are mediated by four pharmacologically and biochemically distinct adenosine receptors (AR), A1, A2a, A2b and A3. A1AR and A3AR generally couple to Gj proteins, whereas A2a and A2b receptors activate Gs proteins. Although, the presence of these receptors has been reported in normal as well as cancer cells, no data is available for breast cancer. Therefore, this study is aimed to investigate the existence and possible role of A3AR in ER+ MCF-7 and ER- MDA-MB468 breast cancer cell lines.
Methods: The cell lines were cultured in RPMI-1640 medium and incubated with different concentrations of IB-MECA (0.1-100 µM), A3 selective agonist, and MRS-1220 (0.1-10µM), a highly selective antagonist, at different times (24-72hr). MTT viability test was used to study the proliferative/cytotoxicity response. mRNA was isolated and reverse transcriptase polymerase chain reaction, RT-PCR, was also applied
Results: IB-MECA, at concentrations > 10µM resulted in a significant cell death ($p<0.05$) which reached the maximum at 48hr, in both cell lines. Pretreatment with MRS-1220, at 0.1 and 1µM, prevented the cytotoxicity effect of IB-MECA (at 30 and 60µM), indicating that A3 receptor is present on both cell lines. MRS-1220 had no effect when used alone. Further confirmation was provided by the application of RT-PCR method.
Conclusion: Since, both cell lines responded to the treatment with A3 agonist and RT-PCR analysis showed the presence of the receptor mRNA, it is concluded that this membrane receptor is present in the breast cancer cell lines, irrespective of ER status.

## P - 37

Different Patterns of Craving and Withdrawal Symptoms During Smoking Abstinence

Teneggi V., Squassante L., Ziviani L., Milleri S., Bye A.
GlaxoWellcome SpA, Medicine Research Centre, Verona, Italy

Little is known about the effects of individual smoker characteristics (sex, age, etc.) on craving and withdrawal symptoms [1, 2]. We show data from 4 double blind, randomised, 3 period, crossover studies, in healthy smokers. In each study, subjects went through three periods of: free smoking, enforced abstinence with an active treatment or placebo. Self-reported questionnaires were administered: the Questionnaire on Smoking Urges-Brief for craving and the Smoker Complaint Scale for withdrawal [3]. In total 117 subjects (66 males, 51 females) were enrolled. The intensity of craving was on average 3.5 during free smoking and 4.8 during placebo, while the intensity of withdrawal symptoms was on average 55.2 and 65 respectively. The increase of craving during placebo was: greater in females than in males, with an effect size [4] of 1.21 (large) and 0.65 (medium) respectively; greater in youngers (18-39 years) than in olders (40-65 years), with an effect size of 1.17 (large) and 0.48 (medium) respectively. The increase of withdrawal symptoms during placebo was: greater in females than in males, with an effect size of 0.74 (large) and 0.27 (small) respectively; greater in olders than in youngers, with an effect size of 0.43 (medium) and 0.20 (small) respectively. References 1. American Psychiatry Association Diagnostic and Statistical Manual of Mental Disorders, 1994 Forth Edition, Washington, DC, P 244 2. Shiffman S, Jarvik ME Smoking Withdrawal symptoms in two weeks abstinence. Psychopharmacology, 1976; 50: 35-39 3. Patten CA, Martin JE Measuring tobacco withdrawal. A review of self report questionnaires.

## P - 38

Effects of Acetylsalicylate on Spinal Reflexes in Rats

[1]Genc O., [1]Turgut S., [1]Turgut G., [2]Kortunay S.
Pamukkale University, Faculty of Medicine, Department of [1]Physiology and [2]Pharmacology, Denizli, Turkey.

The effects of nonsteroidal antiinflammatory drug, acetylsalicylate, on spinal monosynaptic reflexes were tested in spinal rats. Acetylsalicylate was administered orally (50 and 100 mg/kg) via nasogastric tube. Adult rats (n=30) weighing 150-200 g were anaesthetized with ketamine (50 mg/kg, i.m) and artificially ventilated. Animals were spinalized at C1 level. A laminectomy was performed in the lumbosacral region. The ventral roots of segment L5 were isolated and a pouch of skin formed at the site of the dissection to allow the exposed tissues to be covered with liquid paraffin. The temperature was kept at 36±0.5°C with a heating pad. After the dissection of left thigh region, sciatic nerve was isolated. Sciatic nerve was placed on a silver-silver chloride wire electrode for stimulation through an isolation unit. The reflex potentials were recorded from the ipsilateral L5 ventral root, mounted on a silver-silver chloride wire electrode. The systemic dosages of acetylsalicylicate (50 and 100 mg/kg) significantly decreased the amplitude of reflex response ($p<0.05$). According to these results, the cyclooxygenase products of arachidonic acid may play an important role in regulating the reflex potential at the spinal cord level.

## P - 39

Effects of Metamizol (Dipyrone) on Spinal Reflexes in Rats

[1]Genc O., [1]Turgut S., [1]Turgut G., [2]Kortunay S.
Pamukkale University, Faculty of Medicine, Department of [1]Physiology and [2]Pharmacology, Kınıklı, Denizli, Turkey.

The effects of nonsteroidal antiinflammatory drug metamizol (Dipyrone), on spinal monosynaptic reflexes were tested in spinal rats. Metamizol was administered intramuscular (10 and 15 mg/kg). Adult rats (n=30) weighing 150-200 g were anaesthetized with ketamine (50 mg/kg, i.m) and artificially ventilated. Animals were spinalized at C1 level. A laminectomy was performed in the lumbosacral region. The ventral roots of segment L5 were isolated and a pouch of skin formed at the site of the dissection to allow the exposed tissues to be covered with liquid paraffin. The temperature was kept at 36±0.5°C with a heating pad. After the dissection of left thigh region, sciatic nerve was isolated. Sciatic nerve was placed on a silver-silver chloride wire electrode for stimulation through an isolation unit. The reflex potentials were recorded from the ipsilateral L5 ventral root, mounted on a silver-silver chloride wire electrode. The systemic dosages of metamizol (10 and 15 mg/kg) significantly decreased the amplitude of reflex response ($p<0.05$). According to these results, the cyclooxygenase products of arachidonic acid may play an important role in regulating the reflex potential at the spinal cord level.

## P - 40

The Effects of Zizyphus Jujuba Mill. Extractions On Heart Rates And Minute Respiratory Volume Of Rats

[1]Çelik A., [2]Turgut G., [2]Genç O., [2]Turgut S., [3]Altin R., [4]Aydın M., [5]Kortunay S.
Pamukkale University, [1]Department of Biology, Science & Arts Faculty; Faculty of Medicine [2]Department of Physiolgy and [5]Department of Pharmacology, 20017 Denizli, Turkey, Karaelmas University, Faculty of Medicine, [3]Department of Pulmonary Medicine and [4]Department of Cardiology, Zonguldak, Turkey

In this work, we have investigated the effects of *Zizyphus jujuba* extract on rat minute respiratory volume end heart beat rate. For this purpose plant extract was prepared using soxhlet apparatus and given introperitonally to 15 rats seperated into three groups. Animals were first anesthesized using 1.5 mg/kg, i.p. urathane to equip with cannula and electrods to follow minute respiratory volume and heart rate, respectively. Then, each group was given 200 mg/kg, 300 mg/kg and 400 mg/kg of *Z. jujuba* extract in 0.5 ml olive oil intraperitonally. Results have suggested that *Z. jujuba* extract increased the both hearth rate and minute respiratory volume significantly.

## P - 41

A New, Rapid, Fully Automated Method for Determination of Fluconazole in Serum by Column-Switching Liquid Chromatography

Kümmerer, K.
Institute of Environmental Medicine and Hospital Epidemiology University Hospital Freiburg, Germany

Fluconazole is a triazole agent with potent antifungal activity. It plays an important role in the treatment of superficial and systemic fungal infection. Although the concentration of fluconazole in blood after administration of single doses correlates well with the administered dose, there are patients where drug monitoring becomes necessary, e.g. patients undergoing dialysis. Until now only a few methods are available. All reported fluconazole methods need a sample pretreatment. The aim of the present study was to develop a rapid, accurate and sensitive analytical method to determine fluconazole in serum, which allows fast drug-monitoring of systemic Candida infections in clinical routine.

## P 42

Vasoconstrictor Hyporeactivity in Inflammation can be Corrected by Antioxidants

Pleiner J.
Department of Clinical Pharmacology, University of Vienna

Background: Hyporeactivity to catecholamines and other vasoconstrictors is present in inflammation. Since oxidative stress plays a significant role in inflammation, impaired responsiveness may be overcome by antioxidants.
Methods: After IRB approval, in randomized, double blind cross over studies, forearm blood flow (FBF) responses to norepinephrine (NE), angiotensin II (ANG II) and vasopressin (VP) were assessed before and 4 hours after induction of systemic inflammation by low doses of E. coli endotoxin in healthy volunteers. Further, the effect of intra-arterial vitamin C (24 mg/min) or placebo on NE- or ANG II-induced vasoconstriction was studied after LPS.
Results: LPS administration caused systemic and forearm vasodilatation, increased white blood count, elevated body temperature and reduced Vitamin C plasma concentrations. LPS decreased the responses of FBF to NE by 59%, to ANG II by 25%, and to VP by 51% ($p<0.05$, all effects). Co-administration of Vitamin C completely restored the response to NE and to ANG II, which was comparable to that observed under baseline conditions.
Discussion: E. coli-endotoxemia reduced FBF responsiveness to vasoconstrictors. The hyporeactivity can be corrected by high doses of vitamin C, suggesting that oxidative stress may represent an important target for inflammation-induced impaired vascular function.

## P - 43

Effects of Sildenafil Citrate on Ejaculation Process

Bilge S.S., Kesim Y., Kurt M., Aksoz E., Celik S.
Department of Pharmacology, Ondokuz Mayis University School of Medicine, Samsun, Turkey

Purpose: To investigate the effect of sildenafil citrate on ejaculation process in isolated rat vas deferens.
Methods: The effect of sildenafil citrate (Sildegra®, Fako Ilacları A.S, Istanbul, Turkey) on the electrically induced contractions and contractions produced by exogenous Noradrenaline (NA), Adenosine 5'-triphosphate(ATP), a non-selective P2 receptor agonist, alpha,beta methylene ATP (a,b meATP), a selective P2x receptor agonist in Male Wistar rat vas deferens were investigated.
Results: Sildenafil citrate induced concentration dependent inihibition of electrically (40V, 20Hz, 0,5 ms) evoked contractions. Sildenafil citrate (1-100 microM) did not change NA (1microM-1miliM) and a,b meATP (3 microM) induced contractions. At highest concentration (100 microM) sildenafil citrate inhibited the response to ATP.
Conclusıons: These results suggest that sildenafil citrate may be used on patients with premature ejaculation disorder.

## P - 44

Irrational Drug Use in Some Districts of Lithuania

Maciulaitis R., Janusonis T.
Theoretical and Clinical Pharmacology Dpt., Kaunas Medical University, Mickeviciaus, Lithuania

Aim: The aim of this study was to investigate the irrational use of reimbursed drugs in some districts of Lithuania in 2001 by investigating the viewpoints of the physicians to the problems of the irrational pharmacotherapy, possible causes and solutions of them.
Method: This investigation was designed as a qualitative structured questionnaire.
Results: The study was composed of two stages. The personal health records in 2001 of the Siauliai, Panevezys and Utena districts' residents were analysed and the cases of irrational drug use were selected, examined and verified during the first stage. There were 318 personal health's records analysed and 111 cases of irrational drug use verified. The 23 problems of irrational pharmacotherapy were distinguished and classified according to the responsibilities. The viewpoints of the physicians to the problems of the irrational pharmacotherapy were confirmed and analysed during the second stage of the study. 31 physicians were interviewed and responses summarized.
Conclusions: 1. The 23 types of problems of irrational pharmacotherapy can be classified into the 3 main levels according to the responsibility: the level of the administration (institution), the physician and the patient; other problems can be distinguished separately. 2. The most frequently specified by physicians possible reasons of the irrational drug use were the lack of information, the overcharge of the physician and the lack of qualification. 3. The most frequently specified by physicians possible solutions of the irrational drug use were the growth of qualification, the establishment of the algorithms and the increase of the time spent per patient.

## P - 45

Efficacy of Myrrh in Comparison with Anticoccidial Drug Diclazuril ,on Performance of Broiler Chicks

[1]El -Ashmawy I.M., [2]El- Lakany H.,[3,4]Salama O.M.
Departements of [1]Pharmacology and Aquatic Fish ,and [2]Poultry Diseases, Faculty of Veterinary Medicine , Alexandria Univ. , Departement of [3]Pharmacognosy , Faculty ofPharmacy, Mansoura Univ. and [4]Research&Development and Quality Control Division, Pharco Pharmaceuticals , Alexandria , Egypt

Myrrh is an oleo - gum resin obtained from the stem of Commiphora molmol , Family Burceraceae . The present experiment was run to compare the efficacy of crude Myrrh with the anticoccidial Diclazuril on performance of broilers when they are fed to 1 - day - old chickens over a period of 7 weeks at levels of 200 and 1 ppm respectively . At 4 weeks of age , broiler chicks were infected experimently with sporulated oocysts using a local field isolate of Eimeria tenella . The induced infestations were poor body weight gain and low feed conversion . Fecal samples were examined for oocysts at intervals from 5 to 14 days after infection . Myrrh significantly improve growth rates , feed conversion ,shedding of oocysts and reduced lesion scores in comparison with infected non medicated controls . There were no significant differences for weight gains , feed conversion , shedding of oocysts and lesion scores between Myrrh and Diclazuril treated chicks . It could be concluded that Myrrh appeared to be a valuable feed additive for broiler chicks .

## P - 46

Role of Polyphorphic Human CYP2B6 in Cyclophosphamide Bioactivation

[1]Xie H., [1]Yasar U., [1]Lundgren S., [2]Griskevicius L., [3]Terelius Y., [2]Hassan M., [1]Rane A.
[1]Karolinska Institutet, Department of Medical Laboratory Sciences and Technology, Division of Clinical Pharmacology, Huddinge University Hospital, Stockholm, Sweden; [2]Karolinska Institutet, Department of Medicine at Huddinge University Hospital, Division of Hematology, Laboratory of Hematology, Stockholm, Sweden; [3]AstraZeneca R & D Södertälje, Department of Research DMPK, Södertälje, Sweden

The role of polymorphic CYP2B6 in cyclophosphamide (CPA) bioactivation was investigated in human liver microsomes. Sixty-seven human liver specimens were genotyped with respect to the CYP2B6*5 and *6 variant alleles. CYP2B6 apoprotein were assessed by immunoblotting. 4-Hydroxy-CPA and hydroxy-bupropion were quantified by using HPLC and LC-MS, respectively. 7-Ethoxy-4-trifluoromethyl coumarin O-deethylase activity was measured fluorometrically. The frequencies of CYP2B6*5 and CYP*6 mutant alleles were 9.0 and 16.4 %, respectively. CYP2B6 protein expression was detected in 80 % of the samples, with a large variation (0.003-2.234, arbitrary units). There was a high correlation between CYP2B6 apoprotein content and CPA 4-hydroxylation ($n=55$, $r=0.81$, $P<0.0001$). In addition, the *6 carriers had significantly higher CPA 4-hydroxylation ($P<0.05$). CPA 4-hydroxylation also correlated significantly with other CYP2B6 specific reactions ($n=20$, $P<0.0001$). CYP2B6 showed 25-fold higher in vitro intrinsic clearance than previously observed in recombinant CYP2C19.1 and CYP2C9 variants in yeast expression system. Our results demonstrate that the polymorphic CYP2B6 is a major enzyme in the bioactivation of CPA. Moreover, we identified a strong impact of CYP2B6*6 on CPA 4-hydroxylation.

## P - 47

Optimising the Treatment of Burned Patients by Usage of Tibetan Healing Techniques

Fedorov V.M., Strakhov S.N., Philppov A.I., Kostyukova Z.I., Mikhailov A.G., Redkina V.Y.
Regional Burn Centre, Regional Centre of Holistic Medicine, Omsk, Russia

The purpose of research was to optimise the treatment of 17 patients severely burned by flame as a result of oil pipeline explosion. Mean age of the patients was 29.4 years; the square of burns was 30-90% of body surface. All burns were classified as II - III degree lesions. All patients showed vagal shock within the first 48 hours and received standard infusion-transfusion, analgesia and infection prophylaxis. Simultaneously from the $5^{th}$ day after the lesion all patients received daily energetic sessions of treatment with Tibetan Healing Practice Jin-Key-Do as well as curing of the wounds with aseptic bandages with distilled water. The control group consisted of 10 patients that received no energetic healing.
Energotherapeutic sessions caused deep psychophysical relaxation, which led to improvement of somatic status. Haemodynamic indices were stabilised 24-48 hours earlier, than in patients of the control group. We observed stable hour-diuresis and body weight. The algetic threshold was statistically higher in comparison to the control group. This reduced consumption of narcotic analgetics. The time of preparation for the skin autotransplantation was brought down, transplantability was statistically higher ($p<0.005$). Infectious complications among the observed patients were met in 15%, in the control group in 40%. Investigation of influence of Tibetan Healing Practice on the growth of microorganism colonies in the water demonstrated protective activity of energetic techniques.
Thus, usage of Tibetan Healing Technique Jin-Key-Do in severely burned patients allows to reduce the terms of treatment and may be recommended as an effective addition to traditional methods of treatment.

## P - 48

Effects of Chronic Lead Acetate Intoxication on Blood Indices in Male Adult Rat

[1]Noori M.M.H.,[2]Heidari Z., [2]Mahmoudzadeh Sagheb H.R.
[1]Tehran University of Medical Sciences, [2]Zahedan University of Medical Sciences

History and Objective: Environmental pollution is one of the main problems in big industrial cities of the world. Lead as one of these pollutants can threaten the life of living beings in many ways. In this study the hematological effects of chronic toxicity caused by Lead Acetate in male rats were investigated.
Materials and Methods: 45 male Wistar rats were chosen through simple random sampling. During a period of 12 weeks, administration group was given a solution of 1 % Lead acetate solved in 0.4% acetic acetic as drinking water, control and sham control groups were given distilled water and 0.4% acetic acid solution respectively. Then the animals were anesthetized and blood were taken from their hearts. The measurement of Lead concentration was carried out by means of atomic absorption system. Hematological analysis and differential cell count were also conducted.
Results: Lead concentration in the treatment group was significantly higher than the control groups ($p<0.001$). The results also revealed the observation of Basophilic Stippling, Howell Jolly bodies, decreased RBC count (Anemia), Increased leukocyte count (Leukocytosis). Monocytosis , Eosinopenia , Neutrophilia and trombocytosis ($p<0.001$) in the test group.
Conclusion: It seems that microcytic hypocromic anemia can be contributed to the interaction of lead with iron and copper metabolism. Furthermore, increased leukocytes can be attributed to the inflammatory effects of lead on lymphatic organs.
Keywords: Lead, Hematology, Erythrocyte, Leukocyte, Rat

## P - 49

Survival Following Severe Dapson Poisoning

[1]Vessal G., [2]Moiensadat M., [2]Shadnia S.
[1]Department of clinical Pharmacy, Faculty of Pharmacy, Tehran Uiversity of Medical Science, [2]Poisoning center, Loghman-Hakim Hospital, Faculty of Medicine, Shaeed-Beheshti University of Medical Science

Aim: To describe the treatment and successful outcome of a patient who had taken a lethal amount of Dapson tablets.
Case Report: An 18 -year-old lethargic girl was referred to the emergency center after taking 40 tablets of Dapson. Treatment consisted of gastric lavage with water, oral administration of charcoal and sorbitol solution, lactulose, and intravenous administration of sodium bicarbonate, ranitidine, ascorbic acid, methylene blue, ceftriaxone, clindamycine, packed cell, and fresh frozen plasma. Supportive therapy in the Intensive Care Unit was also provided. His clinical course included cyanosis (due to methemoglobinemia), and ichter. Laboratory results showed respiratory alkalosis with a compensatory metabolic acidosis and significantly reduced hemoglobin, hematocrite and platelet levels.
Discussion: Dapson is an antibiotic used for many years to treat leprosy and rare dermatologic conditions. Recently its major use is for prophylaxis against pneumocystis carinii infections. Toxic effects are caused by the P450 metabolites, and include methemoglobinemia, sulfhemoglobinemia and Heinz body hemolytic anemia (1). This patient has apparently ingested what would normally be a lethal amount of Dapson (death has occurred with doses of 1.4 gram and greater), and has signs and symptoms of severe toxicity. He survived following rapid treatment and supportive care. Recommended measures performed rapidly after onset of poisoning may have contributed to survival in this case.
1.Olson, K.R. Poisoning and Drug Overdose. Appleton & Lang, 1999, pp.152-154

## P - 50

Hange-koboku-to (Banxia-houpo-tang) Raises Neuropeptide Levels in Human Plasma and Saliva

Naito T., Itoh H., Takeyama M.
Department of Clinical Pharmacy, Oita Medical University, Oita, Japan

Objective: Hange-koboku-to (Banxia-houpo-tang) (HKT), Chinese herbal Kampo medicine, is prepared from five crude herbs: Pinelliae Tuber, Hoelen, Magnoliae Cortex, Perillae Herba, and Zingiberis Rhizoma. This medicine has been used for improvement of hoarse voice, something foreign in throat and esophagus, etc. One of the mechanisms on those empirical effects is assumed due to changes neuropeptide levels locally. We examined the effects of HKT on neuropeptides, calcitonin gene-related peptide (CGRP), substance P (SP), somatostatin (SS) and vasoactive intestinal peptide (VIP) in saliva and plasma, and salivary secretion in healthy subjects.
Methods: For 5 healthy subjects, a 6.0-g of HKT (EK-16) or placebo was orally administered. Neuropeptides levels in plasma and saliva were determined by a double-antibody enzyme immunoassay. Results: A single oral administered HKT caused significant increases in SP-immunoreactive substance (IS) (40 min), and showed slight tendency of increase in CGRP-IS, SS-IS, and VIP-IS compared with levels of placebo in plasma. In saliva neuropeptides, HKT caused significant increases in SP-IS (20 min) and SS-IS (60 min), and showed slight tendency of increase in CGRP-IS and VIP-IS. However, we could not take the significant effects of the sialosis volume on a single HKT stimulation.
Conclusion: These results might suggest that HKT improves hoarse voice, something foreign in throat and esophagus by stimulation of neuropeptidergic nerves locally.

## P - 51

Comparison Between the Analgesic Effect of Carum Copticum Extract and Morphine in Phasic Pain Modle in Mice

Dashti M.H., Hejazian S.H. , Morshedi A.
Dept of Physiology Sahid Sadughi Medical University, Yazd , Iran

Pain is a universal complaint which needs further investigations for new pain relieving agents. Carum Copticum(Yamani Ajowan) is a plant in Umberella family which is mentioned to have some therapeutic effect on headache and joint pains in Iranian traditional literatures , but there is a little if any scientific reports to prove its effects on pain. So we conducted to design an experimental clinical trail study to assess and compare the analgesic effect of ethanolic extract of Carum Copticum fruit with morphine by using a Tail-Flick analgesiometer device. Our results indicate that the test drug produced significant increase in tail-flick latency during 2 hours post drug administration($p<0.05$). the pick of the effect was observed at 45 minutes after drug injection., which was comparable to that of 1mg/kg morphine (ip). Positive results in this type of analgesiometric test indicate that the antinociceptive action may be of the opoid type. The present study support the claims of Iranian traditional medicine showing that Carum Copticum extract possesses a clear cut analgesic effect. However, further investigations are required to evaluate the efficacy and safety of this herbal medication in man.
KeyWords: pain , Carum Copticum , tail-flick , mice

## P - 52

The Analgesic Effect of Ethanolic Extract of Lactuca Sativa Seeds in Mice

Morshedi A.; Dashti M.H.
Dept of Physiology Shahid Sadughi Medical University, Yazd , Iran

Seed of Lactuca Sativa is an ancient drug that is mentioned by Iranian old physicians as an important drug for treating acute inflammation, chest pain, fever, headache, cough., etc. and It is widely used in old Greek Medicine for nervous disorders. but Seeds of Lactuca Sativa were not scientifically studied for neuropharmacological activities in systemic manners. Therefore, it was planned to study the drug pharmacologically to substantiate an improve its therapeutic uses on scientific basis. In the present study a comprehensive pharmacological screening of the 50% ethanolic extract of Lactuca Sativa Seeds was carried out for its effects on phasic pain. The drug was administered interapretoneally in a dose corresponding to human dose described in Iranian classical literature. Analgesiometer Tail-Flick Test was carried out for detecting analgesia. In this Analgesiometer Test, the test drug did not produced significant increase in the reaction time (Tail-Flick latency) (p=0.453). the present study did not supports the claims of Iranian traditional medicine in this type of analgesiometric test. however It needs further investigations to assess the analgesic effect of this traditional herbal medication in other types of pain models.

Keywords: phasic pain, Lactuca Sativa, Tail-Flick , mice

## P - 53

Commonly Prescribed Chemotherapeutics in Pregnancy in Trabzon, Turkey

[1]Kadioglu M., [2]Yaris F., [1]Ulku C., [1]Kesim M., [1]Yaris E., [1]Kalyoncu N.
[1]Karadeniz Technical University, Department of Pharmacology, [2]Karadeniz Technical University, Department of Family Medicine, Trabzon Turkey

Aims: In our study, we aimed to evaluate the chemotherapeutics which were the most common drugs prescribed in pregnancy by the physicians in our cases.
Methods: The pregnant cases who used drugs have been consulted by the Departments of Pharmacology and Family Medicine of Karadeniz Technical University School of Medicine since 1999. Physicians and families were consulted on the risk levels according to the doses and exposure periods of the drugs and gestation weeks.
Results: 312 (76.7%) of the 405 cases were unaware of pregnancy. 349 (86.0%) cases had used more than one (2-21) drug. Of the 278 kinds of drugs, the most common drug group was chemotherapeutics. Chemotherapeutic drugs were ciprofloxacin(41), ornidazole(37), sultamicillin(28), amoxicillin(27), gentamicin (25), metronidazole + miconazole(20), fluconazole(19), ofloxacin(19), cefuroxime(18), clarithromycin(17), cefazolin(15), trimethoprim+sulfomethoxazole(13), penicillin(13), nitrofurantoin(11), doxycycline(10), isoconazole(9), clindamycin(8), phentyconazole(7), cefprozil(6), levofloxacin(5), cefaclor(5), spiramicin(4), mebendazole(4), cefixime(4), amikacin(3), lincomycin(3), azithromycin(3), sulfisoxazole(3), ceftriaxon(3), metronidazole(3), loracarbef(2), povydoniodure(2), thiamphenicol(2), nifuroxazide(2), roxithromicin(2), pimaricin(2), cephadroxyl(2), cefalexine(1), tetracycline(1), lamivudine(1), albendazole(1), pyrantelpomoate(1), isoniaside(1), rifampicin(1), morfozinamide(1), etambutol(1), bacampicillin(1), fucidic acid(1), acyclovir(1), hydroxychloroquine(1), neomycine(1). 28 high risk cases who used chemotherapeutics combined with some other drugs had therapeutic abortion. One renal congenital anomaly was found in 199 babies exposed to the chemotherapeutics.
Conclusion: Chemotherapeutics were generally prescribed unaware of pregnancy. The probability of pregnancy must be remembered in reproductive women while prescribing for the infections.

## P - 54

Analgesics Prescribed in Pregnancy in Trabzon, Turkey

[1]Kadioglu M., [2]Yaris F., [1]Ulku C., [1]Kesim M., [1]Yaris E., [1]Kalyoncu N.
[1]Karadeniz Technical University, Department of Pharmacology, [2]Karadeniz Technical University, Department of Family Medicine, Trabzon Turkey

Aims: Drug usage in pregnancy is a common problem. In our study, we aimed to evaluate the analgesics prescribed by the physicians unaware of pregnancy.
Methods: The pregnant cases who used drugs have been consulted by the Departments of Pharmacology and Family Medicine of Karadeniz Technical University School of Medicine since 1999. Names, doses of the drugs, exposure periods and gestation weeks were recorded. Physicians and the families were consulted on the risk levels.
Results: 312 (76.7%) of the 405 cases were unaware of pregnancy. 349 (86.0%) cases had used more than one (2-21) drug. Of the 278 kinds of drugs, one of the most common drug groups were paracetamol (121) and nonsteroidal-antiinflamatory (NSAI) drugs (201). NSAI drugs were naproxen sodium (47), diclofenac (36), acetylsalicylic acid (26), nimesulide (23), piroxicam (17), flurbiprofen (11), ibuprofen (6), benzydamine HCl (5), tenoxicam (5), mefenamic acid (4), diflunisal (4), meloxicam (3), etofenamate (3), acemetacine (2), celecoxib (2), etodolac (2), ketoprofen (1), rofecoxib (1), tiaprofenic acid (1), indometacine (1), nabumetone (1). 18 high risk cases who used analgesics combined with some other drugs had therapeutic abortion. No congenital anomaly was found due to the analgesics in the 216 babies born.
Conclusion: Analgesics were generally prescribed for acute diseases and unaware of pregnancy. The probability of pregnancy must be remembered in reproductive women while prescribing analgesics.

## P - 55

GABAergic Mechamisms in Nucleus Tractus Soliarius on Barareflex Sensitivitg in Acut Hypertension Rat

[1]Rafati A., [2]Pourshanazari A.A., [3]Ciriello J.
[1]Shahid Sadughi University of Medical Sciences Isfahan,Iran , [2]Rafsanjan University of Medical Sciences Rafsanjan,Iran , [3]University of Western Ontario,London,Canada

Considerable evidence exists that GABAergic mechanisms have important role in control of blood pressure and heart rate, but there is some controversy about which GABA receptor subtype is involved in cardiovascular regulation within the NTS. In this study the baroreceptor reflex was evaluated in anesthetized rats with microinjection of Bicuculine (GABAA antagonist) and phaclofen (GABAB antagonist) into the nucleus tractus solitaius (NTS). Phenylepherine (PE) (1, 2, 4, 8, 16 microg/kg, i. v.) elicited pressor and bradicardic responses. Extracellular recording of baroreceptive neurons in the NTS during application of PE were monitored in anesthetized rats.Regression analysis of the baroreflex curve, revealed a significantly smaller baroeflex sensitivity in Bicuculine receiving group compared with sham. The baroreflex sensitivity was not affected by phaclofen. In Extracellular recording the firing frequency of baroreceptive neurons in NTS were increased during microiontophoretic application of Bicuculine but not with phaclofen. Bicuculine exited 71 of 86 (83%) NTS neurons without affecting the remaining 13 neurons (17%). These result demonstrate that GABAA receptors are involve in baroreflex sensitivity and spontaneous discharge in the great majority of the NTS baroreceptive neurons.

## P - 56

Anti Nociceptive Effect of Carum Copticum in Mice

Hejazian Yazdy S.H.
Dept of Physiology Shahid Sadughi Medical University, Iran

The Carum Copticum is a species of Umbeliferae family that its effective agents are an essence which is obtained from its fruits. This essence is colorless or mildly brownish and smells as thymole. The fruit of this plant have been traditionally used in many societies as an anti- inflammatory and pain relevant agent but there is no scientific report about these effects. So we designed an experimental study to investigate the effect of alcoholic extraction of Carum Copticum fruit on tonic pain induced by formalin in mice. Our result showed that 10 mg/kg of this extract decreased the pain in 2nd phase, but not in first phase of formalin test. This effect in 2nd phase was not significantly different from that of 1mg/kg morphine.

## P - 57

The Comparison between the Anti Nociceptive Effect of Chamomile Extract and Morphine in Mice

Vahidi Mehrjardi,A.
Dept of Physiology Shahid Sadughi Medical University, Iran

Chamomile is a plant in which many traputic effects has been mentioned since all time .one of its usage in Iranian traditional medicine was to relieve spastic pain since there is a little scientific documents to prove its effectiveness in relieving pain. We conducted to study the effect of its extract on tonic pain induced by formalin in mice our result showed that 2mg/kg Chamomile extract (I.P) attenuated the pain score in both phase of formalin test which was more prominent in 2nd phase and was comparable that of morphine 1mg/kg (I.P) in conclusion Chamomile extract may act as an antinociceptive in a manner which resemble morphine analgesia

## P - 58

Esrrogen Regulation of GABA Response in Nucleus Tractus Solitarii of Rats

[1]Pourshanazari A.A., [2]Alaei H.A., [3]Rafati A., [4]Ciriello J.
[1]Rafsanjan University of Medical Rafsanjan,Iran , [2,3]Isfahan University of Medical Rafsanjan,Iran , [4]University of Western Ontario,London,Canada

Electrophysiological recording of parabrachial nucleus(PBN) neurons were used to investigate that which subtype of GABA receptors participate in the role of estrogen as a modulator of cardiovascular information through the nucleus tractus solitarii(NTS). Experiment were done in anaesthetized(Urethan;150gr/100g bw) male and ovarectomized female rats supplemented for 7 days prior with either 17beta-estradiol(OVX-E2) or saline (OVX-S). A portion of the right cervical vagus was isolated for the electrical activation (0.8Hz,2ms duration) of visceral afferents. The evoked single and multi-unit activity was recorded via a recording electrode in the PBN. Exogenous microinjection of 17beta-estradiol (0.1, 0.25, and 0.5microM; 200 nl) into the NTS produce a significant, dose-dependent attenuation in the magnitude of visceral afferent activation-evoked responses of neurons recorded in the PBN in both male and OVX-E2 groups. No effect on evoked PBN activity was observed following injection of estrogen into the NTS of OVX-S animals. Co-injection of estrogen with the GABAA receptor antagonist, bicuculine (0.1 μM;200nl) but not phaclofen(GABAB; 0.1,0.5or 1 microM;200nl) resulted in an increased in the evoked thalamic response in male(61±13%)and OVX-E2 female(72±18%)rats. These studies suggest that estrogen via an interaction with the GABAA receptor inhibits neurotransmission in the NTS to modulate the visceral information to the PBN.

## P - 59

On GABAA Receptor to Increase Baroreflex Sensitivity in Rats

[1]Alaei H.A., [2]Pourshanazari A.A., [3]Eslami H.R.
[1]Isfahan University of Medical Sciences Isfahan,Iran , [2,3]Rafsanjan University of Medical Sciences Rafsanjan,Iran

The nucleus tractus solitarii (NTS), the termination site of baroreceptor afferent fibers has been shown to be involved in the regulation of cardiovascular reflexes. In this study subthreshold electrical stimulation( 5s,50Hz,0.5ms.50microA) was applied into the NTS in anesthetized rats(150mg/kg ketamin and 0.1mg/kg rampon) and baroreflex sensitivity was evaluated after microintophoretic injection of bicuculine (a GABAA receptor antagonist 0.1 microM;200nl). Canulation were used for femoral vein and artery and with stereotaxix instrument, NTS site was distinguished according to paxinos atlas. Monopolar stainless steel electrodes(150 microm diameter) were inserted into NTS for electrical stimuilation(ES). Blood pressure(systolic, diastolic and mean arterial pressure, MAP) and heart rate(HR)were recorded by physiograph before , during and after application of ES. Phenylephrine(16microg/kg iv)elicited dose-dependent pressor and bradycardic responses. The results showed that application of ES into NTS had no effected on HR or MAP, but baroreflex sensitivity ($\Delta$HR/$\Delta$MAP) was increased immediately and 30 min after application of ES into NTS in comparison with normal state .Microinjection of bicuculine into NTS decreased baroreflex sensitivity to normal level. It is concluded that application of ES into NTS may potent GABA neurotransmition which act on GABAA subtype receptor and increase baroreflex sensitivity.

## P - 60

Prescribing Pattern of Antipsycotic Drugs in Patients with Schizophrenia

[1]Chinellato A., [1]Salvato C., [1]Terrazzani G., [1]Pullia G., [1]Serraglia D., [2]GiustiP., [3]Lucioni C., [4]Haycox A., [4]Walley T.
[1]Local Health Authority Treviso Italy, [2]Department of Pharmacology University of Padua Italy, [3]ADIS International/Health Economics, Milan Italy, [4]Department of Pharmacology University of Liverpool UK

Atypical antipsychotic drugs (clozapine C, olanzapine O, risperidone R and quetiapine Q) are reported to have a better compliance than typical antipsychotics and therefore to be more effective compared to older typical agents (haloperidol H), since they improve the negative as well as the positive symptoms of schizophrenia and exhibits diminished tendency to cause unwanted motor side-effects and prolactin release. We investigated the use of antipsychotic drugs for schizophrenic outpatients in the local health authority of Treviso (Italy) to examine compliance and health care use.
Methods: Pharmaceutical, hospitalisation and psychiatry department databases were used to identify patients beginning any antipsychotic therapy for the first time between 1/7/2000 and 30/6/2001 and followed for 1 year. We used the numbers of Average Daily Quantities ADQ dispensed for each patient to calculate compliance.
Results: The numbers of patients prescribed each drug were: 16C, 142R, 104O, 29Q, and 84H. The ADQ prescribed for each was 242.81 mg C, 3.32 mg R, 8.85 mg O, 240.96 mg Q, 3.85 mg H oral and 3.5 mg H depot. Compliance was better for H (75% of expected ADQ) followed by Q (65%), O (57%) R (49%) and C (29%). The average numbers of days in hospital was similar for each drug.
Conclusions: despite current medical opinion, haloperidol offers better compliance than atypical antipsychotics in schizophrenic outpatients.

## P - 61

Some Degradation Pathways Affecting the Biological Activity of IFN Alpha 2b, Interleukin 2 and Epidermal Growth Factor

Ruiz L., Zurita M., Reyes N., Duany L., Gerónimo H., Aroche K., Hardy E.
Center for Genetic Engineering and Biotechnology, Havana, Cuba

DNA technology has permitted the commercial production of biologically active proteins during the last two decades. Some of these products have exhibited many problems because of their instability. These degradative reactions may affect the biological activity of the protein. In this work we induced some degradation pathways on interferon alpha 2b, interleukin 2 and epidermal growth factor, and characterized them by physical, chemical and biological techniques. Active ingredients were purchased by CIGB, Havana, Cuba. Degradation pathways were induced by heating samples at 37 °C during at least 30 days. All reagents used to prepare each formulation were of analytical grade. Degradation products were purified by RP-HPLC using the adequate gradient, and then analized by SDS/PAGE, Western blot, ELISA and Biological activity assay. We found that some degradation routes (e.g. oxidation) did not affected biological activity of the evaluated cytokines, but other modifications such as aggregation or deamidation significantly affected this property. In addition we determined that immunodetection were dramatically affected when proteins degraded which was in agreement with that previously reported. Basically we found that degradation pathways significantly affected both, biological activity of the proteins and their immunoidentification.

## P - 62

The Influence of Some Formulation Factors on the Protein Stability

Ruiz L., Reyes N., Aroche K., Sotolongo J., Pujol V., Hardy E.
Center for Genetic Engineering and Biotechnology, Havana, Cuba

Some therapeutic proteins have been produced at the Center for Genetic Engineering and Biotechnology (CIGB, Havana, Cuba). However, a great challenge has been to identify the storage conditions preserving the protein stability. The aim of this study was to investigate the effect of different factors on the stability of three therapeutics proteins produced at CIGB. Evaluated proteins were EGF, IL-2 and IFN-alpha-2b. Evaluated factors were active ingredient concentration, freeze-drying process, stressing agents, pH, buffer composition, ionic strength and interactions between auxiliary additives. Samples were stored at 37°C and analyzed by RP-HPLC, SDS/PAGE, ELISA and antiviral titration. We found that the biological activity was retained better at higher concentrations of the active ingredient, freeze-dried process must be achieve in the presence of other auxiliary additives, and the increase on the concentration of the preferentially excluded additives can augment the protein degradation in the presence of small stressing molecules. Here we find some factors that must be taken into account to preserve the stability of, at least, the three proteins evaluated here. Additionally we found that these factors can be taken into consideration for the designing of formulations containing other therapeutics proteins.

## P - 63

A Bioavailability/Bioequivalence Study of Generic Fluoxetine Tablets

Jovanovic D., Maksimovic M., Todorovic V., Srnic D., Stojšic D., Ciric B., Vehabovic M., Potogija N.
National Poison Control Centre, Belgrade, Serbia and Montenegro and Bosnalijek, Pharmaceutical and Chemical Industry, Sarajevo, Bosnia and Herzegovina

The pharmacokinetics and relative bioavailability of fluoxetine capsules (reference) and tablets (test), manufactured by two different pharmaceutical factories (Eli Lilly, USA and Bosnalijek, Bosnia and Herzegovina), were studied in 24 healthy subjects of both sexes after a single 20 mg oral dose of fluoxetine. A single-blind (for the analytical staff) cross-over design with a three week washout period between each dose was applied. Serum samples, obtained before dosing and at various appropriate time points up to 72 hours, were analyzed for fluoxetine content by a sensitive liquid chromatographic-mass spectrometic method with positive ion electrospray ionization and selected ion recording. ANOVA, power analysis, 90% confidence intervals, and two one-sided tests were used for the statistical analysis of pharmacokinetic parameters. Since both 90% CI for the log-transformed AUC and Cmax geometric mean ratios were included in the 80% to 125% interval proposed by the FDA, test drug (Oxetin tablets) was considered bioequivalent to the reference one (Prozac capsules) according both to the rate and the extent of absorption.

## P - 64

Development of Formulations of Interleukin 2 with a Long-Term Stability

Reyes N.
Center for Genetic Engineering and Biotechnology, Havana, Cuba

Interleukin 2 (IL-2) has been investigated as an adjuvant for the therapy with antiviral drugs in HIV patients. The biological activity of this cytokine, is an essential characteristic for the treatment. For IL-2, the major degradation routes are oxidation and aggregation, which may decrease the therapeutic potential of the product and also increase an immune response against this cytokine. The aim of this work was to investigate the stability of IL-2 produced at the Center for Genetic Engineering and Biotechnology (CIGB), when stressing factors were applied to this molecule. IL-2 was diluted to 0.4 or 1.0 mg/mL in sodium acetate buffer. Glycine, alanine, PEG 8000, sucrose, raffinose, EDTA, methionine, polisorbate 80, EDTA and dextran were added in different combinations. Samples were stored at 37°C and periodically analyzed by the in vitro proliferation of CTLL-2 cells, RP-HPLC and SDS/PAGE. Resulted formulation was evaluated in a long-term stability study. As judged by the techniques used here, resulted formulation keeps the IL-2 stability during long periods at 4°C (more than fifteen months, at least, while the stability study stills in course).

## P - 65

Development of New Albumin-Free Formulations of Interferon Alpha 2b for Clinical Purposes

Hardy E.
Center for Genetic Engineering and Biotechnology, Havana, Cuba

In the past two decades, and even today, many investigators have searched the storage conditions able to maintain the biological activity of Interferon alpha 2b (IFN&2b). One of the most widely used stabilizers to improve IFN&2b stability has been human serum albumin (HSA). Unfortunately the use of blood-derived HSA to stabilize rec-IFN-& 2b has many inconvenients (e.g the potential risks of viral contamination). The aim of this study was to obtain an albumin-free formulation, through key pre-formulation and formulation studies. The effect of experimental factors on IFN&2b was evaluated at 37°C. Evaluation was achieved by ELISA, antiviral titration, RP-HPLC and SDS/PAGE. Factors were: additives (sucrose, raffinose, dextran, PEG 8000, glycine, trehalose, PVP, mannitol, sorbitol), buffers (citrate, phosphate, acetate and citrate-phosphate), protein concentration (1, 10, 50 and 100 M IU/mL) and freeze-dry process. Formulations finally designed, were analyzed in a long-term stability study. Two new lyophilized (sucrose/PEG 8000) and liquid (Tween 80/benzyl alcohol) formulations of IFN&2b were designed. These two albumin-free formulations retained the stability of IFN&2b during more than 24 months at 4°C. These formulations have a greater safety for patients and regulatory agencies.

## P - 66

How Prevalent and How Rational is the Prescription of more han one Benzodiazepine to the Same Patient?

[1]De Las Cuevas C., [2]Sanz E.
[1]Clinical Pharmacology, [2]Psychiatry, School of Medicine, University of La Laguna, La Laguna, Tenerife, Spain

The use of multiple psychotropic drugs in psychiatric treatments is increasingly common and usually is made by using two or more drugs to treat discrete clusters of symptoms or diagnoses (combination treatment) or adding one or more drugs to an existing drug to potentiate an increase the effectiveness of the primary drug (augmentation treatment).
In order to estimate the prevalence, characteristics and risk factors associated to the prescription of more than one benzodiazepine to the same patient, a representative sample (n=1048) of patients currently receiving benzodiazepine treatment for 1 month or longer (mean 38,2±52 months, range 1-360 months) was studied. Patients were administered the Severity of Dependence Scale (SDS) as screening test to detect benzodiazepine dependence.
Copharmacy with two or more benzodiazepines was present in 17,4% of patients using benzodiazepines. Clorazepate, lorazepam and clotiazepam were the benzodiazepines more involved in copharmarcy. Prescriptions made by psychiatrists registered higher rates of copharmacy with benzodiazepines than corresponding figures of general practitioners (21,4% vs 13,8%). According to the SDS, 41,6% of patients using one benzodiazepine showed a behavioural dependence to these active ingredients, whereas in those using more than one benzodiazepine the behavioural dependence rate rise to 73,6%.

## P - 67

Effect of Antioxidant Vitamins on Serum Paraoxonase Activity and Lipid Peroxidation in Women With Type 2 Diabetes

Gorshunska M., Karachenzev Y.
Kharkiv Medical Postgraduate Academy, Kharkiv, Ukraine

Increased oxidative stress and damage to lipoproteins may enhance vascular risk in Type 2 diabetes. High density lipoprotein-associated paraoxonase (PON) seems to play a determinant role in the protection of low density lipoprotein against peroxidation. The study was conducted to evaluate the impact of antioxidant vitamins supplementation (AVS) on lipid peroxidation and antioxidant defence parameters, in particular, serum PON activity in Type 2 diabetic women (DW). Twenty nine DW (age: 53.0±1.1 yrs; diabetes duration: 5.3±0.9 yrs, fasting blood glucose: 8.5±0.5 mmol/l, HbA1c: 7.2±0.9%) controlled by diet alone or oral antidiabetic agents were treated with AVS (DL-a-tocopherol 600 mg+vitamin C 500 mg/day per os during the meal) for 1 month. PON activity was measured using paraoxon as substrate. AVS induced a significant decrease in serum malonic dialdehyde by 24.5% ($p<0.01$) and conjugated dienes concentrations by 25.4% ($p<0.05$). There was also a significant increase in serum catalase activity ($p<0.01$), reduced glutathione concentrations ($p<0.02$) and PON activity (85.52±4.20 U/L vs 77.38±3.45 U/L, $p<0.01$). AVS had no significant effect on glycemic control indices. But the favorable effect of AVS in DW did not result in full rehabilitation of lipid peroxidation and antioxidative defense parameters as compared with health controls ($p<0.001$). We conclude that DL-a-tocopherol+vitamin C supplementation in women with Type 2 diabetes reduces oxidative stress through decreasing of lipid peroxidation and increasing of antioxidant defense parameters, in particular, serum paraoxonase activity. Thus it may be beneficial in the prevention of vascular complications related to diabetes.

## P - 68

Loratadine Bioequivalence Study

Jovanovic M., Vuksanovic J., Ivezic S., Segrt Z., Maksimovic M., Jovanovic D.
National Poison Control Centre, Belgrade, Serbia and Montenegro

The bioequivalence of two loratadine tablet formulations was assessed in 24 healthy volunteers who received a single 20 mg dose of each loratadine formulation, and a new sensitive method for the quantification of loratadine, and its active metabolite descarboethoxyloratadine (DCL), in human serum was developed. The study was conducted using an open, randomized, two-sequence, two-period crossover design with a 2-week washout period. Serum samples were obtained over a 48-hour period and analyzed by combined liquid chromatography coupled to mass spectrometry (LC-APCI-MS). A multiplicative/additive statistic model was used for the comparison of pharmacokinetic parameters describing the rate and the extent of bioavailability. For loratadine, the respective 90% CI of the individual ratio geometric means were 91.2 to 103.9 for AUC(0-inf.) and 86.9 to 107.8 for Cmax, while the corresponding 90% confidence limits for DCL were 102.9-113.6 [AUC(0-inf.)] and 101.1-135.0 [Cmax], respectively. Since both 90% CI for the log-transformed AUC and Cmax geometric mean ratios were included either in the 80%-125% interval, or in the wider 70%-143% range, test drug (Pressing tablets, Hemofarm) was considered bioequivalent to the reference (Claritine tablets, Schering-Plough).

## P - 69

Comparative Bioavailability of Two Oral Formulations of Nitrazepam in Healthy Volunteers

Jovanovic D., Jovanovic M., Maksimovic M., Kilibarda V., Vehabovic M., Potogija N.
National Poison Control Centre, Belgrade, Serbia and Montenegro and Bosnalijek, Pharmaceutical and Chemical Industry, Sarajevo, Bosnia and Herzegovina

The aim of the study was to compare the pharmacokinetic profile of two nitrazepam tablet formulations, Mogadon tablets (ICN Iberica, Spain) and Trazem tablets (Bosnalijek, Bosnia and Herzegovina) in 12 healthy volunteers. An open, randomized clinical trial designed as two-sequence, two-period crossover with a 14-day washout between the single 5-mg oral doses was employed. Serum samples for HPLC-UV determination of nitrazepam content were collected over 96 h after administration. No adverse effect was reported for any of the formulations administered.The following pharmacokinetic parameters were calculated: AUC(0-96 h), AUC(0-inf.), Cmax, Tmax, Ke, T1/2 and MRT. The 90% confidence intervals (CI) for the mean test/reference individual ratios were 97.8-100.3 for AUC(0-inf.) and 99.7-103.0 for Cmax. Since both 90% CI for the log-transformed AUC and Cmax ratios were within the 80%-125% interval proposed by the Food and Drug Administration, it is concluded that the test drug (Trazem) is therapeutically equivalent to the reference formulation (Mogadon) for both the rate and the extent of absorption.

## P - 70

6-Mercaptopurine Metabolites in Patients with Inflammatory Bowel Disease

[1]Derijks L.J.J., [2]Gilissen L.P.L., [2]Engels L.G.J.B., [1]Lohman J.J.H.M., [3]van Deventer S.J.H., [3]Hommes D.W., [1]Hooymans P.M.
[1]Department of Clinical Pharmacy and [2]Gastroenterology, Maasland Hospital Sittard; Department of [3]Gastroenterology and Hepatology, Academic Medical Centre, Amsterdam, The Netherlands

The efficacy and myelotoxicity of 6-mercaptopurine (6-MP) is based on the formation of 6-thioguaninenucleotides (6-TGN), whereas 6-methylmercaptopurineribonucleotides (6-MMPR) is associated with hepatotoxicity. Patients with variant alleles for thiopurine S-methyltransferase (TPMT) develop high 6-TG levels and are at risk for leukopenia. We evaluated 6-MP pharmacokinetics, including genetic background for TPMT, in inflammatory bowel disease (IBD) patients. Metabolite levels were measured in 30 IBD-patients at t=0, 1, 2, 4 and 8 weeks after start of treatment with 6-MP 50 mg once daily. Mean age of the patients was 41 years (range 19-68), 20 were male 10 were female. TPMT genotype was *1/*1 in 20, *1/*3A in 2, TPMT*1/*3C in 2 patients and *3A/*3A in one. Steady state levels were reached after 4 weeks and measured 368 pmol/8x108 RBC (CI95%:284-452) for 6-TG and 2837 (CI95%:2101-3573) for 6-MMP respectively. No correlation was found between dose/kg bodyweight and metabolite levels. Only for leukopenia, a significant correlation with TPMT background was observed with an increase in relative risk (RR) of 12.0 (CI95%: 1.7-92.3) for patients with variant TPMT alleles. Notably, first week 6-TG levels in all 4 patients with leukopenia were above 300. Based on our results, therapeutic drug monitoring of 6-MP may be useful.

## P - 71

High Serum Concentrations of the Acyclovir Main Metabolite 9-Carboxymethoxymethylguanine in Renal Failure Patients with Acyclovir-Related Neuropsychiatric Side Effects: An Observational Study

[1]Helldén A., [2]Odar-Cederlöf I., [3]Diener P., [4]Barkholt L., [2]Medin C., [1]Svensson J.O., [1]Säwe J., [1]Ståhle L.
[1]Division of Clinical Pharmacology, Department of Medical Laboratory Science and Technique, Karolinska Institutet, Huddinge University Hospital, Stockholm, Sweden, [2]Department of Nephrology, Karolinska University Hospital, Karolinska Institutet, Stockholm, Sweden, [3]Department of Neurology, Huddinge University Hospital, Stockholm, Sweden, [4]Center for Allogenic Stem Cell Transplantation, Huddinge University Hospital, Karolinska Institutet, Stockholm, Sweden

Background : Acyclovir (ACV)- related neurological adverse side effects have occurred during ACV-treatment in patients with renal failure, but the cause of the symptoms remains unknown. We hypothesized that increased concentrations of the ACV main metabolite 9-carboxymethoxymethylguanine (CMMG) correlated to these symptoms.
Method : We conducted an observational study from 1991 to mid 1999 based on samples sent for analysis of ACV concentration from various hospital departments in Sweden. Patients with neuropsychiatric symptoms (NS+, n = 49) were compared with patients without symptoms (NS-, n = 44). ACV and CMMG concentrations were analyzed by HPLC.
Results : The serum CMMG levels were significantly higher in the NS+ group (mean = 34.1 µmol/L, 95% confidence interval 23.4 to 46.1) compared to the NS- group (mean = 4.7 µmol/L, 95% confidence interval 3.3 to 6.6; P<0.001). CMMG was the strongest predictor in a receiver-operating-characteristics curve analysis (ROC), based on 77 patients, of ACV-related neuropsychiatric symptoms. The ROC curve for CMMG demonstrated that neuropsychiatric symptoms could be predicted with a sensitivity of 91 per cent and a specificity of 93 per cent with the use of a cut-off value of 10.8 µmol/L of CMMG. Haemodialysis reduced CMMG and ACV levels and relieved the symptoms.
Conclusions : The determination of CMMG levels in serum may be a useful tool in supporting the diagnosis of ACV-associated neuropsychiatric symptoms. Furthermore, the monitoring of CMMG levels may prevent the emergence of symptoms.

## P - 72

The Effect of Chamomill Extract on Phasic Pain in Mice

Mirvakili M., Dashti M.H., Vahidi A., Morshedi A.
Dep. of Physiology Shahid Sadughi Medical School Yazd Iran

Pain is an almost universal experience. not surprisingly ,its mechanisms of induction, transduction and sensation and the way to relief or attenuate pain sensation have been the object of considerable attention not only by neurophysiologist but also by philosophers, theologians and physicians since old time .due to wide spread use of antinociceptive , therapeutics and suggested their side effects recently more attentions have been focused on traditional alternatives. Chamomill sp is referred to as a pain relief herbal therapeutic in Iranian traditional medicine literatures. We conducted to study the effect of Chamomill extract on phasic pain induced by noxious thermal stimulus by using a tail flick analgesiometer device in Syrian male mice weighting 32-38 grams. Percent of analgesia index (%AI) was measured as indicated by D-Amour in 1941 in both test and control groups. Our results indicate that Chamomill extract significantly attenuated pain sensation during a range of 60-90 minutes after intrapretoneal injection ($p< 0.05$). This analgesic effect was also compared with doses of 0.5, 1and 2mg/kg injected subcutaneously which was comparable to 1mg/kg morphine after 60 minutes following injections. We concluded that Chamomill extract induce a relatively powerful analgesic effect on phasic pain.

Key words:Chamomill Extract ,Phasic pain ,Morphine ,Tail Flick ,Mice

## P - 73

Effects of Exposure to Selective Serotonin re-uptake Inhibitors During Pregnancy on Infant Outcome

Laine K., Heikkinen T., Ekblad U., Kero P.
University of Turku, Dept. of Pharmacology and Clinical Pharmacology, Turku, Finland

There seems to be an increased risk for neonatal adaptation problems after exposure to SSRIs in late pregnancy. We investigated the perinatal sequelea of infants exposed to SSRIs during their fetal life and the relationship of these symptoms with the cord blood monoamine concentrations. Twenty mothers taking 20 to 40 mg daily either citalopram or fluoxetine during pregnancy and their infants as well as 20 prospectively matched controls for confounding obstetric characteristics were followed. Maternal, cord blood and infant SSRI concentrations, and cord blood monoamine and prolactin concentrations were measured. The newborns were subjected to standard clinical examination and specific assessment of serotonergic symptoms during the first 4 days of life and at the age of 2 weeks and 2 months. There was a significant ($p=0.0078$), 4-fold, difference in the serotonergic symptom score during the first 4 days of life between the SSRI group and the control group. The most prominent symptoms in the newborns included tremor, restlessness, rigidity and hyperreflexia, but they were essentially resolved by the age of two weeks. Citalopram or fluoxetine was detected in all mother-infant pairs. The SSRI-exposed infants had lower cord blood 5-HIAA concentrations ($p=0.015$) and an inverse correlation ($r=-0.66$, $p=0.0073$) was seen between the serotonergic symptom score and umbilical vein 5-HIAA concentrations. In conclusion, infants exposed to SSRIs during late pregnancy were at increased risk for serotonergic central nervous system adverse effects and the severity of these symptoms was significantly related with cord blood 5-HIAA levels.

## P - 74

Tauredon and Wobenzym Combination in Treatment of Rheumatoid Arthritis

[1]Shalamberidze L., Gongadze N., [1]Kartvelishvili E., Chapichadze Z.
Georgian Society of Pharmacology, [1]Scientific-Practical Center of Rheumatology, Tbilisi, Georgia

The aim of the study was the improvement of basic treatment of rheumatoid arthritis and osteoporosis by the combined use of gold and enzyme drugs. The open controlled study was conducted in 60 pts with rheumatoid arthritis during 24 months. Two patient groups (I- active and II- control) were comparable by all parameters. The pts of I group received Wobenzym (Mucos Pharma, Germany) 7 tabs tid during 6 months, then 3 tabs tid during 18 months and also Tauredon (Byk Gulden, Geormany) in increasing dosage till 1500 mg, than 1000 mg monthly during 2 years. The pts from the II group received only Tauredon according the same schedule. The basic therapy in both groups included diclofenac 150 mg daily and prednisolone (60% of pts) from 5 to 15 mg. A number of cellular and humoral immunity, and clinical parameters were evaluated before, after 6, 12 and 24 months. X-ray, ultrasound investigation and ultrasound densitometry was performed before and after the study. Our results show that the positive effects were detected in both groups (in patients of group I improvement and significant improvement was detected in 80,0% of pts and in 63,4% pts of the II group), but remissions were achieved earlier and the number of adverse effects was lower in the I group. X-ray and ultrasound indicators of disease progression was absent in 53.3% of pts of the I group and 40.0% of the II group. Thus, the combinatedl basic therapy of Tauredon and Wobenzym increased the treatment efficacy and significantly loweredthe progression of this pathology and osteoporosis.

## P - 75

Treatment with Selective Cyclooxygenase 2 Inhibitor Rofecoxib in Mice Model of Parkinson's Disease.

[1]Przybylkowski A., [1]Joniec I., [2]Ciesielska A., [1]Kurkowska-Jastrzebska I., [1]Czlonkowski A., [1,2]Czlonkowska A.
[1]Department of Pharmacology, Medical Academy, Warsaw, Poland, [2]2nd Department of Neurology, Institute of Psychiatry and Neurology, Warsaw, Poland

Cyclooxygenase (COX) 1 and 2 are indicated as a factors playing important role in many neurological disorders. 1-Methyl-4-phenyl-1,2,3,6-tetrahydropyridine (MPTP) is a neurotoxin which causes neuropathological, behavioral and biochemical changes that closely mimics Parkinson's disease. We investigated the expression of COX1 and COX2, prostaglandins (PGs) production, dopamine(DA) depletion in stria of C57Bl/6 mice after MPTP administration. We also examined if therapy with rofecoxib a selective COX2 inhibitor after MPTP intoxication would cause changes in COX expression, tyrosine hydroxylase(TH) protein expression, PGs production and striatal DA concentration. We observed overexpression of COX2 protein and transcript reaching maximum level at 7th day after MPTP and lasted until 21st day with cox-1 expression not altered. PG production raised significantly only 24 hours after MPTP and thereafter returned to the level of a control group. Changes in prostaglandins production do not correspond to changes in COX2 expression. Rofecoxib (10 mg/kg) treatment being started 24 h after MPTP and lasted 14 days did not influence striatal TH expression and decreased DA concentration. These results together suggest that COX2 may be involved in MPTP induced neuronal degeneration and regeneration and may become in the future a target for therapeutic interventions in patients suffering from Parkinson's disease.

## P - 76

Effects of Cimetidine on Male Reproductive System

Takzaree A.R., Takzaree N., Rezayat M., Akbari M., Yarmohammady K.
Tehran University of Medical Sciences, Faculty of Medicine, Dept of Anatomy

In the present study the effect of cimetidine on male Reproductive system and sperm motility. 60 mature male rats divided in 3 groups: Control group, received normal saline and test I group received cimetidine 100 mg/kg/day for one week. Test II group received cimetidine 100 mg/kg/day for five weeks. The result revealed that sperm count was decreased in the test compared to control groups and non motile sperms were increased in test compared to control groups. t-test was done and Pvalue < 0.05 showed significant decrease in sperm counts. Then the testises were excised from body and after weighing we studied then microscopically. Results revealed lower testicular weights in test II group. Atrophy of spermatic germ cells and hypoplasia of spermatic germinal layer of seminiferous tubules were observed microscopically. We concluded that the above changes may be due to the direct effect of cimetidine on the seminiferous tubules which is reversible.

Key Words: Cimetidine, male reproductive system, sperm

## P - 77

OCP Intake During Pregnancy and Its Side Effects Leading to Anomalies

Takzaree N., Yarmohammady K., Takzaree S., Rezayat S.M.
Tehran University of Medical Sciences, Faculty of Medicine, Dept of Anatomy

Some researchs have reported the risks of OCP intake during pregnancy. Using progestinal drugs before 20th week of gestational age because of some androgenic effects can cause male pattern anomalies in the females external genitalia. Somethimes women are not aware of pregnancy and may continue OCP intake for weeks after getting pregnant. In this research we studied the effects of OCPs containing estrogen and progestron on reproductive system diffrentiation. 10 female virgin rats of the same age and weight were used for our research. After the rats getting pregnant and observing vaginal plaque the day zero of pregnancy was determined. Then we divided the rats randomly into case and control groups. The rats of the case group were feeded with water soluble OCPs from the first day. After 20th day of pregnancy the embryos were delivered by cesarian and then were studied. In female embryos some changes were seen in the external genitalia. Because of androgenic effects of progestinal hormones. Clitoris has grown more and a small scrotom like sac was seen between Anus and external genitalia. In male rats undescended testis and small penis was observed. In statistical analysis, significant difference was seen between case and control groups (P value < 0.05).

Key words: Oral contraceptive, Anomalies, Genital system

## P - 78

Teratogenic Effects of Diazepam Intake During Pregnancy Leading to Visual System Anomalies

Takzaree N., Yarmohammadi K., Takzaree A.R., Rezayat M., Akbari M.
Dept. of Embryology, Tehran University of Medical Sciences, Faculty of Medicine, Tehran Iran

Diazepam is un sedetive that belongs to Benzodiazepines. It has been increasingly used recently. Itshould be noticed that Diazepam consumption during pregnancy may have teratogenic effects on embryo. Pregnantwomen use this drug in pregnancy pica, shortsleeping or necesserily in psychologic and neurologic disease. So inthis research we have studied Diazepam intake during pregnancy and its side effects leading to cleft lip, cleft palate-and anopsia. In our study the virgin rats of known age weight have been selected. After being pregnant they weredivided in three groups: Control group: 10 rats (injection of sterile water) First case group: 10 rats (sterile water andDiazepam 3 mg/kg Second case group: 10 rats (sterile water and Diazepam 8 mg/kg). These three groups took thedrugs daily, after embryonic period pregnant rats have been killed and their embryos have been divided also in thesame three groups. After being studied macroscopically the embryos were observed microscopically. This sowed thatsome anomalies have been appeared in some cases. After analysing there were significant differences between caseand control groups (P value > 0.05). So it was proved that Diazepam is teratogen and is dangerous for pregnantwomen.

Key Words: Diazepam, Teratogen, Cleft palate, Cleft lip

## P - 79

The Effect of Ginger on Hyperglycemia and Hyperlipidemia Induced by Cyclosporin a Drug in Male Rats

Taghizadehafshari A.
Departement of Nephrology,Imam khomini hopital, Urmia,Iran

Cyclosporine A is one of immunosuppressive drugs that is widely used to prevent ransplant rejection. Some of its imporant complications are increasing of blood sugar and lipids. In this study the effect of ginger on cyclosporin inducedhyperglycemia and hyperlipidemia was investigated. To do this research 40male albino wistar rats were selected. Before using the drug serum levels of glucose and triglyceride were measured (T1). Then 25 mg/kg cyclosporin was given orally to the rats, for a period of 30 days. Then blood sampling was done to measure serum glucose and triglyceride (T2). Eighteen rats which showed serum glucose and triglyceride increase were divided into two equal groups, namely control and experiment groups. In control group, rats received only cyclosporin for another 30 days, but in experimental group, rats received cyclosporin plus ginger in a measure of %7 of the diet. At the end of study blood glucose and triglyceride levels were measured (T3). The results showed that in control group serum glucose and triglyceride levels were ascending in all the T1, T2, and T3 experiments, statistically this increase was significant (P<0.05). But in experimental group serum glucose and triglyceride levels were significantly high in T2, compared to T1 (P<0.05), although this increase stopped in T3 compared to T2, comparing to T2 in T3 there was a significant decrease in glucose and triglyceride level (P<0.05). After all it can be concluded that ginger can have a decreasing affect on the hyperglycemia and hyperlipidemia induced by cyclosporin.

## P - 80

The Effect of Garlic On Cyclosporin a Induced LDL Changes

Shirpoor A.
Department of Physiology, Faculty of Medicine Medical University of Urmia,Jaddeh Nazloo Urmia, Iran

Cyclosporin A is a very potent immunosuppressive drug which is used to prevent transplant rejection. In spite of this beneficial effect, this drug has dangerous side effects such as LDL rise. This increase in LDL results in cardiovascular problems in subjects receiving allograft transplanation. In this study the effect of garlic on cyclosporin induced LDL rise was investigated. Forty male wistar rats weighing 250gr, and with the age of 10 month were chosen. The rats were given cyclosporin 25mg/kg orally for 30 days. Then blood sampling was done and their LDL levels assayed. Rats with LDL increase were divided into two groups of eight namely control group and experimental group. Experimental rats received garlic tablet with the dose of 400mg and cyclosporin with the same dose for 30 days. Control group received normal diet with cyclosporin. At the end of experiment, blood samples were taken and they were assayed for LDL level. In control group, seven rats showed significant increase comparing to the previous 30 days ($p<0.02$). In experimental group LDL level was decreased but in four rats this decrease was more than 50% and it was significant. This study showed that alicine(the effective substance in garlic) caused LDL reduction and this reduction can be a useful way for patients receiving transplant.

## P - 81

Dispensing Habits of The Community Pharmacists in Ümraniye Distiict Of Istanbul, Turkey

[1]Toklu H., [2]Akıcı A., [1]Sezen S., [3]Calı Ş., [2]Oktay S., [1]Keyer-Uysal M.
Marmara University [1]Faculty of Pharmacy, Department of Pharmacology; [2]School of Medicine, Departments of Pharmacology & Clinical Pharmacology and [3]Public Health

Introduction Irrational drug use is a common problem in many countries. Since the pharmacists play an important role in promoting rational use of drugs, we have investigated the dispensing habits of the community pharmacists.

Methods Eighty four community pharmacists at Ümraniye district were evaluated with a questionnaire and a simulated case scenario. The average dispensing time, stock availability and adequate labelling of the drug were used as rationality indicators.

Results Only 40.5 % of the prescriptions were dispensed by the pharmacists. Almost half (44.5 %) of the pharmacy employees had primary school degree and 90.5 % of the pharmacists believed their employees were satisfactory in dispensing drugs by their own. However, the stock availability was 81.0%; the average dispensing time for the prescriptions was 149.07 to 72.8 seconds, and 42.8% of the drugs were adequately labelled. Interestingly, only 2.6% of the dispensers warned the patients about potential drug interactions.

Conclusions It appears that rationality indicators for dispensing drugs were unsatisfactory in most of the community pharmacies evaluated at this study. Therefore, continuing education seems to be urgent and essential for pharmacists and pharmacy employees in promoting rational use of drugs.

## P - 82

Evaluation of Childhood Respiratory Tract Infections' Treatment

[1]Akıcı A., [2]Kalaça S.; [1]Uğurlu Ü., [1]Oktay Ş.
Departments of [1]Pharmacology & Clinical Pharmacology, and [2]Public Health, Marmara University School of Medicine, Istanbul, Turkey

In the present study, prescribing behavior of general practitioners (GPs) was investigated in the example of childhood upper and lower respiratory tract infections (URTI and LRTI). A questionnaire was given to 352 parents admitted to primary health care centers for their children diagnosed URTI or LRTI, and a total of 331 prescriptions were analyzed according to rational use of drugs (RUD) principles. Almost 8 % of the patients were not examined by the physicians, but directly prescribed medicine. The physicians did not tell the diagnosis to 25.3 % of the patients/parents; did not inform 41.2 % of them about the drugs, 95.7 % about the side effects, 42.6 % about drug use instructions, 83.5 % about the warnings, and 81.2 % about non-drug treatment. Only 26.3 % of the prescriptions were easily readable. Although URTI and LRTI are usually viral diseases, the majority of the patients were given antibiotics, penicillin+beta lactamase inhibitors being the first. In conclusion, this study revealed that irrational prescribing is quite common among GPs working at primary health care level which might have serious consequences regarding children's health.

## P - 83

The Effect of Rational Pharmacotherapy Training on Therapeutic Competence of Interns and General Practitioners

[1]Akıcı A., [2]Kalaça S., [1]Uğurlu Ü., [3]Akkan G., [1]Karaalp A., [1]Gören Z., [1]Demir D., [1]Oktay Ş.
Departments of [1]Pharmacology & Clinical Pharmacology and [2]Public Health, Marmara University School of Medicine and [3]Department of Pharmacology, Istanbul University Cerrahpaşa School of Medicine, Istanbul, Turkey.

Therapeutic competence of final year medical students (interns) and general practitioners, who had and had not received systematic training in rational pharmacotherapy (RP) was compared. Upper respiratory tract infection and hypertension were selected indications as an acute and a chronic disease, respectively. Subjects of this study were interns of Marmara University Medical School (MUMS) and Istanbul University Cerrahpaşa Medical School. Problem-based RP training program has been implemented in the curriculum of the former Institution in 1996. General practitioners working at health care centers who had not received such training were also included in the study. Participants were asked to fill a questionnaire, plan the management and prescribe for the written cases of the selected indications. According to the questionnaire, all participants declared a positive attitude towards applying the RP principles. However, when they were asked to manage the simulated cases, MUMS interns were found to be more rational particularly in terms of spending effort to make the patient understand the instructions and allocating time for this approach. Prescription analysis also revealed better results for MUMS interns concerning the number of drugs/prescription, suitability and cost of the treatment. These results indicate the benefit of a problem-based RP course in undergraduate medical curriculum.

## P - 84

Comparison of Osce and Unstructered Oral Examination to Assess Therapeutic Competence

[1]Akıcı A., [2]Kalaça S., [3]Kocabaşoğlu Y. E., [1]Demir D., [1]Oktay Ş.
Departments of [1]Pharmacology & Clinical Pharmacology and [2]Medical Education, Marmara University, School of Medicine, Istanbul, Turkey, and [3]Department of Clinical Pharmacology, Groningen University School of Medicine, Groningen, The Netherlands.

Objective Structured Clinical Examination (OSCE) is an objective evaluation measure to assess various components of clinical competence. In this study, it was aimed to compare the scores of medical students evaluated with two different methods: unstructured oral examination and OSCE. Sixty-eight clinical teachers from Akdeniz University Medical School (AUMS) were presented four videos of simulated examination records of four students who had been asked to plan pharmacotherapy for simulated patients. Teachers were asked to assess performance of the first 2 students as if they were doing an unstructured oral examination, and the last two by using a detailed OSCE score sheet. Teachers were also applied a questionnaire to learn about their perception on OSCE.
The difference between the expected and observed scores (error score) was significantly smaller when the students were evaluated by OSCE ($p < 0{,}05$). Interestingly, although OSCE was not a method of assessment used at AUMS and the teachers were happy with and used to classical oral examination methods, most of them (% 97.9) evaluated OSCE as being more objective compared to unstructured oral examination. The results demonstrated the superiority of OSCE in objective and reliable assessment of pharmacotherapy competence even if the scorers are not experienced.

## P - 85

On the Pathophysiology of Schizophrenia

[1]Bjerkenstedt L., [1]Farde L., [1]Terenius L., [2]Edman G., [3]Venizelos N., [4]Wiesel F. A.
[1]Department of Clinical Neuroscience, Karolinska Institute, Stockholm, Sweden; [2] Department of Psychiatry, R&D Section, Danderyd's Hospital, Danderyd, Sweden; [3] Department of Caring Sciences, Division of Biomedicine, Örebro University, Örebro, Sweden; and [4] Department of Neuroscience, Psychiatry Ulleråker, Uppsala University, Uppsala, Sweden

Tyrosine is an essential amino acid and the precursor in the biosynthesis of pamine. Tyrosine is transported by the L- and A-systems. The brain is the only organ for which amino acid transport is limited and competition for transport over membranes occurs at physiological plasma concentrations. In schizophrenic patients, basal levels of ten plasma amino acids, most of them competing for transport with tyrosine, have been shown to deviate from corresponding levels in a control group. Alanine, methionine, valine, isoleucine and phenylalanine were elevated, but not tyrosine. A negative relationship was found in the schizophrenic group, but not in the control group, between the dopamine metabolite homovanillic acid (HVA) in the cerebrospinal fluid and the plasma amino acids methionine, valine isoleucine, leucine, phenylalanine, the higher levels of these plasma amino acids the lower level of HVA. Furthermore, the HVA level was reduced in the schizophrenic group as compared to the controls. In vitro studies using fibroblasts have demonstrated an intact L-system but nevertheless a reduced tyrosine transport in schizophrenia as compared to controls. The reduced tyrosine transport into the brain and the elevated plasma levels of phenylalanine in schizophrenic patients (see above) might accordingly disturb protein synthesis within the brain and thereby influence brain development and brain structure. In summary, the pathophysiology of schizophrenia is suggested to be primarily a disturbance in the periphery resulting in reduced central dopamine synthesis and possibly a reduced brain growth.

## ORAL

Which Factors Affect Hypertension Management in Diabetic Patients?

Denig P., Schaars C.F., Kasje W.N., Haaijer-Ruskamp F.M.
Clinical Pharmacology, University of Groningen, Netherlands.

Introduction: Tight blood pressure control significantly reduces morbidity and mortality in diabetic patients, but current hypertension management seems far from
optimal. Objective: We aimed to assess the quality of hypertension care in patients with type 2 diabetes and to identify patient, physician and organisational factors associated with suboptimal care in general practice.
Methods: Analysis of process and outcome measures, including check of blood pressure in the previous year, treatment of hypertension, and achievement of target blood pressure levels. ACE-inhibitors were considered as the optimal treatment for patients diagnosed with hypertension or with average blood pressure levels above 135/85 mmHg. Data from 895 randomly selected diabetic patients were extracted from the computerised medical records of 95 general practitioners (GPs). A short survey was used to collect additional physician and organisational characteristics. Results: For 652 of the 895 patients (73%) one or more blood pressure measurements were recorded in the last year. Of these patients only 132 (20%) reached a target level of 135/85 mmHg. In total, 595 patients were classified as having hypertension, 192 of whom received no treatment (32%), 193 received treatment with an ACE-inhibitor (32%), and 210 received other antihypertensives. Patients visiting a special diabetic service, being recently referred to a specialist, or being overweight had better recordings of their blood pressure. Suboptimal treatment was higher in older patients and smoking patients.
Conclusion: Interventions aimed at improving the quality of hypertension management in diabetic patients should focus more on specific patients groups than on specific doctors.

## P - 86

Differential Effect of Cyclophosphamide on the Expression and Activity of Cytochromes P450

[1]Xie H., [1]Mirghani R., [1]Yasar Ü., [3]Terelius Y., [1]Lundgren S., [1]Rane A., M [2]Hassan M. [1]Department of Laboratory Medicine, Division of Clinical Pharmacology, and [2]Department of Medicine, Division of Hematology, Laboratory of Hematology at Huddinge University Hospital, Karolinska Institutet, Stockholm, Sweden; [3]AstraZeneca R & D Södertälje, Department of Research DMPK, Södertälje, Sweden.

The present study was to clarify the effect of cyclophosphamide on the expression and activity of cytochromes P450 (CYP). Single doses of cyclophosphamide (either 40 or 200 mg/kg) were administrated intravenously to Wistar/Fu male rats. Specific mRNAs for CYP2B1, 2B2, 2C11, 3A1 and 3A2 were quantified from liver samples by Real-time RT PCR; CYP2C and 3A activities were estimated by losartan oxidation and quinine hydroxylation in liver microsomes, respectively, at 4 h, 8 h, 16 h, 24 h, 48 h and 120 h after the cyclophosphamide treatment and at zero time as control (n=4 or 5 for each time point). In the low cyclophosphamide dose group, the mRNAs of CYP2B1, 2B2, 2C11 and 3A2 were significantly induced up to 218-, 6.7-, 5.8- and 5.0-fold, respectively; while CYP3A1 mRNA was decreased significantly by 6.1-fold. In the high dose group, mRNA of CYP2B1 was significantly induced 4838-fold, followed by mRNAs of CYP2B2, 3A2, 2C11 by 52, 22 and 5.5-fold of induction, while CYP3A1 was decreased significantly by 6.0-fold. Activities of CYP3A and 2C11 were significantly increased up to 1.7- and 2.4-fold at both low and high dose cyclophosphamide groups. Our data showed the induction of cyclophosphamide on CYP2B1, 2B2, 2C11, and 3A2 whereas CYP3A1 expression was decreased. This will add important information on efficacy and toxicity of cyclophosphamide therapy, as well as cyclophosphamide related drug interaction.

## P - 87

Drug Treatment After Acute Myocardial Infarction in Estonia

[1]Marandi T, [2]Thetloff M.
[1]North Estonia Regional Hospital, [2]Estonian Health Insurance Fund.

The aim of the study was to analyse the drug treatment and outcome of patients suffered from myocardial infarction (MI) in Estonia during one year from admission to hospital due to an acute MI. Methods. Inpatients admitted to hospital due to an acute MI during the year 2000 were selected from Estonian Health Insurance database. Data about drugs reimbursed were collected during one year from index hospitalisation. Mortality data were obtained from Health Insurance and Population Registry. Results. During the year 2000 2350 patients suffered from acute MI - 1307 men and 1043 women. Mean age ± SD were 65 ± 12 and 73 ± 10 years, respectively. 0.36 million euros were spent for reimbursement of cardiovascular drugs during one year from index episode in population studied. One year after MI 327 (25%) men and 370 (36%) women were dead. Analysis of drugs reimbursed revealed no patients with identical treatment scheme among patients discharged after index episode (n=1997). Nitrates were used in 1587 (80%), betablockers in 1337 (67%), ACE inhibitors in 1176 (59%), diuretics in 756 (38%) and statins in 500 (25%) patients. However, at least six prescriptions, usually for two months period, were reimbursed for the following numbers of patients discharged - nitrates 449 (23%), betablockers 271 (14%), ACE inhibitors 242 (12%), statins 98 (5%) and diuretics 41 (2%). In conclusion, drug treatment strategies after acute MI need more attention and standardising according to international guidelines and local resourses.

## ORAL

Early Exposure To Ciprofloxacin in A Bioequivalence Study

Macedo T.R.A., Neta C., Martins F., Marques H., Silva J., Morgadinho M.T., Fontes Ribeiro C.A.
Association for Innovation and Biomedical Research on Light and Image (AIBILI), Coimbra, Portugal

Bioequivalence between a test (T) and a reference (R ) substance signifies their closeness regarding the rate (Cmax and tmax) and extent (AUC) of absorption. When it is necessary a rapid absorption or early exposure to the drug to achieve a therapeutic effect, the AUC0-tmax could be a better parameter. Our aim was to evaluate and correlate, in a bioequivalence study, the rate and extent of absorption, and the early exposure to ciprofloxacin. An open, randomised, two-phase and crossover study was carried out with a single dose of 500 mg ciprofloxacin. Blood samples were collected and ciprofloxacin measured by a validated HPLC method. T and R were bioequivalent. However, the 90% confidence interval (CI) of lnT/R for AUC0-tmax (early exposure to the drug) was not within 0.80-1.25. Moreover, r2 for AUC0-tmax vs Cmax and for AUC0-tmax vs tmax were 0.13 and 0.23 for T, and 0.22 and 0.33 for R, respectively. Cmax tmax AUC0-t AUC0-inf AUC0-tmax (mg.L-1) (h) (mg.L-1.h) (mg.L-1.h) (mg.L-1.h) T 1.61±0.46 1.6±0.5 7.38±2.33 8.15±2.28 R 1.60±0.55 1.5±0.6 7.10±2.62 7.86±2.60 90%CI T/R 0.91-1.10 0.91-1.16 0.98-1.10 0.98-1.09 0.86-1.19 90%CI ln T/R 0.93-1.10 - 0.98-1.11 0.99-1.10 0.71-1.03 (mean±SD; n=27 (healthy volunteers)) In conclusion, in spite of the bioequivalence between the two formulations of ciprofloxacin (rate and extent of absorption), there was not bioequivalence regarding early exposure to the drug. For drugs with a narrow therapeutic index this can have relevant clinical implications.

## P - 88

Correlation Between Busulphan Concentration and Transplantation Related Toxicity in Patients Undergoing Stem Cell Transplantation

Hassan M., Aschan J., Hassan Z., Ringden O., Winiarski J., Nilsson C., Öberg G.
Laboratory of Hematology, Division of Hematology, Department of Medicine Departments of Allogenic Stem Cell Transplantation (CAST) and Pediatrics Huddinge University Hospital, Stockholm, Sweden

Busulphan is still one of the main components in the preparative regimen for patients undergoing allogeneic as well as autologous stem cell transplantation (SCT) but toxicity is still a problem. In the present study we have retrospectively evaluated 450 patients transplanted between 1987 and 2001. Patients were treated with SCT for both haematological and non-haematological malignancies as well as genetic disorders. Busulphan concentrations were calculated as the trough levels based on at least 10 measurements (one level prior to each administered dose). Acute toxicity e.g. Veno-occlusive disease (VOD), interstitial pneumonia (IP) and hemorrhagic cystitis (HC) was evaluated to day 100 post transplantation. VOD was diagnosed according to Jones criteria. Busulphan concentrations were significantly (p<0.001) higher (782 ± 250 ng/ml) in patients who developed VOD compared to the mean concentration of the population (603 ± 221 ng/ml). In patients who developed IP the trough levels of busulphan were 890 ± 291 ng/ml that is significantly (p<0.001) higher compared to the mean concentration of the population. No difference was found between gender and the occurrence of toxicity. The incidence rate of VOD in patients transplanted between 1987 and 1995 was 21% (45 of 212 patients) and the incidence of IP was 14 % (29 of 212 patients). In 1995 therapeutic drug monitoring and dose adjustment of the drug was introduced. The incidence of acute toxicity in patients treated between 1995 and 2001 was: VOD 7% (16 of 238 patients) and the IP 4% (10 of 238 patients). We conclude that busulphan levels correlate with both veno-occlusive disease as well as interstitial pneumonia.

## P - 89

Accelerated Healing of Chronic Nonhealing Pressure Ulcer in a Patient Induced by The Lipid Calf Thymic Extract

Majsimovic D., Pitic L., Beleslin D.B.
Galenika a.d., Institute, Biomedical Research Center, Batajnicki drum bb, 11080 Belgrade, Serbia and Montenegro

Investigations on wound healing effects of thymic peptides in healing-impaired animal models and humans are still scarce and not well understood. In addition, indications for healing-impaired wounds are not yet well defined. In this investigation lipid calf thymic extract was topically applied in a patient with chronic nonhealing pressure ulcer unsuccessfully treated with conventional treatment for 3.7 years. Lipid calf thymic extract was spread evenly on the entire surface twice daily during a 20-week treatment period. An approximately 30% decrease in wound size was observed after three weeks of treatment. Thereafter the healing process advanced further, and by the end of 13 weeks the hard-healing wound defect disappeared. Twenty four month following the treatment with the extract neither excessive scarring nor malignant alterations were observed. However, at the end of the twenty second month a new pressure ulcer appeared about 5 cm from the healed wound. In conclusion, the topical application of lipid calf thymic extract locally accelerates the healing of chronic nonhealing pressure ulcer and prevents relapse for at least two years, protecting the cutaneous tissue approximately 5 cm around the wound.

## P - 90

Comparison of the Rate and Extent of Absorption of Nimesulide Contained in Tablets and Granules

Fontes Ribeiro C.A., Neta C., Martins F., Marques H., Silva J., Macedo T.R.A.
Association for Innovation and Biomedical Research on Light and Image, Coimbra, Portugal

The rate of absorption is influenced by the dissolution of a drug which in turn is dependent on the pharmaceutical formulation. This work aimed to compare the rate and extent of absorption of 100 mg nimesulide (Aulin®) contained in tablets and granules in single-dose sackets. Each formulation was administered to 25 healthy volunteers during fasting. Plasma was collected and nimesulide measured according to a validated HPLC method.

| | Cmax | tmax | AUC0-24h | AUC0-inf | t1/2 | (mg.mL-1) | (h) | (mg.mL-1.h) | (mg.mL-1.h) | (h) |
|---|---|---|---|---|---|---|---|---|---|---|
| Tablets | 6.20 | 1.71 | 34.074 | 37.310 | 5.22 | ±1.66 | ±0.53 | ±10.479 | ±11.776 | ±2.82 |
| Granules | 5.81 | 2.81 | 50.462 | 54.780 | 4.70 | ±1.73 | ±1.25* | ±26.563* | ±32.238* | ±1.88 |

Results obtained through software Kinetica2000 (InnaPhase Corporation, USA mean±SD (n=25 for each group) *P<0.05 (ANOVA and Student´s t test and/or Wilcoxon test) It appears that tablets but not granules did not dissolve readily, affecting bioavailability. If the effect of nimesulide is concentration-dependent, the efficacy of nimesulide administered in granules may be higher than that obtained after the ingestion of tablets. In conclusion, the extent of absorption of nimesulide contained in sackets with granules is significantly higher than nimesulide in tablets.

## P - 91

Analysis of Roscovitine Using Novel High Performance Liquid Chomatography and Uv-Detection Method: Pharmacokinetics and Tissue Distribution of Roscovitine and Its Major Metabolite in Rat

[1]Fernanda Vita M., [2]Meurling L., [2]Pettersson T., [1]Cruz M., [1]Sidén Å.,[3]Hassan M.
[1] Department of Neurology, [2] Department of Clinical Pharmacology, TDM laboratory, [3] Department of Medicine, Division of Hematology, Laboratory of Hematology, Huddinge University Hospital, S-141 86 Stockholm, Sweden

Roscovitine is a potent and selective inhibitor of cyclin-dependent kinases (CDKs). It inhibits cell proliferation; induces DNA fragmentation and causes cell cycle arrest in S phase. Its stability and toxicity are not fully known. A liquid chromatography method was developed to measure roscovitine in human and rat plasma and to study the pharmacokinetics of the drug and its major metabolite in rats. Roscovitine was administered as a bolus injection (25 mg/kg body weight), blood and tissue samples were obtained after 5, 10, 20, 30, 60, 120, 180 minutes and analysed by HPLC method.
The limit of quantitation was 100 ng/ml and the inter-day precision and accuracy were (6.49 ± 3.30) % and (-3.25 ± 0.65) %, respectively. The stability of the drug after 24 hours was 91 % at room temperature. The recovery of roscovitine from plasma was 84 % at 750 ng/ml. The pharmacokinetic analysis showed that roscovitine is fitted to a two-compartment openmode with a biphasic elimination half-life (6 and 26 minutes respectively), short half-life was seen in the tissues. The distribution volume was determined to 3.5 L/kg and the clearance was 29.5 ml/min.
Roscovitine is cleared very rapidly from the blood circulation after i.v. (bolus) injection and it is highly distributed to other organs. A metabolite appeared in plasma and various tissues immediately after i.v. injection of roscovitine.
roscovitine.

## P - 92

Time Course of Platelet Aggregation and Inhibition of Thromboxane and Prostacyclin Biosynthesis after Administration of Different Single Oral Doses of Aspirin in 48 Male Healthy Subjects

Becker A., Kornberger R., Völker M., Grossmann M.
IKP GmbH

Objective: The time course of inhibition of thromboxane and prostacyclin biosynthesis and platelet aggregation after single doses of Aspirin (100, 300, 500 and 1000 mg) was determined.
Methods: In 12 male healthy volunteers each dosing group, platelet aggregation induced by arachidonic acid, serum TXB2 concentrations and plasma 6-keto-GF1alpha concentrations were measured predose to 168 h after application (a.a.). Results: For all doses of Aspirin serum TXB2 concentration was decreased from 1 h till 72 h a.a. but less pronounced for the 100 mg group. No statistically significant changes of 6-keto-PGF1alpha were found. Reduction of platelet aggregation was over 90 % from 1 h a.a. until 24 h a.a. for 100 mg and 72 h a.a. for all other doses. Conclusions: Analgesic oral doses of Aspirin reduce the platelet function for three to four days, but only 24 h for 100 mg Aspirin. Gastric protection by 6-keto-PGF1alpha seem to be fully sustained after a single dose of ASA, because its level are steady.

## P - 93

Identification of a Novel G816A SNP in the Human MRP1 Gene Using a LightCycler Technique

[1]Oselin K., [2]Mrozikiewicz P.M., [1]Pähkla R., [2]Roots I.
[1]Institute of Pharmacology, Tartu University, Estonia [2]Institute of Clinical Pharmacology, University Medical Centre Charité, Berlin, Germany

The human multidrug resistance-associated protein 1 (MRP1/ABCC1) comprises 1531 amino acids and is encoded by the MRP1 gene. Using a LightCycler technique, we established PCR assay for T825C SNP in the MRP1. Unexpectedly, a novel silent mutation G816A (Pro272Pro) was identified, with an allele frequency of 4.1%. The derivative melting curves on LightCycler are highly reproducible under constant conditions. Shifts greater than 1°C from the characteristic melting curve suggests the presence of two mismatches. Using the sensor (position at 813-834 bp) for T825C genotyping, we determined 4 individuals with atypical melting curves. Subsequent sequencing showed that all these individuals, but not subjects with typical melting curves for T825C, were heterozygous GA at position 816. Hence, the G816A substitution destabilized the binding of the long T825C sensor. A new, shorter sensor (position at 817-834 bp) for T825C detection, and another pair of hybridization probes for G816A detection were designed. When designing hybridization probes to recognize the G816A and T825C polymorphisms, oligonucleotides that cover the both mutation sites should be avoided. Mutations affecting MRP1 expression could influence the pharmacokinetic properties of drugs that are substrates for MRP1. The potential impact of the G816A SNP in the MRP1 requires further studies.

## P - 94

Euro-Med-Stat: Monitoring Expenditure and Utilisation of Medicinal Products in the European Union Countries. A Public Health Approach

Van Ganse E., Pietri G.
On Behalf of the EURO-MED-STAT

Group Background: There is uncertainty about the level of utilisation and expenditure for medicines in the European Union,so our aim is to develop indicators for price, expenditure and utilisation of medicinal products in the EU, to facilitate comparisons.
Methods: There are 4 major tasks (T); T1: to catalogue data sources and available data in each EU Member State; T2: to assess the reliability and comparability of data among the EU Member States by ATC/DDD on country coverage, reimbursement, prescriptions, price category and composition, and private vs. public spending; T3: to develop Standard Operating Procedure for data management and to define the proposed indicators; T4: to pool, compare and report the validated data according to the established indicators, using cardiovascular medicines as an example.
Results: Preliminary results from T1 & T2 demonstrate methodological difficulties in comparing data from different countries. Multiple data sources have to be used. These cover different populations, and refer to different prices or costs. Nevertheless, useful data can be derived, illustrated by the example of lipid lowering drugs: the data shows that only 5 products are commonly available in all countries (simvastatin, pravastatin, fluvastatin, atorvastatin, cholestyramine). There may be substantial differences which can hinder comparison such as wide pack size variations , from 10 up to 112 tablets. Utilisation of statins shows high usage in Scandinavian countries and least in Italy (60 vs 12 DDD/1000Inh/day in Norway and Italy respectively).
Conclusion: The preliminary results show wide differences in availability and use of medicines across Europe; they illustrate the complexity of European transnational comparisons.

## ORAL

Community Pharmacy Survey of Diabetes Patients

[1]Bauguil G., [1]Catala O., [2]Van Ganse E., [2]Travier N., [1]Chamba G.
Faculty of Pharmacy, Claude-Bernard University, Lyon, France [2]Pharmacoepidemiology Unit, CHU-Lyon, France

Background : A significant part of diabetes-induced morbidity can be prevented with adequate care. In France, Community pharmacists (CPs) are well positioned to contact diabetes patients and to collect data on disease management.
Objectives : To identify a sample of type 2 diabetes patients visiting CPs and to record exhaustive data on disease management.
Methods : Community pharmacists invited type 2 diabetes patients who were known users of the pharmacy to complete a questionnaire on knowledge of diabetes, lifestyle, frequency of clinical and biological follow up, and therapy (diabetes and co-morbid conditions). For each patient, prescribed and OTC medications were retrieved from pharmacy records.
Results : 528 patients were identified (58.5 % males) by 71 CPs; 74% of patients had regular visits with General Practitioners (GPs) and 26 % visited a specialist for their diabetes in the past year. Patients were treated with 1 (42 %), 2 (43 %), 3 (8 %) oral antidiabetic medications, or insulin (7 %); 71 and 49% of patients had cotherapy with cardiovascular or lipid lowering agents, respectively. Side-effects were reported by 45% of patients using oral agents and by 62% of insulin users. More than 90% of patients reported a good adherence to therapy; this will be verified with dispensing records. Only 28 % of patients were immunised against influenza.
Conclusion : The survey suggests that the management of type 2 diabetes was not optimal at the time of study. Segments of care were identified where interventions are needed , e.g., by community pharmacists.

## ORAL

Tolerance of Antihypertensive Therapy : The Ota Study, Design and Overall Data

[1]Van Ganse E., [2]Girerd X., [3]Larguier J.S., [3]Alamercery Y. , [1]Laforest L., [3]Mistretta F.
[1]Pharmacoepidemiology, CHU Lyon, [2]Cardiology, CHU Lyon [3]RCTs, France.

Background & Objectives. Few studies have investigated the tolerance of antihypertensive medications in post-marketing conditions. OTA is a PMS that compared the tolerance profile of rilmenidine (R), a new a2-central agonist, with other antihypertensive agents, in actual conditions of use.
Methods. The study is conducted from GP sites in France. Each investigator identified up to 12 patients treated with antihypertensive agents [R, diuretics (D), beta-blockers (BB), calcium channel blockers (CCB), ACE-inhibitors, AT-receptors antagonists (ARA II), other classes (O), fixed combinations (FC)]. Patients were included in a 12-month follow-up observational study; 1/3 of them had to be treated for <2 months at inclusion. The primary outcome was any change in therapy (interruption, substitution, changes in prescribed doses, additional prescriptions) explained by the GP as being due to side effects.
Results. 6,319 hypertensive patients (mean age: 65.9 yrs, 44.9% males, mean disease duration: 7.7 yrs) were included in the study by 550 GPs, corresponding to 10,557 treatments (48% monotherapy, mean N medications/patient: 1.7). Treatment distribution was: ARA II: n=825; CCB: n=825; FC: n=825; O: n=640; BB: n=784; D: n=818; R: n=795; ACEI: n=807. On average, each GP prescribed 5 to 6 classes of antihypertensive agents. We contacted 340 patients: 79.1% considered their blood pressure to be well-controlled and 84.6% mentioned a change in therapy in the last 3 months. Altogether, according to care-givers, 5 to 10 percent of patients had a change in therapy due to side effects.
Conclusions. The data confirm that in hypertension, the selection of therapy is primarily determined by patients' history.

## P - 95

Medicated Chewing-Gum : Formulation for Prevention of Dento- Periodontal Diseases

Belgun – Florea S.
Lagep, UCB Lyon 1 - ESCPE Lyon, Bât.308G, Boulevard du Novembre 1918

Prevention of oral plaque-related diseases (caries, gingivitis and periodontitis) relies on the use of antimicrobial agents, which are valuable additives to the mechanical therapy. Medicated chewing gums have been described as convenient and effective means in delivering oral active products. Controlled - release formulations aim to achieve prolonged local active concentrations of antimicrobial agents incorporated therein. Triclosan (2,4,4'-trichloro-2'-hydroxydiphenyl ether),a broad-spectrum non-ionic, liposoluble antibacterial agent, with anti- inflammatory proprieties, lacks the staining effect of cationic agents. Triclosan was encapsulated in micro- particles using an acrylate-methacrylate copolymer (Eudragit RS 100 and/or RL 100) by the emulsification - solvent evaporation method. The obtained micro-particles had a mean size ranging between 80-110 µm (varying between 10 - 300 µm) and a triclosan loading between 15% and 34% (w/w). Micro- particles were included in a medicated chewing gum by a compression manufacturing process. Progressive and sustained release profiles of encapsulated triclosan, included in the chewing gum, were observed in an in vitro dissolution solution, with 40 - 60 % triclosan being released after 30 minutes.

## P - 96

Telomeres and Telomerase in Pediatric Patients with Acute Lymphoblastic Leukemia (T-All)

[1]Kleideiter E., [2]Bangerter U., [1]Schwab M., [2]Niethammer D., [2]Greil J., [1]Klotz U.
[1]Dr. Margarete Fischer-Bosch Institute of Clinical Pharmacology, Stuttgart, Germany and [2]University Children's Hospital Tübingen, Germany

Shortened telomeres and high telomerase activity or expression of its catalytic subunit hTERT are apparently characteristic features of hematologic neoplasias such as high-grade lymphomas and relapsing leukemia indicating that their measurement might be useful to monitor disease conditions or clinical outcome. In order to investigate their prognostic potential we analyzed in T-ALL cells derived from 19 leukemic patients (age range 1-17 years) telomere length (TRF) by Southern blotting, hTERT at the mRNA level by real-time TaqMan PCR and telomerase activity by a modified TRAP assay. TRF varied widely (3.5 - 7.9 kB; mean +/-SD: 6.4 +/- 1.2 kB) and was significantly shorter ($p<0.0001$) than that of age-matched controls (8.3 +/- 0.4 kB; n=19). Likewise, expression of hTERT demonstrated a wide interindividual variability (range 141-424000 normalized units). In patients with T-ALL TRF was not affected by age and no relationship with hTERT was found. Both, TRF and hTERT did not correlate with the clinical outcome of the investigated patients limiting their prognostic potential for pediatric T-ALL. (supported by the Reinhold Beitlich Foundation Tübingen and the Robert Bosch Foundation Stuttgart)

## P - 97

Assessment of Drug-Induced Gastrointestinal Diseases in Sugery University Hospital Hippius J.M., Hegenbart U., Hoffmann A.
Department of Clinical Pharmacology

The use of drugs is always accompanied by the risk of adverse drug reactions (ADRs). Particularly important are serious ADRs (bleedings and ulcer diseases) that require hospital admission. We evaluated all individual medical files in viszeral, vascular, and accidental surgery in the year 2000. Side-effects were classified according to their severity, duration, symptomatology, pathogenesis. The frequency was studied with regard to age, sex, kind of surgery department. Out of the 4.976 evaluated patients, 319 showed gastrointestinal disorders. 122 patients had 168 ADRs, 36 patients with serious disorders. We analyzed 72 patients (42.9%) with gastric, 52 patients (30.9%) with intestinal ulcerations, 18 (10.7%) with upper gastrointestinal bleedings, 26 patients (15,5%) with unclarified bleedings. The average age was 66.8 in men, 69.5 years in women (1.7% of them was below 40). In 20% of the patients analgetics were the reason for ADRs. Advancing age is apparently associated with polypharmacy and multiple pathology, and this complex inter-relationship makes it difficult to conclude that age itself is a causative factor for ADR. Surgeons had not enough time to analyze ADRs as one part of different risk factors.

## ORAL

Eradication of Helicobacter Pylori (Hp) by Short-Term Lansoprazole Quadruple Therapy in Caucasians Depends on CYP2C19 Genotype

Schwab M., Schäffeler E., Treiber G., Klotz U.
Dr. Margarete Fischer-Bosch Institute of Clinical Pharmacology, Stuttgart, Germany

Eradication of Hp can be best accomplished by combined treatment of proton pump inhibitors such as lansoprazole (L) with 2 or 3 antibiotics (e.g. amoxicillin /A, clarithromycin /C, metronidazole /M). As L is metabolised by the polymorphic CYP2C19 we determined whether in Caucasians eradication success depends on the CYP2C19 genotype of patients who had been treated for 5 days with L (30mg bid), A (1g bid), C (250mg bid) and M (400mg bid). In addition, trough steady state serum concentrations (min Css) of L have been monitored. Among the 131 initially Hp positive patients we found 3 (2.3%) homozygous mutant carriers (*2/*2), 42 (32.1%) heterozygous patients (*1/*2) and 86 (65.6%) wildtype (wt) subjects. Overal eradication rate (ITT) of Hp averaged 86%. Differentiation according to the CYP2C19 genotype resulted in significant ($p< 0.01$; OR : 10.8) differences between the wt group (80.2%) and heterozygous (97.6%) or homozygous (100%) patients. These differences were associated with significant corresponding changes in min Css of L: median values were 27,83 and 753ng/ml for wt, heterozygous and homozygous patients, respectively. In conclusion, when standard doses of L are administered in a short-term quadruple regimen eradication rates of Hp depend also in Caucasian patients on their genotype of CYP2C19. Patients with wt of CYP2C19 might benefit from higher dosage of proton pump inhibitors for a more complete Hp eradication. (supported by the Robert Bosch Foundation Stuttgart)

## P - 98

Influence of Genetic Polymorphisms on Rifampicin-Mediated Induction of MRP2 (ABCC2) mRNA Expression

Cascorbi I., Haenisch S., Gießmann T., Dazert P., [1]Hecker U., Kroemer H.K., Siegmund W.
Peter Holtz Center of Pharmacology and Experimental Therapeutics, [1]Dept. of Internal Medicine, Ernst Moritz Arndt University, D-17487 Greifswald, Germany

The multidrug resistance protein 2 (MRP2; ABCC2) has an excretory protective role by transporting conjugated endogenous and xenobiotic substrates and can be induced by rifampicin via PXR binding elements. Some hereditary mutations of the MRP2 gene are linked with the Dubin-Johnson syndrome, however a number of polymorphisms have been identified with yet unknown function. We have genotyped the six most frequent MRP2 SNPs C-24T in the 5?-UTR, G1249 (Val417Ile), C2302T (Arg768Trp) and C2366T (Ser789Phe), C3972T (Ile1324Ile), and G4348A (Ala1450Thr) in 196 German unrelated subjects using conventional PCR/RFLP methods. Intestinal mRNA was isolated from duodenal biopsy specimens of 28 healthy subjects included in drug interaction studies with rifampicin. MRP2 mRNA was quantified using TaqMan rt-PCR. The following allelic frequencies were assessed: C-24T 31.6%, G1249A 44.4%. C3972T 62.2%. C2302T, C2366T, and G4348A could not be confirmed. Basal mRNA levels were not affected by any SNP. 13 samples were induced by rifampicin (3.2-fold, p= 0.013 Wilcoxon test), however a pronounced induction was detectable only in ten carriers of -24CC (2.85-fold) but not in the three carriers of CT (0.73-fold). The induction was 1.5-fold in six 1249GG, but 5.76-fold in six GA, and 5.15-fold in six 3972CC-subjects and 1.36-fold in six CT-genotypes. However, due to the small number, these differences were statistically not significant. In conclusion, the SNPs investigated do not have a considerable functional impact on basal MRP2 expression, but possibly on the extent of induction in presence of PXR ligands.

## P - 99

Embryotoxicitic Effects of Ranitidine

Nassrollazadeh B., Lalaney M., Onsory D.
Department of Anatomy, School of Medicine, Tehran University of Medical Sciences, Tehran, Iran.

In this work, we tried to know something more about the embryotoxicity effects of the doses of 50, 200, 400 mg/kg/day of ranitidine of (H2 antihistaminic agent) by intraperitoneal administation in mice. The studies were performed on albino mice kept under specific conditions and a constant dark- light cycle at 24+1 C and 55+ 5% relative humidity. Generally, the animals were acclimatised for four weeks before mating. Two female mice at 12-14 weeks of age were placed overnight with a male of proven fertility. The day on which a vaginal plug was found, was taken as day one of pregnancy. Also the vaginal smear was prepared for further proof. Treatment of pregnant females was started from day 7 and continued up to the 15th day of gestation and then on day 18 they were necropsied for routine teratological observations. Resorption plus dead fetuses less than 6mm of length were designated early death and dead fetuses of more than 6mm of length were consequently called late death. One- third of the fetuses were fixed in bouin's fluid to detect visceral malformations by the rasor- section technique. There was no significant difference in the frequency of late death between the control groups and the groups given ranitidine. Differences were observed in the number of implantation sites except for 400mg/kg/day. Data pooled from all experimental groups clearly show that pig tail, deformed cranium, low body weight and skeleton, unshaped external ear and jaw and polydactyly are the most common external abnormalities. Results of this study show the hazards of ranitidine used during early pregnancy in mice.

## P - 100

Evaluation of Contraceptive Effects of Trimethoprim and 2,4-Diamino - 5 (3,4-Dichlorophenyl6- Isopropyloxmethyl Pyrimidine in Male Rats

Sadeghipour Roudsari H.R.
Tehran University of Medical Sciences

With the problems resulting from the rapid trend of population growth, the development of procedures capable of decreasing the population growth rate, to inhibit and stagnate this condition is a necessity. It is obvios that without the contribution and sense of responsibility of men, population control programs and family planning will be unsuccessful. In the present study, attempts have been made to evaluate a newly synthesized analogue of diamino prymidines compounds with the chemical name of 2,4-diamino - 5 (3,4-dichlorophenyl) -6-isopropyloxymethyl) pyrimidine, (IPO) and trimethoprim (TRI) on male rats. This study indicates that the compound without any toxic effects, important side effects or serum testosteron changes decreases the fertility of rats. Also IPO significantly decreases the sperm motility (SM), percent of viable sperm, daily sperm production (DEP) and epididimal sperm reserve (ESR) but TRI decreases the SM and ESR.

Key Words: 1) Male contracptive 2) Isopropyloxymethyl pyrimidine 3) Trimethoprime 4) Rat

## P - 101

Efavirenz Plasma Concentrations in HIV-Infected Patients: Inter- and Intraindividual Variability and Clinical Effects

Ståhle L., [1]Moberg L., Svensson J.O., [1]Sönnerborg A.,
[2]Departments of Clinical Pharmacology, [1]Infectious Diseases and [2]Clinical Virology, Huddinge University Hospital, Karolinska Institute, SE14186 Huddinge, Sweden.

Efavirenz is a drug subject to extensive metabolism, mainly by the cytochrome P-450 isoenzyme CYP2B6, known to exhibit extensive interindividual variability. The aim of the present study was two-fold: to investigate the relation between plasma concentration and clinical effects of efavirenz and to investigate the extent of the inter- and intra-individual variability of the plasma concentration measurements. From an open clinic, 68 HIV-positive patients on efavirenz-containing treatment were recruited. From each patient 1-5 samples were collected, 43 had more than one sample taken Most samples were taken 10-24 hours after the latest dose. Efavirenz was analysed by high-performance liquid chromatography with UV-detection. The data were analysed by the variance component model analysis of variance. Efavirenz concentrations were reproducible and intraindividual variability constituted only 16% of the total variance, thus 84% of the variance was attributed to interindividual variability. The incidence of primary treatment failure was related to low plasma concentrations with a geometric mean concentration of 6.1 μM compared to 8.7 μM in those responding to therapy ($p<0.05$). Using a cut-off of 7 μM 10 of 13 failing to respond were below this level compared to 15 of 45 in those responding. It is concluded that efavirenz plasma concentration measurement gives reproducible results predictive of primary treatment failure. We propose a lower bound for the therapeutic level of 7 μM while data from other authors suggests that an upper level of 13 μM may be applied.

## P - 102

Activity of CYP3A Determined by Quinine Hydroxylation in Pregnant and non Pregnant Women Infected with Plasmodium Falciparum

[1]Mirghani R.A., [2]Elagib I., [1]Hellgren U., [2]Adam I., [2]Elghazali G., [2]Elbashir M.I., [1]Gustafsson L.L.
[1]Karolinska Institutet, Department of Medical Laboratory Sciences and Technology, Division of Clinical Pharmacology and Division of Infectious Diseases at Huddinge University Hospital, SE-141 86 Stockholm, Sweden.
[2]Department of Biochemistry, Khartoum University, Khartoum, Sudan.

We used quinine as a probe to investigate he difference in the activity of CYP3A between pregnant and controls during infection and after treatment. Nine pregnant and eight non-pregnant women in their second or third trimester were included. All subjects were diagnosed as severe Plasmodium falciparum malaria cases and treated by a combination of quinine and artemether. Quinine hydrochloride, 10 mg /kg body weight was given as a constant infusion during two hours on admission (phase I) followed by 4 doses of 1.6 mg/kg artemether intramuscularly 12, 24,48 and 72h post quinine. Seven days later they received a second infusion of quinine (phase II). Blood samples were collected at different time points post quinine dose. Total quinine (Q) and 3-hydroxyquinine (3OHQ) concentrations were determined in plasma by HPLC. The metabolic ratio (MR), which is Q/3-OHQ, was determined at 12 h post dose. There was a 1.7-fold increase in the mean MR in both groups during infection (20.1 vs. 11.8 in pregnant and 16.4 vs. 9.8 in controls). There was no significant difference in the mean MR between pregnant (20.1±18.4) and controls (20.3±10.5) during infection. No significant difference in the mean MR was observed between the two groups after treatment (11.0±8.2 in pregnant vs.8.9±3.2 in controls. Our results indicate reduced activity of CYP3A during p. falciparum infection and not changed during pregnancy.

## P - 103

Pilot-Analysis of Pharmacogenetic Polymorphisms in Patients with Gastrointestinal Carcinoma

[1]Farker K., [1]Merkel U., [2]Wedding U., [2]Höffken K., [1]Hoffmann A.
[1]Department of Clinical Pharmacology and [2]Clinic of Internal Medicine, Friedrich Schiller University Jena, Germany

Genetic polymorphisms of xenobiotic metabolising enzymes may influence the risk for the development of different cancers. In a pilot investigation, the frequencies of selected polymorphisms involving NAT2 and CYP2D6 were prospectively compared in 42 Caucasian patients with advanced gastrointestinal carcinoma and 42 age/sex-matched controls. Polymorphisms were determined by using PCR/RFLP. The frequency of slow acetylators was not significantly higher among cancer patients compared with controls (59.5% versus 47.6%; P=0.274). Also the frequency of poor metabolisers did not change between both (9.5% versus 11.9%; P=0.724). These first results do not indicate an association between the investigated genetic polymorphisms and susceptibility to gastrointestinal carcinoma. At this stage of investigation we neither can exclude nor support the possibility that gastrointestinal cancer risk may be modulated by the combined effect of genotype and exposure to environmental carcinogens. Within a second step we will include large numbers of subjects as well as validated estimates of exposure to environmental factors. The project was founded by German Cancer Aid (Grant AZ 70-2445-Hö3).

## P - 105

The Priorities in Prescription of Ukrainian Cardiologists

Sharayeva M.L., Victorov O.P., Khomenko Z.A.
Institute of Cardiology Ukrainian Academy of Medical Sciences, State Pharmacological Center, Kyiv, Ukraine

We scored the results of anonym questionnaires of 80 physicians - members of Kyiv Cardiological Society due to professional experience (up to five - more than ten years working). Such factors as the results of randomized trials, frequency of prescription, adverse effects and costs of medications were evaluated. The results of approved guidelines were authorial mostly for experienced physicians (78,5%) and for young ones (52,5%). Adverse effects are of great importance for more than half of professionals. The costs of medications are dominated in generic prescription due to economic hardship. The variety of antihypertensive treatment has been shown for all cardiologists: while ACE inhibitors prevail in elder physician's prescriptions (48%), young ones most commonly prescribed diuretics (38%), followed by beta-blockers and ACE inhibitors (34,8%). Only few (4%) respondents start with combination therapy. All cardiologists approved main classes of antianginal therapy, lipid therapy was ranked the last one. Amiodarone was ranked as first in antiarrhythmic therapy due to lack of effective available medications at the domestic market. Our data estimated a good compliance to the international guidelines and high adherence to "evidence-based medicine" for almost all respondents.These findings suggest that physicians can provide a good level of appropriate cardiovascular treatment.

## P - 104

Autoimmune Thyroiditis in Patients with Chronic Hepatitis C during Treatment with Combination Therapy (Interferon Alfa Plus Ribavirin)

[1]Nesic Z., [2]Delic D., [1]Prostran M., [1]Vuckovic S., [1]Todorovic Z., [1]Stojanovic R. [1]Department of Clinical Pharmacology, School of Medicine Belgrade, and [2]Institute for Infectious and Tropical Diseases, CCS, Belgrade, Serbia and Montenegro

Interferon alfa (IFN) has important immunomodulatory properties and some patients with chronic hepatitis C during or after therapy develop autoimmune thyroiditis. We treated 67 (46 male and 21 female) patients with combined therapy (IFN-alfa, 3 MU, three times a week plus ribavirin 1000-1200 mg per day during), last year in our Hepatology Department. In all patient thyroid function test (T3, T4 and TSH levels in serum) before treatment were normal and antithyroid antibody were negative. During treatment four patient (1 male and 3 female) developed autoimmune symptomatic thyroiditis. Two female (age 27 and 42) complained of cold intolerance, paresthesias of the hand and feet, dry skin, facial puffiness, periorbital swelling and menometrorhagias. High TSH serum level and slightly decreased levels of T3 and T4 were detected. In addition, positive titer of antithyroid antibodies (antimicrosomal, anti-TSH receptors and antithyroid peroxidase antibodies) were detected. Other two patients (39-year old male and 23-year old female) complained of nervousness, weight loss, insomnia and weakness. Laboratory analysis showed low level of TSH, increase level of T3 and T4 in serum, and positive titer of antithyroid antibodies. In all four cases, treatment with combination therapy was discontinued permanently and patients had spontaneous resolution of thyroiditis.

## P - 106

The Influence of Caffeine Preparations Intake on Pharmacodynamic Effects of Propranolole

[1]Brajovic T., [2]Raskovic A., [1]Boljevic A., [2]Jakovljevic V.
[1]Faculty of Medicine Podgorica, [2]Dept of Pharmacology, Toxicology and Clinical Pharmacology, Faculty of Medicine Novi Sad, Serbia and Montenegro

The age of urbanization and industrialization has resulted in a fast lifestyle, fatigue and stress, and it has led to an increase in the number of cardiovascular diseases and imposed the need for a larger intake of caffeine preparations. The aim of the paper was to investigate the influence of caffeine on pharmacodynamic effects of propranolole in adult health voluntaries. First group of them ($G_1$), does not take any caffeine preparations, while second group ($G_2$) includes voluntaries who take caffeine preparations, which contain about 50 mg of caffeine per day. In the first part of study, voluntaries have taken propranolole (40 mg), and blood presure and ECG changes were observed before and after propranolole treatment. In the second part, they have drunk a cup of coffee (about 20 mg of caffeine), 30 minutes before propranolole (40 mg). Results show that propranolole causes significant decrease of heart frequency, $p<0.05$, in the first group, but only without caffeine pretreatment. There were not significant changes in ECG and blood presure in voluntaries which consume caffeine preparations no consider to caffeine pretreatment. On the basis of the results obtained, we can conclude that chronical use of caffeine prevents changes which appear after single propranolole treatment.

## P - 107

Impaza - a New Promising Remedy for Erectile Dysfunction: Placebo-Controlled Trial

Martyushev-Poklad A.V., [1]Smolenov I.V., [1]Petrov V.I., Dugina J.L.,.Sergeeva S.A, Epstein O.I.
"Materia Medica Holding" Research-and-Production Company, Moscow, Russia [1]Volgograd Medical Academy, Volgograd, Russia

According to earlier experimental studies, a novel antibody-based remedy impaza (oral ultra-low doses of antibodies to endothelial NO synthase) stimulates NO-cGMP pathway in penile cavernous tissue through increase in activity of NO synthases. In a double-blind placebo-controlled randomized trial, we evaluated efficacy and safety of impaza in 90 patients with erectile dysfunction (ED) of organic, psychogenic, or mixed causes. Impaza was given in a 12-week course, 3-4 times weekly, without strict adherence to sexual activity. Placebo group included 30 men. Patients of a parallel, randomized open-label group received sildenafil (25 mg). We assessed efficacy according to the International Index of Erectile Function (IIEF), and a global-efficacy question. Impaza effect (IIEF scores), more pronounced on course treatment, differed significantly ($p<0.001$) from placebo, and on 12-week treatment approached the effect of sildenafil. On global-efficacy doctor's assessment, 83,4% of impaza patients demonstrated excellent or good response (20% in placebo group, and 83,5% in sildenafil group). Unlike sildenafil, impaza caused no adverse effects requiring cessation of treatment (10% in sildenafil group). Some impaza patients showed rise in serum testosterone after course treatment. The findings indicate that impaza is a promising, effective and safe treatment for ED.

## P - 108

Artrofoon in Treatment of Rheumatoid Arthritis Patients: A Pilot Randomized Clinical Study

Petrov V.I., Babaeva A.R., Tcherevkova E.V., Martyushev-Poklad A.V., Sergeeva S.A., Epstein O.I.
Volgograd Medical Academy, Volgograd, Russia; "Materia Medica Holding" Research-and-Production Company, Moscow, Russia

In an open randomized clinical study we assessed efficacy and safety of Artrofoon (ultra-low doses of oral anti-TNF alpha antibodies) in rheumatoid arthritis (RA) patients in comparision with a reference NSAID (diclofenac). The study covered thirty patients with classic or definite RA (aged 29-60, RA duration 5-22 years) to receive artrofoon (8 lingual tablets/day) or diclofenac (100 mg/day) for 6 months. After 6-month treatment, patients of artrofoon group unlike those of diclofenac group showed statistically significant net improvement in 5 of 8 clinical indices: joint pain (reduced in 86,7% of artrofoon as against 40% of diclofenac patients), duration of morning stiffness (more than 30-min reduction in 93,3% of artrofoon and 40% of diclofenac), Ritchie index (reduced by >=3 in 80% of artrofoon and 33,3% of diclofenac), joint swelling and joint circumference (in 60% of artrofoon and 20% of diclofenac patients). C-reactive protein levels reduced in 80% of artrofoon and 27% of diclofenac patients. None of artrofoon patients developed any clinical or laboratory changes calling for temporary withdrawal or reduction of artrofoon dose. In diclofenac group, 27% of patients revealed NSAID gastropathy. Artrofoon was shown effective and safe in RA, it excelled diclofenac in efficacy and safety.

## P - 109

Tissue Pharmacokinetics of Metronidazole

[1]Pähkla R., [2]Karjagin J., [2]Starkopf J.
[1]Department of Pharmacology and [2]Clinic of Anesthesiology and Intensive Care, University of Tartu, Estonia

Metronidazole is an antimicrobial agent used in the treatment and prophylaxis of anaerobic bacterial infections. Plasma pharmacokinetics of metronidazole has been characterized in detail but few data exists about the pharmacokinetics of metronidazole in tissues. The aim of the present study was to evaluate the pharmacokinetics of intravenous metronidazole in muscular tissues using in vivo microdialysis technique. Six female patients participated in the study. Microdialysis catheters were placed into the m. vastus lateralis. Metronidazole 500 mg was given intravenously by infusion over 10 min. Microdialysis and plasma samples were collected during ten hours after drug administration. Perfusion speed was 2 ml/min. Metronidazole concentrations were analysed by validated HPLC method. Maximum metronidazole concentration in plasma was 16.45±4.62 mg/l. In muscle maximum concentration 6.93±2.23 mg/l was achieved at 60 min. AUC0-10h values were 76.04±19.37 mg/lxh for plasma and 54.08±10.72 mg/lxh for tissue, respectively. Present data demonstrate that metronidazole penetrates well into the muscular tissue. Tissue concentrations reach values far greater than reported MIC90 for susceptible anaerobic bacteria and persist at such high level for more than 10 hours.

## P - 110

Anaferon - A Novel Therapeutic For Influenza in Children: Clinical Efficacy and Immunomodulation

Martyushev-Poklad A.V., Drinevskiy V.P., Osidak L.V., Dugina J.L., Kotelnikova M.P., Sergeeva S.A., Epstein O.I.
"Materia Medica Holding" Research-and-Production Company, Moscow, Russia Influenza Research Center, Russian Academy of Medical Sciences, St-Petersburg, Russia

Earlier experimental data showed that Anaferon, a novel antibody-based remedy (oral ultra-low doses of antibodies to IFN-gamma) has immunomodulatory, IFN-inducing and antiviral activities. A controlled double blind clinical study of anaferon efficacy and safety involved 160 children aged 0.5-14 years with confirmed influenza infection. Anaferon (placebo in reference group) was administered on days 1-10 of infection perorally 3-7 times daily with background conventional symptomatic and/or antibiotic drugs (where necessary). Major clinical signs of influenza were significantly ($p<0.05$) less severe and prolonged in patients of anaferon versus reference group: duration of fever reduced by 40%, intoxication - by 48%, rhinitis - by 21%, cough - by 29%. No adverse effects were registered along the study. Positive clinical outcome was accompanied by recovery (to age-specific range) of peripheral blood lymphocyte subpopulations: of CD3+ cells - in 75% of children (40% in reference group), CD4+ - in 78% (reference - 40%), CD20+ - in 64% (reference - 35%), CD16+ - in 100% (reference - 65%). Thus, anaferon was found highly effective in children with influenza. When administered early, anaferon reduced duration of all signs of the infection. Anaferon was well tolerated and compatible with conventional therapy. Anaferon alleviated some peripheral blood signs of immunodeficiency typical of influenza patients.

## P - 111

Anxiolytic and Antidepressant Action of Proproten: Experimental and Clinical Study

Voronina T.A., Molodavkin G.M., Krylov E.N., Dugina J.L., Sergeeva S.A., Epstein O.I.
"Materia Medica Holding" Research and Production Company, Moscow, Russia Research Institute of Pharmacology under the RAMS, Moscow, Russia

The aim of this research was to study anxyolitic and antidepressant activity of proproten (oral ultra-low doses of antibodies to S-100 protein) in experiments and in alcohol addicts during withdrawal syndrome. All experiments were carried out on male outbred rats (230-280 g). Standard methods of evaluation of anxiolytic (Vogel conflict test, elevated plus-maze test, open field method), antidepressant (models of behavioral despair by Pellow, forced swimming test by Nomura) and myorelaxant activity (rotarod test) were used. Antidepressant and anxiolytic effects of proproten (2,5 ml/kg) revealed in these tests equaled those of amitriptylin (10 mg/kg) and diazepam (2 mg/kg) respectively. Unlike conventional antidepressants and tranquilizers proproten caused no sedation, drowsiness or muscle relaxation. Notably, anxyolitic activity of proproten was higher in the group of low active rats as compared to highly active ones. Anxiolytic effects of proproten were proved to involve GABA-ergic system. In open-label comparative trial, a total of 256 alcohol addicts received proproten (8 tablets/day) versus phenasepam (2 mg/day) plus amitryptilin (10mg/day) plus standard detoxification therapy. Anxiolytic activity of proproten was almost equal to phenazepam, and antidepressant exceeded that of amitriptylint.Thus, proproten should be considered as a promising drug for treatment of anxiety and depression.

## P - 112

Ketoconazole Increases Venlafaxine Plasma Concentrations Regardless of CYP2D6 Pheno/Genotype

[1]Lindh J., [1]Annas A., [1]Meurling L., [2]Dahl M.L., [1]AL- Shurbaji A.
[1]Department of Medical Laboratory Sciences and Technology, Division of Clinical Pharmacology, Karolinska Institutet at Huddinge University Hospital, Stockholm and [2]Department of Medical Sciences, Clinical Pharmacology, University Hospital, Uppsala, Sweden

Objective: To study the influence of CYP3A4 inhibition by ketoconazole on venlafaxine disposition in individuals with different CYP2D6 pheno- and genotypes. Methods: 21 healthy volunteers with known CYP2D6 pheno- and genotype (14 EM, 7 PM) were given a single oral dose of venlafaxine. Plasma and urine levels of venlafaxine and its metabolites were measured and the pharmacokinetics of venlafaxine were determined. Later, subjects were treated for two days with ketoconazole starting one day before the administration of venlafaxine; and the procedure was repeated as above.
Results: There was a good correlation between the debrisoquine metabolic ratio and the ratio between venlafaxine and O-desmethylvenlafaxine AUC ($R_s$=0.93, $P<0.002$). The majority of subjects showed higher plasma levels of venlafaxine and O-desmethylvenlafaxine upon co-administration of ketoconazole; irrespective of CYP2D6 phenotype. AUC of venlafaxine significantly increased by 36% and that of O-desmethylvenlafaxine by 26% ($P<0.01$). Cmax increased by 32% and 18%, respectively. The elimination half-life of venlafaxine was unaltered. Three PMs displayed marked increases in AUC (81, 126 and 206%) and Cmax (60, 72, 119%) of venlafaxine while the other three showed small or no changes.
Conclusions: Ketoconazole affects the disposition of venlafaxine irrespective of CYP2D6 pheno/genotype. The mechanisms underlying this interaction remain to be elucidated.

## P - 113

Population Kinetic Analysis of the Interactions Between Lamotrigin and Inducers and Inhibitors of Glucuronidation

Böttiger Y., Ståhle L.
Clinical Pharmacology, Karolinska Institutet, Huddinge University Hospital. SE-14186, Stockholm, Sweden

Background: Lamotrigin is known to interact with valproic acid and with the enzyme inducing antiepileptics phenytoin, carbamazepine and phenobarbital. We analysed the quantitative impact of these interacting drugs on the population pharmacokinetic parameters of lamotrigine clearance. Such data are valuable in Bayesian estimation of individual parameters.
Method: A total of 212 samples from 107 individuals formed the basis of the analysis. We applied non-linear mixed effect modelling (NONMEM), and used a first order absorption, one compartment model, estimating inter-individual variance of clearance and volume of distribution. The clearance model was simply a basal clearance, with one term added for valproic acid (i.e. subtracted) and one term added for the three inducers. More complicated models did not improve the fit to any substantial degree. The variance terms were all exponential, which was essential to avoid negative clearances.
Result: The absorption rate constant was 2.59 and the volume of distribution was 67.7 L, with an inter-individual CV of 200% (i.e. very large). The clearance was 2.16 L/h, which was reduced by 1.54 L/h by of valproic acid treatment, and increased by 1.36 L/h with concomitant treatment with an inducer. The remaining inter-individual CV of clearance was 38%. The residual CV was 24%. An interesting observation is that the effects of inducers and valproic acid almost precisely cancelled one another. Conclusion: On average, valproic acid co-treatment should result in a dose reduction by 75% of lamotrigin, while inducers should be associated with an averagage increase of the lamotrigine dose by 65%.

## P - 114

Anar in the Treatment of Opiate Withdrawal Syndrome

Bohan N.A., Abolonin A.F., Dugina J.L., Sergeeva S.A., Epstein O.I.
Research Institute of Mental Health, Siberian Branch of the Russian Academy of Medical Sciences, Tomsk, Russia; "Materia Medica Holding" Research and Production Company Moscow, Russia

Clinical efficacy of anar (ultralow doses of antibodies to morphine) in the treatment of opiate withdrawal syndrome (OWS) was studied. Therapy started on subjects, who had been opiate-free for 7 days, after reduction of acute OWS. A total of 107 opiate addicts aged from 15 to 35 years old (mean age - 23,5±4,1) were included in the 5-week trial. Patients were randomly divided into two groups: 67 of 107 patients (anar group) received anar 5-8 tablets/day for the first 2 weeks, then 4-6 tablets/day. The rest (40 patients, reference group) were assigned to conventional therapy including individual prescription of amytriptiline, tofisopam, periciazine, thioridazine, chlorprothixene, piracetam or proroxan. The resolution of OWS symptoms was achieved in 20,9% of patients in anar group within 7 days of treatment (none in reference group); within 10 days - 65,7% in anar group (17,5% in reference group); within 16 days - 79,2% in anar group (82,5% in reference group). Compared to conventional treatment anar monotherapy was associated with a more rapid reduction of affective symptoms and insomnia (1,6 and 1,3-fold faster, respectively). No side effects occurred during treatment in anar group. Thus anar appears to be an effective and safe therapy of choice for OWS.

## P - 115

### Knowledge of Patients about Prescribed Drugs

[1]Akıcı A., [2]Kalaça S., [1]Uğurlu Ü., [3]Altunbaş-Toklu H., [1]İskender E., [1]Oktay Ş.
Departments of [1]Pharmacology & Clinical Pharmacology and [2]Public Health, School of Medicine, and [3]Department of Pharmacology, Faculty of Pharmacy, Marmara University, Istanbul, Turkey.

Providing adequate information to the patients about their drugs is an essential principle of rational pharmacotherapy. Knowledge of patients on prescribed drugs was evaluated in this study. A total of 1618 patients who applied to health-care centers in Istanbul were asked about the number, name(s) and effect(s) of the drug(s) on their prescriptions. Factors that might influence the background knowledge and perception of patients such as sociodemographic characteristics, drug-use habits and physicians' attitude were also questioned. Information provided by the patients were compared with the prescriptions. Patients knew little about their prescriptions. Level of education had a positive effect on their knowledge about the drugs. Patients who applied for a refill prescription, with a chronic disease, and who had used these drugs previously reported more accurate information ($p<0.05$). Only 42.5 % of the patients stated that they were informed by the physician about drug-effects. In conclusion, although some findings might be attributed to the problems regarding primary health care system, the present study indicates an urgent need for education not only for the physicians but also to increase the level of knowledge of the population about drugs and patient's role in rational pharmacotherapy.

## P - 116

### Lack of Effect of Age, Weight and Body Mass Index on Trough and Peak Indinavir Plasma Concentrations in HIV-Infected Patients Treated with Different Indinavir Boosted Regimens

[1]Zouai O., [1]Poirier J.M., [2]Meynard J.L., [2]Lacombe K., [3]Guiard-Schmid J.B., [2]Girard P.M., [1]Jaillon P.
[1]Department of Pharmacology, Saint-Antoine University Hospital,Paris, France, [2]Department of Infectious Diseases, Saint-Antoine University Hospital, Paris, France, [3]Department of Infectious Diseases, Tenon University Hospital, Paris, France.

Background : In a subset study from the Athena Cohort (1), the demographic factors associated with highest risk of urological symptoms for the HIV-patients treated by indinavir, were low weight and low lean body mass.
Methods : To assess the effects of demographic variables such as age, weight and body mass index (BMI), trough (Cmin) and peak (Cmax) of indinavir (IDV) and ritonavir (RTV) plasma concentrations were retrospectively analyzed in 52 HIV-patients receiving different IDV/RTV bid dosing regimens with two nucleosides analogues : 800/100 mg (n=14), 600/100 mg (n=24) and 400/100 mg (n=14).
Results : No statistically significant effect of age (<66 yr) and body mass index was observed for IDV and RTV Cmin.and Cmax. Despite patients with lower body weigh had significant higher RTV Cmax ($p<0.05$) at 600 and 800 mg IDV dosing regimens, IDV Cmax was independent from body weight.
Conclusion : None of the demographic factors explored in this small retrospective study was predictor of IDV plasma concentrations. (1) Dieleman JP, Sturkenboom MCJM, Jambroes M et al. Risk factors for urological symptoms in a cohort of users of the protease inhibitor indinavir sulfate. The Athena Cohort. Arch Med Int 2002, 162 : 1493-1501

## P - 117

### Identification and Characterisation of Novel SNPs in the 5'-Flanking Region of the CYP2C9 Gene

[1]Sandberg M., [2]Bloethner S., [2]Malmebo S., [1]Rane A., [2]Johansson I., [1]Eliasson E.
[1]Division of Clinical Pharmacology, Karolinska Institutet, Huddinge University Hospital, 141 86 Stockholm, Sweden and [2]Division of Molecular Toxicology, IMM, Karolinska Institutet, 171 77 Stockholm, Sweden

In DNA samples from 27 Caucasian subjects, 16 SNPs were identified in 3.5 kb of the CYP2C9 gene 5'-flanking region. HeLa cells were transfected with reporter constructs including the 5'-flanking region, and the variant with both -1537A and -981A showed 38 % lower expression than -1537G/-981G. The allele frequencies in 195 Caucasian subjects were 7.2% for both SNPs. All subjects carrying CYP2C9*3 alleles also carried one or two -1537A/-981A alleles, suggesting a linkage between these three SNPs. The median metabolic ratio of losartan was significantly higher in subjects with the genotype -1537G/A/-981G/A or -1537A/A/-981G/A as compared to subjects carrying -1537G/G/-981G/A or -1537G/G/-981G/G (2.5 ± 1.4 and 1.1 ± 0.72, respectively). In summary, the data suggest that the SNPs at -1537 and -981 influence expression of the CYP2C9 gene, and that the -1537A/-981A combination might contribute to the decreased activity observed in individuals carrying CYP2C9*3.

## P - 118

### Bufrenorphine Treatment in Heroin Addicts

Guglielmino L., Vigezzi P., Silenzio R., De Chiara M., Corrado F., Marzorati P., Cocchi L., Cozzolino E.
Public out-patient Addiction Unit ( Ser.T), 25 via Boifava, A.S.L. Città di Milano, Italy.

Aim: To evaluate efficacy of buprenorphine treatment in heroin addicts in a public addiction Center since 2001 to 2002.
Population: 88 (69 males) patients (pts.) consecutively assigned to overall 95 treatments with mean age 34 ± 6 years and dependence mean time 11± 6 yrs.
Treatments: 44 treatments came from MMT. 156 days (range: 1-581) was the mean period of treatment and 11± 6 mg./die the mean max. dosage. 17 were short-term treatments ( ≤30 days ), 39 medium-term (> 30 ≤180 days ) and 39 long-term ( > 180 days). 40% were psico-social integrated treatments.
Result : Urine examinations resulted negative in 83,5% for opiate and in 82,2% for cocaine; the rate of positive opioid and cocaine samples significatively decreased from the baseline during the treatment ( ANOVA; P=0,0257 - P=0,0309).
62 pts. are still in treatment, 7 therapies were succesfully completed, 13 dropped-out, 8 shifted to MMT, 3 continued in jail and 2 in other addiction Centers.
Treatment outcomes between two groups with a maximum dosage > or ≤ 10 mg./die resulted significatively different (P< 0,05); in the first group the drop-out was less than in the lower dosage group (P< 0,05).
Conclusion: Retention treatment rate was 73,2% after one year; it risulted different between the pts. coming from MMT - 87,2% - and from heroin - 61,7%; and between groups with different dosage: 82,9%( > 10 mg.) and 65,9% (≤ 10 mg./die).

## ORAL

Lowering of LDL and Raising of HDL by High-Dosage Itraconazole in Men

[1]Lütjohann D., [2]Gerdsen R., [1]Lindenthal B., [1]Locatelli S., [3]Diczfalusy U., [3]Björkhem I., [4]Neuvonen P., [2]Bieber T., [1]Von Bergmann K.
[1]Department of Clinical Pharmacology and [2]Dermatology, University of Bonn, Germany. [3]Department of Medical Laboratory Science and Technology, Division of Clinical Chemistry, Karolinska Institute, Huddinge University Hospital, Sweden. [4]Department of Clinical Pharmacology, Helsinki University Central Hospital, Finland.

Lowering of LDL-cholesterol and raising of HDL-cholesterol is thought to lower the risk of coronary heart disease. It has been demonstrated previously that ketocanozole, an inhibitor of cytochrome P450 (CYP) mediated 14alpha-demethylation of the cholesterol precursor lanosterol, and reduced serum concentrations of total and LDL-cholesterol. The effect of another antifungal azol agent, itraconazole, on concentrations of lipoproteins and surrogate serum markers of cholesterol and bile acid synthesis was investigated within a prospective controlled exploratory trial. Eight male patients, with diagnosed onychomycosis, were treated with 400 mg itraconazole once daily for one week. This therapy resulted in a significant decrease of total (-11%; $p < 0.01$) and LDL-cholesterol (-20%; $p < 0.001$), while HDL-cholesterol was raised by 16.2% ($p < 0.01$). The ratio of LDL-C to HDL-C, also denoted atherogenic index, was decreased by 32%. There was a high correlation between the serum concentrations of itraconazole and its metabolite hydroxyitraconazole and the ratio of LDL-C/HDL-C ($r = 0.571$; $p < 0.01$). Concentrations of the cholesterol precursor lanosterol and dihydrolanosterol increased twenty- and two-hundred-fold, respectively, while the ratio of serum lathosterol to cholesterol, an indicator of endogenous cholesterol synthesis, remained unchanged. Serum concentrations of the brain specific cholesterol metabolite 24S-hydroxycholesterol as well as its ratio to cholesterol increased slightly, but significantly ($p < 0.01$). These results were reproducible in a second treatment cycle after a three week wash-out period. High-dosage itraconazole (400 mg/day) lowers the ratio of LDL-/HDL-cholesterol and presumably lowers hepatic degradation of 24S-hydroxycholesterol.

## P - 119

Ezetimibe Effectively Reduces Serum Plant Sterols in Patients with Sitosterolemia

[1]Lütjohann D., [1]Von Bergmann K., [2]Salen G., The Multicenter Sitosterolemia Study Group
[1]Department of Clinical Pharmacology, University of Bonn, Bonn, Germany. [2]UMD, New Jersey Medical School, Newark, NJ, U.S.A.

Sitosterolemia is a recessively inherited disorder that results from a gene mutation in either ABCG5 or G8 transporter proteins with hyperabsorption and decreased hepatic excretion of plant sterols and cholesterol. As a consequence of markedly elevated plasma and tissue sitosterol and campesterol levels premature atherosclerosis develops. In this multicenter, double-blind, randomized, placebo-controlled study, we examined whether treatment with ezetimibe, an inhibitor of cholesterol absorption, reduces plant sterol levels in patients with sitosterolemia. After a 3-week placebo run-in, 36 patients were randomized to receive placebo ($n = 7$) or ezetimibe 10 mg/day ($n = 29$) for 8 weeks. Sitosterol concentrations decreased by 21% in patients treated with ezetimibe compared with a 4% rise in those on placebo (between group $p < 0.001$). The reduction in sitosterol from baseline was progressive with greater decline observed at each subsequent biweekly visit. Campesterol also progressively declined with a mean decrease after 8 weeks of 24% with ezetimibe and a mean increase of 3% with placebo treatment (between group $p < 0.001$). The reductions in plant sterol concentrations were similar irrespective of whether or not patients were on concomitant treatments (resin or statin). Reductions in total sterols and lipoprotein apo-B were also observed. Ezetimibe was well tolerated with no serious treatment-related adverse events or discontinuations due to adverse events being reported. Ezetimibe produced significant and progressive reductions in plasma plant sterol concentrations in patients with sitosterolemia, consistent with the hypothesis that ezetimibe inhibits the intestinal absorption of plant sterols as well as cholesterol, leading to reductions in plasma concentrations.

## P - 120

Use of Non-specific Intravenous Human Inmunoglobulins, Need for a Hospital Protocol

Cabrera García L., Ruiz A.S., Antorán B.R., Valderas M.S., [1]Torralba A., Solá C.A.
Clinical Pharmacology Deparment. [1]Pharmacy Deparment . University Hospital Puerta de Hierro, Madrid

A recent revision by EMEA on the authorised indications of Non-specific Intravenous Human Inmunoglobulins (IgIV), has motivated the need to develop a utilisation protocol. It included the indications authorised by EMEA (group 1), those indications non authorised but with accepted supported (group 2) and finally the indications non-accepted (group 3), which follow a compassionate use procedure. In addition patient's data, indication, type and batch numbers of IgIV are registered in the Pharmacy. Objective: To assess the feasibility of the protocol and the measures of control developed. To describe the utilisation of IgIV since the implantation of the protocol. Methods: The data were obtained from the systematic review of the Inmunoglobulins controlled medication request during the four first months after the protocol was implemented. The compliance with the form of IC was evaluated for those cases established by the protocol.

Results: During the study period, 60 requests (corresponding to....different patients) were sent to the Pharmacy Department: a 70% were authorised indications, amongst these the most frequent were Bone Marrow Transplant (30%) and Idiopathic Trombocytopenic Purpura (13,1%). The non-authorised but well supported indications accounted for 27% of requests: Myasthenia Gravis (10%) and Multifocal Motor Neuropathy (10%) were the most frequent ones in this group.

Conclusions: A substantial proportions (70%) of the requests were authorised indications (group 1). In-group 2 and 3, the IC was obtained in an important number of cases (83%). The implementation of the protocol has been well accepted.

## P - 121

Lead and Cadmium Content of Korbal Rice in Northern Iran

[1]Bakhtiarian A., Gholipour M., Ghazi-Khansari M.
Department of Pharmacology, School of Medicine, Tehran University of Medical Sciences, P.O.Box 13145-784,Tehran, Iran

Every year the entrance of factory wastes such as Shiraz Petrochemical Complex, Marvdasht sugar cube factory, and Charmineh factory, and other industrial units into the Kor and Sivand rivers and also the entrance of the Marvdasht and Zarghan city sewer system wastes into the Kor river and the use of their water in the cultivation of the rice has caused a significant increase in the lead and cadmium content of the grains of rice. To study the effect of the Kor river's pollution on the lead and cadmium content of the grains of rice, 57 samples of 6 different types of were prepared in 19 different stations in the Korbal region and also 18 samples of 6 different types of rice, cultivated with unpolluted water, were prepared in the National Institute of Rice Research (Gilan). A comparison of the pollution level of the Korbal and Gilan rice samples shows a significant difference and indicates the significant effect of the pollution of the river on the lead and cadmium content of the Korbal rice samples. The results of the study show that the lead and cadmium content of the hybrid, prolific, and late rice sample types were greater than that of unprolific and early types, such that the amount of these two elements was highest in the Hassani type (the lead content was 0.9625 ppm and the cadmium content was 0.0793 ppm), whereas the Gasroddashti type which blooms earlier and is long seeded has the lowest amount of these two elements.

## P - 122

Replacement Therapy With L-Thyroxine Plus Triiodothyronine (14:1) Is Not Superior to Thyroxine Alone with Respect to the Psychical and Physical Wellbeing of Patients with Hypothyroidism

[1]Siegmund W., [2]Spieker K., [1]Giessmann T., [4]Jasmann D., [1]Modess C., [5]Engel G., [3]Kirsch G., [4]Hamm A., [2]Meng W.
Departments of [1]Clinical Pharmacology [2]Internal Medicine, [3]Nuclear Medicine and [4]Psychology, [5]Hospital Pharmacy, University of Greifswald, Germany

There is evidence (NEJM 1999;340:424) that replacement therapy of hypothyroidism with thyroxine (T4) combined with triiodothyronine (T3) may improve the wellbeing of patients. However, the study is still subject of controversial debate. Therefore, 23 patients (3 males, age 23-69 years, 21 after surgery/radioiodine, 2 autoimmune thyroiditis) on long-term replacement with 100-175 µg T4 were randomly allocated to a double-blind, two-period, cross-over trial to confirm superiority of a 12 weak replacement therapy with a physiological mixture of thyroid hormones (bioavailable molar T4/T3 ratio; 14 : 1) relative to T4 alone with regard to psychological and physical wellbeing and cognitive performance as assessed by psychological standard tests.
Results: The neuropsychological examinations revealed no significant differences between the treatments (Table):

| | | T4 | T3/T4 |
|---|---|---|---|
| TSH | (mU/L) | 1.5 ± 1.3 | 0.5 ± 0.6 (p < 0.001) |
| Subjects with TSH = 0 | (N) | 2 | 8 |
| Digit Span Test | (N) | 12.13 ± 2.46 | 12.39 ± 2.78 |
| Visual Scanning Test | (sec) | 61.61 ± 28.14 | 64.76 ± 28.69 |
| Global Mood Score | | 11.04 ± 9.62 | 12.26 ± 13.35 |

Conclusions: Replacement therapy with a physiological combination of L-thyroxine with triiodothyronine (14 : 1) is not superior to thyroxine alone.

## ORAL

COX-2 Selective Inhibitors Rofecoxib and Celecoxib Protect Against Colorectal Adenomas Occurrence and Recurrence. A Nested Case-Control Study.

Rahme E., Barkun A.N., Toubouti Y., LeLorier J., Bardou M.
McGill University Montréal

Background and aims: Colorectal cancer (CRC) is one of the leading causes of cancer death. Most are believed to develop from colorectal adenomas (CRA).
Objective: To examine the effect of non-selective NSAIDs, aspirin, acetaminophen and the selective cyclooxygenase-2 inhibitors, rofecoxib and celecoxib on CRA. Methods: A nested case-control study, using data from a government insurance database on patients 65 years and older who underwent a diagnostic test or procedure for CRA/CRC between January and June 2001. Logistic regression models were used to determine the effect of exposure to the drugs of interest for at least 3 months on the occurrence or recurrence of CRA, and/or CRC.
Results: The control group included 2,568 patients found to be free of either CRA or CRC; 730 patients were diagnosed with CRA, and 179 with CRC. Patients more likely to have CRA (odds ratio, 95% confidence interval) were those diagnosed with CRA (4.12, [3.27, 5.18]) or CRC (3.74, [2.32, 6.03]) in the previous 1-3 years, and those with hemorrhage of rectum or unspecified anemia in the prior month (3.19, [2.46, 4.12]). Exposures to rofecoxib, and non-selective NSAIDs were both found to reduce the risk of CRA (0.67, [0.45, 0.98], and 0.41, [0.21, 0.83], respectively). Exposures to non-selective NSAIDs, rofecoxib and celecoxib were all protective against all neoplasia (CRA or CRC combined; OR 0.47 [0.23, 0.86], 0.64 [0.45, 0.91], and 0.73 [0.54, 0.99] for NSAIDs, rofecoxib and celecoxib respectively, as compared to non-exposed patients).
Conclusion: The non-selective NSAIDs and the coxibs, rofecoxib and celecoxib, appear to protect against the development of CRA or CRC.

## P - 123

Disposition of Oral Carvedilol Is Inducible by Rifampicin Mainly Dependent on Up-Regulation of Intestinal P-Glycoprotein and MRP2

Siegmund W., Giessmann T., Zschiesche M., [1]Hecker U., [2]Kunert-Keil C., [2]Warzok R., [3]Engel G., Dazert P., Cascorbi I., Kroemer H.K.
Peter Holtz Research Center of Pharmacology and Therapeutics, Departments of [1]Internal Medicine and of [2]Pathology and [3]Hospital Pharmacy, University of Greifswald, Germany

There is evidence for disposition of R(+)- and S(-)-carvedilol to be dependent on CYP2D6 genotype and on CYP450 enzymes and transporter protein which are susceptible to PXR-type enzyme induction. Therefore, we measured the pharmacokinetics of intravenous (5 mg) and chronic carvedilol (25 mg, 7 days) before and after comedication of rifampicin (600 mg, 6-9 days) in 12 healthy subjects (3 females; 21-29 years; 6 PM and 6 EM of CYP2D6) in dependence on duodenal MDR1- and MRP2-mRNA (Taqman®) expression and content of P-glycoprotein and MRP2 (immunostaining).
Results: Rifampicin induced P-glycoprotein and MRP2 manifold. MRP2- but not MDR1-mRNA correlated with the enzyme content ($r_s$=0.78, p<0.001). The following pharmaco-kinetic data (means) were assessed (Wilcoxon, p<0.05; *vs control, °vs R(+), #vs PM):

| | | before rifampicin | | | | after rifampicin | | | |
|---|---|---|---|---|---|---|---|---|---|
| | | PM | | EM | | PM | | EM | |
| | | R(+) | S(-) | R(+) | S(-) | R(+) | S(-) | R(+) | S(-) |
| AUC | (ng/ml×h) | 230 | 62.9° | 93.9# | 32.7#+ | 70.2* | 18.0*° | 32.6 #* | 14.9*+ |
| F | (%) | 48.3 | 24.4° | 24.0# | 14.5#° | 15.3* | 6.98* | 9.13#*° | 6.39* |
| $CL_{iv}$ | (ml/min) | 494 | 959° | 698 | 1103° | 662* | 1034° | 889# | 1166 |

Serum concentrations of intravenous and oral carvedilol were highly correlated to intestinal expression of MRP2, in part also to P-glycoprotein.
Conclusions: Carvedilol disposition in controlled by P-glycoprotein and MRP2. Their up-regulation by rifampicin leads to significantly lower oral bioavailability independent of chirality and CYP2D6 genotype.

## P - 124

Postoperative Analgesia After Traumatic and Orthopaedic Surgery: a Methodological Qualitative Systematic Review

Montané E, Vallano A, Aguilera C, Laporte JR.
Unitat d'assaigs Clínics i Farmacoepidemiologia. Fundació Institut Català de Farmacologia. Departament de Farmacologia Clínica. Hospital Universitari Vall d'Hebron. Barcelona. Spain.

Objectives: Analgesic drugs have been evaluated in a number of clinical trials on the treatment of postoperative pain after traumatic and orthopaedic surgery (TOS), but their methodological quality has not been systematically assessed yet. The methodological quality of those trials was systematically reviewed.
Methods: Randomised trials (RCTs) on opioids or NSAIDs drugs after TOS in adult patients were included. Trials on anaesthetic drugs, preemptive analgesia and spinal drug administration were excluded. Quality was assessed according to Jadad scale and CONSORT statement recommendations.
Results: 299 published studies were identified and 86 were included. The control group received placebo in 36 RCTs (42%). Forty-four trials (51%) assessed a single-dose, 18 (21%) reported methods for allocation, 71 (83%) were double-blind but masking was described in 47 (55%), the primary outcome was clearly defined in 8 (9%), sample size calculation was described in 6 (7%), the flow of patients and withdrawals were described in 29 (34%) and analysis was by "intention to treat" in 28 (33%). Most of RCTs (84; 98%) analysed pain intensity and global pain assessment (53; 62%) but rating scales were not homogeneous. The mean (SD) Jadad scale and CONSORT statement scores were 3.43 (1.01) and 10.21 (2.63) respectively.
Conclusions: Evidence from RCTs on the treatment of postoperative pain after TOS is inadequate for clinical decision taking. Problem oriented assessment of interventions in this condition should evaluate composite interventions in representative populations, and should be based on longer observation periods, agreed clinically relevant outcomes, adequate allocation and blinding methods, and other methodological improvements.

ORAL

Proton Pump Inhibitors Used as High Dose Intravenous Infusion Decrease Both Re-Bleeding and Mortality in High-Risk Patients with Acute Peptic Ulcer Bleeding: a Series of Meta-Analyses.

Bardou M., Toubouti Y., Benhaberou-Brun D., Rahme E., Barkun A.
McGill University, Montréal, Canada

Objective. To assess the role of pharmacological treatments in the management of patients with acute ulcer bleeding.
Data Sources: Comprehensive searches of the MEDLINE and EMBASE databases from 1990 to August 2002 and scanning of references of the identified articles
Study selection: Randomized trials that assessed the efficacy of pharmacological treatments on re-bleeding (RB), surgery (S), and mortality (M). Pharmacotherapy was categorized into four groups: high dose intravenous proton pump inhibitors (HD IV-PPI, 80 mg bolus followed by 6-8 mg/h constant infusion), PPI (all routes and doses except high dose IV-PPI), H2-receptor antagonists (H2RA) and somatostatin and octreotide studied together.
Data extraction: Outcomes measured were the decrease of RB, S and M rates according to treatment groups. Data synthesis: A total of 30 studies involving of 3530 high-risk (Forrest Ia to IIb) patients were included in the meta-analyses. Pharmacotherapy of any type compared to placebo, significantly decreased RB (risk difference -12.2%; 95% confidence interval [-16.6%, -7.8%]) and M (-1.9%; [-2.6%, -1.2%]). HD IV-PPI, most often initiated following endoscopic therapy, significantly decreased RB compared to H2RA (-20.0%; [-21.4%, -19.0%]) and placebo (-15.6%; [-16.1%, -15.1%]). HD IV-PPI was also associated with a decrease in M compared to placebo (-2.8%; [-4.5%, -1.1%]). Compared to placebo, PPI (HD IV-PPI excluded) were associated with a significant decrease in both RB (-19.7%; [-23.4%, -15.8%]) and M (-2.4%; [-2.5%, -2.4%]) rates.
Conclusions: This study found a PPI-induced reduction in mortality in high risk patients with acute peptic ulcer bleeding.

P - 126

Real Time RT-PCR: A method for the Assessment of Immun-Response on mRNA Level. A case study on fosfomycin.

[1]Joukhadar C., [1]Jilma B., [1]Müller M., [2]Wagner O., [1,2]Marsik C.
[1]Department of Clinical Pharmacology, Division of Clinical Pharmacokinetics University of Vienna Medical School, Vienna; Austria [2]Institute of Medical and Chemical Laboratory Diagnostics, Vienna, Austria

Background: An established in-vitro endotoxin model was used to elicit an inflammatory reaction in human leukocytes. In the present study we explored the immuno-modulatory effects of fosfomycin, a broad spectrum antimicrobial agent frequently used in septic patients.
Methods: Whole blood from eight healthy volunteers was incubated with 50 pg/ml endotoxin and 100 µg/ml of fosfomycin or physiological sodium chlorite for a period of four hours. Total cellular RNA from whole human blood was extracted using the QIAmp RNA Mini Kits. For mRNA quantification the TaqMan Human Cytokine Card, a research tool for profiling human cytokine gene expression using the comparative CT method of relative quantification. Real time RT-PCR was performed on an Abi Prism 7700.
Results: Endotoxin incubation of human leukocytes increased tumor necrosis factor alpha (TNF-alpha) and interleukin-1 alpha (IL-1 alpha) mRNA levels up to several thousand fold. mRNA levels of interleukin-10 (IL-10) and M-CSF were enhanced by 500-1000 fold compared to baseline. However, addition of fosfomycin at therapeutically relevant plasma concentrations reduced TNF-alpha, IL-1 alpha and IL-10 cytokine expression by 30-50% after four hours. Expression of other cytokines was less pronounced ($p>0.05$). Levels of mRNA for IL-3, IL-5, IL-12p40, IL-13, IL-17, G-CSF and GM-CSF were not significantly affected by endotoxin and fosfomycin incubation.
Conclusion: Fosfomycin extensively decreased expression of pro-inflammatory cytokines in human leukocytes in vitro. The broad anti-microbial coverage of fosfomycin and its immuno-suppressive effects could be clinically useful, particularly in patients with known overwhelming immune response to bacterial pathogens.

P - 125

Intra- and Inter-Individual Variability in Losartan Metabolic Ratio, a Specific Marker of CYP2C9 Activity in Vivo

Eliasson E., Sandberg M., Christensen M., [1]Dahl M.L., [2]Yasar Ü.
Karolinska Institutet, Clinical Pharmacology, Huddinge University Hospital, SE 141 86 Stockholm, Sweden [1]Present address: Uppsala University Hospital, Sweden, [2]Present address: Hacettepe University, Ankara , Turkey

The angiotensin II receptor antagonist losartan is subject to CYP2C9-dependent oxidation, with the formation of a carboxylic acid metabolite, E-3174. Based on results from experiments performed in vitro and in vivo, we have proposed that losartan might serve as a CYP2C9-specific phenotyping agent, sensitive to CYP2C9 genotype and the hepatic level of CYP2C9 expression (1, 2). We here present further work on losartan in vivo, using the metabolic ratio (MR) between losartan and E-3174 in 0-8 hour urine samples after oral intake of 25 mg losartan. The intra-individual variability in CYP2C9 appears to be low, with a significant correlation between MRs measured at two different occasions (up to 6 months apart) in the same individual (3). Losartan was given to 137 healthy volunteers of Caucasian origin, as part of a cocktail with 4 other CYP-isozyme specific probe drugs. A significantly higher losartan MR in individuals hetero- (n=20) or homozygous (n=2) for the CYP2C9*3 allele was observed, but there was a marked variation even among individuals with the same genotype. The genetic basis for this variation is currently under investigation.

ORAL

Microdialysis: An Innovative Method for the Assessment of Penetration Properties of Antimicrobial Agents into Target Tissues in Humans

Joukhadar C., Zeitlinger M., Müller M.
Department of Clinical Pharmacology, Division of Clinical Pharmacokinetics University of Vienna Medical School, Vienna; Austria

Objective: The microdialysis (MD) technique is capable of measuring unbound concentrations of antibiotics in the interstitial space fluid (ISF) in select tissues. Measurement of ISF concentrations of antimicrobial agents is of particular importance as this compartment represents the relevant target site for antimicrobial therapy. We set out to assess the scope of this technique for pharmacokinetic (PK) and pharmacodynamic (PD) studies in patients and healthy volunteers.
Methods: MD was used to measure ISF concentrations (ISFCs) of several classes of antibiotics, i.e. ß-lactams, fosfomycin, fluoroquinolones, macrolides, oxazolidinones, ketolides and aminoglycosides following drug administration to healthy volunteers or patients. In addition, a new approach was developed to simulate in-vitro the antimicrobial effect of antibiotics at the target site based on in-vivo PK data obtained by MD.
Results: In healthy volunteers ISFCs of ß-lactams, oxazolidinones, fluoroquinolones and fosfomycin were in the range of unbound plasma concentrations. For macrolides, ketolides and aminoglycosides ISFCs were considerably lower than corresponding total plasma concentrations. Local inflammation exerted no influence on ISFCs, whereas capillary leakage associated with sepsis significantly affected ISFCs of all antibiotics. Using a combined PK/PD approach we could show that therapeutic success and failure in antimicrobial therapy may be explained by PK variability in ISFCs.
Conclusion: It is concluded that MD allows for the study of penetration properties of antimicrobial agents into select tissues in humans. The use of a PK/PD method permits the prediction of the antimicrobial effect of antibiotics at the target site.

## P - 127

Are We Participants or Bystanders?

[1]Milan Stanulovic, [2]Vid Stanulovic, [3]Dusan Duric
[1]Department of Pharmacology, Toxicology and Clinical Pharmacology, Medical School, University of Novi Sad, Yugoslavia, [2]Ingenix Pharmaceutical Services, Yugoslavia, , [3]ZORKAPharma, Yugoslavia

International Conference on Harmonization of Technical Requirements for Registration of Pharmaceuticals for Human Use (ICH) guidelines offer the mainframe for drug development. They were designed by and for the pharmaceutical industry and regulatory agencies with only the E6 Topic: GCP being more widely known to the medical-clinical community. The guidelines offer increasing guidance for specific study populations, indications, and aspects of early to final phases of development. An aspect the guidelines failed to consider, as being a non-technical requirement, is clinical drug development in the developing countries. This is being covered by other guidelines. The fifth revision of the Declaration of Helsinki on ethical principles for research involving human subjects, adopted in 2000, requires that at the conclusion of the study, every patient should be assured of access to the best therapy identified in the study. This statement raises the question how to project the optimal treatment in relation to socioeconomic status. CIOMS, Council for International Organizations of Medical Sciences, published its own International Ethical Guidelines for Biomedical Research Involving Human Subjects. As a body affiliated with WHO, CIOMS shares its broad global concern, including the developing world. Taking CIOMS recommendation as a model, developping countries can develop their guidelines on clinical trials being performed in their region, still retaining concordance with Helsinki declaration and the guidelines developed in rich countries and embodied in ICH documents.

## P - 128

Assessment of Opiates and Cocaine Consumption During Pregnancy by Self-Reported Questionnaire and Meconium Analysis

Pichini S., Zuccaro P., Marchei E., Pellegrini M., , Perez-Alarcón E., Puig C., Vall O., Pacifici R., Ordobas L., García-Algar Ó.
Istituto Superiore Di Sanita

The accurate assessment of fetal exposure to drugs of abuse through the objective measure of biomarkers could provide the basis for appropriate treatment and follow-up of new-borns, which can present symptoms of drug withdrawal. Furthermore, information regarding the real prevalence of drugs of abuse use during pregnancy could also be disclosed. Within the framework of "Meconium Project" aimed to estimate chronic fetal exposure to pharmaceuticals, drugs of abuse and tobacco smoke in Italy and Spain, we assessed the use of opiates and cocaine during pregnancy by maternal structured interview and meconium analysis. Structured interview was recorded the delivery day and meconium of 24 and 48 hours was collected and analysed by standardised liquid-chromatography-mass spectrometric methodologies. Up to now, 117 of the 1500 meconium samples of 24 and 48 hours, planned to be analysed during 2003-2004, have been examined. Only one case of opiates and two cases of cocaine consumption were disclosed by maternal interview. Conversely, analysis of 24 hours meconium detected 7(6.0%) cases of opiates consumption and 10 (8.5%) cases of cocaine consumption. The 48 hours meconium confirmed those findings. The high sensitivity of meconium analysis and the ease of collection make this test ideal for perinatal drug screening.

## P - 129

Resistance to Ceftriaxone in two Periods: First of Restricted Usage and Second of Unrestricted Usage

Knezevic A.,Dobrovic K., Morovic M.
General Hospital Zadar, Zadar, Croatia.

Despite more than 15 years of clinical use, ceftriaxone remains an effective and safe therapy for patients with infections caused by common Gram-pos. cocci and Gram-neg. bacilli. Until September 1999 it was on the regimen of reserve antibiotics and its utilisation in our hospital was restricted. That month it was released in free usage and in 2001 its utilization was five time higher than in 1999. The aim of this abstract is to analyse whether this higher utilisation in a two-year period increased ceftriaxone resistance in our hospital. This study was conducted in Zadar General Hospital, a 480 bed hospital with well-developed medicine and surgical wards. We analysed ceftriaxone susceptibility for the most commonly isolated Gram-neg. bacteria:E.Coli,Klebsiella sp,Proteus mirabilis and group of Enterobacter sp, Citrobacter sp and Serratia sp.Isolates from all sources and from all inpatients in two-six month periods (before and after free usage of ceftriaxone) in 1999 and 2001 were included.The sample of other bacteria was too small and not suitable for any analyses. In 1999 resistance for E.Coli was 3,08% vs. 1,27% in 2001,for Klebsiella values vere 5,97% vs. 1,89%, for group of Enterobacter, Citrobacter and Serratia it was 22,22% vs. 13,51%. In the same periods utilization of ceftriaxone was 0,66 DDD/100 pt days vs. 3,52 DDD/100 pt days. Different patterns of ceftriaxone usage in two six-month periods (restrictive and unrestrictive) in spite of five time higher utilisation rate did not increase Gram-neg. bacteria resistance on ceftriaxone. Could this resistance pattern be associated with lower usage of ceftazidime is the question to be answered.

## P - 130

Effects of the Administration Schedule of Oral Salmon Calcitonin on Bone Resorption Markers

[1]Bucher M., [1]Buclin T., [1]Cosma M., [2]Azria M., [2]Attinger M., [2]Mcleod J., [1]Biollaz J., [1]Burckhardt P.
[1]Division Of Clinical Pharmacology And Toxicology, Department Of Medicine, University Hospital, Lausanne, And [2]Novartis Pharma Inc., Basel, Switzerland.

A specific absorption promoter confers sufficient bioavailability (~1%) on calcitonin to design oral regimens for the treatment of bone disorders. To optimise the dosing schedule of this preparation, 12 healthy male volunteers (age 24±2y, weight 76±7kg) were included in a crossover study comparing three regimens : 0.5mg bid, 1mg qd and 1mg bid. Each treatment was given for 8 days, with 2-week washout between periods. On baseline and days 1 and 8 of each period, serial blood and urine measurements were performed to assess bone metabolism (urine and serum C-terminal telopeptide CTX, calcium and phosphate), plasma calcitonin and biological safety markers. All calcitonin doses markedly reduced bone resorption during subsequent hours, with a moderate difference between 0.5mg and 1mg (nadir plasma CTX: $p<0.0001$); evening doses were less effective than morning doses ($p<0.0001$); there was no response decrease between days 1 and 8, whatever the regimen. The overall daily effect on bone resorption tended to be larger under 1mg bid than 0.5mg bid and 1mg qd (AUC of plasma CTX: $p=0.08$). All doses had hypocalcemic, calciuretic and phosphaturic effects, without clearcut differences between regimens. Over all study periods, 105 mild/moderate adverse events were recorded (42 hot-flushes, 32 gastro-intestinal-symptoms), tending to be dose-related and to decrease over treatment periods. In conclusion, the effects of oral calcitonin in healthy subjects appear related to unitary dose and dosing frequency, however only to a limited extent. There was no evidence of escape phenomenon after one week. These observations may help optimise therapeutic regimens for the treatment of chronic conditions associated with bone loss.

## P - 131

Nociceptin Levels During the Cluster Headache Period

[1]Ertsey Cs., Hantos M., [1]Bozsik Gy., Tekes K.
[1]Department of Neurology and Department of Pharmacodynamics, Semmelweis University, Budapest, Hungary

The trigeminal innervation of the dura and its vessels has a prominent role in the pathomechanism of cluster headache. Nociceptin, an opioid neuropeptide, is the endogenous ligand of OP4R, a novel member of the opioid receptor family, with both algesic and analgesic properties depending on the site of action. Localisation studies have confirmed the presence of nociceptin and the OP4R in cells of the trigeminal ganglion where they colocalized with CGRP, a marker peptide of the trigeminovascular neurons. In an animal model, nociceptin has been found to inhibit neurogenic dural vasodilatation, a phenomenon related to trigeminovascular activation. To explore the possible involvement of nociceptin in cluster headache,we studied circulating levels of nociceptin when attack-free during the cluster period, using radioimmunoassay. In fourteen cluster headache patients nociceptin levels were significantly lower than in age-, and sex-matched controls (4.91±1.96 vs. 9.58±2.57 pg/ml, $p<0.0001$). Nociceptin levels did not correlate with age, disease length or episode length This finding suggests that there is a defective nociceptin- mediated regulation of trigeminal activity during the cluster period which may contribute to the genesis of the attacks.

## P - 132

Efficacy and Safety of Cizolirtine Citrate in the Treatment of Acute Pain Caused by an Attack of Renal Colic.

[1]Abadías M., [2]Suchı J., [1]Sust M., [3]Toufarová P., [4]Villoria J., [1]Bartlett A.
[1]Laboratorios Dr. Esteve, S. A. Av. Mare de Deu de Montserrat, 221 Barcelona - Spain, [2]Urologické oddělení. Fakultní Tomayerova Nemocnice [3]Urologické klinika. Fakultní nemocnice Plzeň [4]PRA International Literature

Objectives: to compare the analgesic efficacy and safety of cizolirtine citrate, an inhibitor of the release of the substance P, versus sodium metamizol to treat acute pain.
Method: sixty four patients presenting with acute pain from suspected renal colic were randomized to a single intravenous dose of either 350 mg of cizolirtine citrate or 2.500 mg of sodium metamizol. Pain was assessed throughout 6 hours by means of visual analogical (VAS) and categorical scales.
Results: renal colic was confirmed in all patients randomized. After 30 minutes, pain adjusted mean scores (100 mm VAS) were (LSM±SEM) 39.203±4.4 mm and 30.155±4.2 mm in the cizolirtine and metamizol groups, respectively ($p=0.1203$). Although not significant, means differed by less than 10 mm, and the proportion of patients showing satisfactory pain relief (decrease of pain intensity ≥50%) at 30 minutes in the cizolirtine group was high (64.5%).
Discussion: achievement of analgesic activity by systemic blockade of substance P release is an interesting finding as blocking NK-1 receptors did not achieve analgesia in former studies. However, efficacy was lower than that of the comparator, an established treatment. Cizolirtine could be more effective to prevent the sensitization of dorsal spinal horn than as a plain analgesic.

## P - 133

Heavy Users of NSAIDs in Finland. A Prescription Database Study

Huupponen R., Helin-Salmivaara A., Klaukka T.
Dept. of Pharmacology and Clinical Pharmacology, University of Turku; Finnish Medical Society Duodecim and The Social Insurance Institution, Finland.

The intensity of NSAID use was investigated in a systematic sample of 500 000 persons taken from the Finnish Population Register linked with the nation-wide prescription database. In 2000, the total and reimbursed use of NSAIDs was 61.2 and 31.2 DDD/1000 inhabitants/day, respectively. The annual pre- valence of low (<30 DDD/year), moderate (31-181 DDD/year)and heavy (>182 DDD/year)use of reimbursed NSAIDs was 7.6, 8.0 and 1.5 %, respectively. Of the heavy users, 27.7 % had continuously used NSAIDs >182 DDD over the preceding 4 years. In subjects without rheumatoid arthritis (RA), the prevalence of NSAID use increased with age, and females used NSAIDs more than men in all age groups. In RA patients the NSAID use was independent of age and gender. Forty-one per- cent of RA patients were heavy users in 2000, and 46 % of them had been heavy users during all preceding four years. Extrapolation to the whole population indicates that in the year 2000 there were about 60 000 non-RA heavy users of NSAIDs in Finland. This group includes especially females over 50 years of age. They are at risk for upper gastro- intestinal bleeding which should be taken into account when promoting rationale drug prescribing.

## ORAL

Initial Drug Therapy of Hypertension in Estonia

[1]Irs A., [2]Thetloff M.
[1]Division of Clinical Pharmacology, University of Tartu, Estonia, [2]Estonian Health Insurance Fund

The prevalence of cardiovascular disease is high in Estonia. This is reflected in expenditures for treatment of cardiovascular diseases. At the same time, control of blood pressure in hypertensive patients remains poor and the complications of hypertension are frequent. Our aim was to study the initial treatment of hypertension in Estonia and evaluate its clinical and economic soundness. A prescription database study was carried out. 2.5 million prescriptions from 01.01.2001 to 31.12.2002 for cardiovascular drugs were extracted, prescriptions for hypertension (ICD 10 diagnosis codes I10,11,12,13) from 01.05.2001 to 01.07.2002 were chosen to allow for pre- and post-prescription monitoring. 84 825 persons started pharmacotherapy for hypertension. 67 649 (80%) were treated by a GP and 17176 (20%) by a specialist. 77204 were treated with one agent, 7621 (9%) received combination therapy as their 1st treatment. ACE inhibitor was prescribed to 35% of patients, calcium channel blockers to 32% and beta-blockers to 29%. Diuretics were the first therapy in 2%. There were no major differences between the GPs and specialists. The initial therapy of hypertension in Estonia generally follows the current treatment guidelines, but is economically questionable. Marginal use of diuretics as first-line agents was detected. Further studies of co-morbidity and age distribution of patients are needed to judge the treatment decisions.

## P - 134

Chronic Ethanol Consumption and Papillary Muscle Responses to Nifedipine

[1]Rasic A., M.Prostran, [1]Stevanovic H.L., Todorovic Z., Vuckovic S., Stojanovic R., Nesic Z.
[1]Department of Physiology, Department of Clinical Pharmacology, School of Medicine, Belgrade, Yugoslavia

The aim of this study was to investigate the effect of the chronic ethanol (Eth) consumption on the inotropic effect of nifedipine (N). Five percent Eth in drinking water was given to male rabbits for six weeks; control (C) rabbits were given tap water. At the end of this period, response of the isolated papillary muscle (Pm) was studied (for details see Prostran et al., Cardiovasc.DrugsTher.2002, 16, Suppl.1, P440). In a continuously stimulated Pm with 0.1 Hz, a sudden change to 1 Hz produced a significant increase in the amplitude of the isometric contractions (IC) in both C- and Eth-group. Increase in the amplitude of the IC was more pronounced in the Eth-group in comparison with C-group (65% vs. 34%). In the presence of N (1.3 µmol; 45 min), a sudden change to 1 Hz produced a depression of the IC in both groups. A three-fold increase in Ca+2 concentration did not reverse this effect of N. A continuous ES (1 Hz for 20s) after 2, 4 and 8s pause, respectively, produced the post-rest-stimulation; the highest amplitude of the single IC was recorded after 8s pause, in both groups. N produced a depression of the IC, but did not change this phenomenon neither in C- nor in Eth-group. In both groups, a three-fold increase in Ca+2 concentration could not restore the amplitude of IC. In conclusion, chronic Eth consumption did not change the effect of N on the isolated ES rabbit Pm.

## ORAL

Considerations When Investigating Association between Drug Exposure and Hepatic Function.

Ghahramani P., Lennon S.M.
Roche Products Ltd, Welwyn Garden City, UK.

In many pharmacokinetic studies drug exposure is correlated with the concentrations of liver enzymes, using the conventional regression analysis, to calculate the slope of the relationship as a guide for dose adjustment based on hepatic function. For example, Kovarik et al (2001) related AUC of everolimus with bilirubin, reporting an increase in AUC of 56 (95% CI: 37-76) ng.h/ml per unit increase in bilirubin. Conventional regression analysis of a dependent variable (Y) on an independent variable (X) assumes that random variability in X is negligible. However, bilirubin has a large within individual CV of 20%. If despite a considerable variability in X the conventional regression analysis is applied, the slope and its 95% CI will be underestimated. Therefore, more sophisticated statistical techniques (Knuiman et al, 1998) must be applied to perform the regression analysis and more information is required with regard to the variability of X. In the example given above, if we adjust for the variability in X, using the method described previously (Ghahramani et al, 2001), the increase in exposure to everolimus is 85 (95% CI: 63-107) ng.h/ml per unit increase in bilirubin. This is significantly different (p<0.0001) from the estimates reported by Kovarik et al (2001) using the conventional regression analysis. These results suggest that the variability in indices of hepatic function (eg, bilirubin) must be considered and accounted for, if necessary, when assessing the relationship between exposure to a drug and indices of hepatic function.

## P - 135

Investigation of the Pharmacokinetics and Metabolism of Promegestone in Healthy Female Volunteers Following Single Oral Administration of 1 Mg Promegestone

[1]Gualano V., [1]Geneteau A., [1]Chassard D., [1]Fordham P., [2]Schatz B.
[1]Aster-Cephac, 3/5, Rue Eugène Millon, 75015 Paris, France [2]Laboratoire Aventis, 46 Quai De La Rapée, F-75601 Paris Cedex 12, France

A single 1 mg oral dose of promegestone (Surgestone®, 2x0.5 mg) was given to 12 healthy pre menopausal women. The aims were to determine the concentrations of promegestone and its metabolites and their pharmacokinetic parameters. Blood and urine samples were followed until 96 hours post dose. To avoid any interference with natural hormones, promegestone was given between day 7 and 10 of the menstrual cycle. Clinical safety and tolerability were good. Most of the minor adverse events observed were estimated possibly linked to the study drug (menstrual disorders) because classically related to progestins therapy. In addition, no clinically relevant biological modifications were observed. There was a stereoselective metabolism of promegestone in favor of the 21S hydroxy-promegestone, the main circulating compound in plasma (AUC ratio S/R of about 21). Levels of 21S hydroxy-promegestone are about twice greater than that of unchanged promegestone. The plasma levels of the second metabolite, i.e. 21R hydroxy-promegestone are far below these of either promegestone and 21S hydroxy-promegestone. Promegestone, 21S hydroxy- and 21R hydroxy-promegestone are not excreted in urine. About 3% of the dose was recovered in urine as sulfo and/or glucuro-conjugate 21S hydroxy-promegestone and about 1% of the dose as sulfo and/or glucuro conjugate 21R hydroxy-promegestone

## P - 136

Chemotherapy for Lung Cancer: Rationalization of Costs

Cervellino J.C., Araujo C.E., Fligman M.D., Pires E.A.
Chair of Pharmacology, School of Medicine, University of Buenos Aires (Argentina).

The development of new drugs for non-small cell lung cancer could be a big success in the treatment of this disease, improving objective response rate and quality of life. To cope with this formidable challenge, interest seems to be focused exclusively in the development of new molecules. But, what about the well-known old agents combinations? Are they not useful anymore? Generally speaking, modern cancer chemotherapy includes combination of new drugs exclusively. However, recent results are often quite similar to those achieved in the past at low cost and with mild toxicity. Comparison with the national history of the disease could shed some light to the actual value of trials' result. According to P. Bunn (ESO Monograph, 1991), median survival (MST) for non-small cell lung cancer was 27 weeks, which is quite similar to most data reported in the last 20 years (Table). If the therapeutic benefit over old treatments is null, is the benefit obtained from an economic analysis? Again, the answer is negative (Table), Considering the higher cost of new drugs and their severe toxicity, the cost-benefit relationship does not seem to be better.

| Chemotherapy | OR (%) | MST (mo) | Six cycles cost (US$) |
|---|---|---|---|
| Gemcitabine + DDP | 30 | 9.8 | 30,006 |
| Paclitaxel + carboplatin | 32 | 9.9 | 40,200 |
| Ifosfamide + epirubicine | 51 | 12.0 | 16,938 |
| Cyclophosphamide | 38 | 9.0 | 504 |

Probably a smarter approach could be to combine both old and new agents, in order to achieve better results when analyzed from the patient's point of view.

## P - 137

Pentoxifylline: Pharmacokinetics of an Acqueous Oral Solution and Influence on PTH Secretion in Healthy Volunteers.

Rochat M.C., Buclin T., Decosterd L.A., [1]Sanderson P., Biollaz J.
Division of Clinical Pharmacology, University Hospital, Lausanne, Switzerland; [1]Aventis, Romainville, France.

Recent research shows that daily subcutaneous injections of parathyroid hormone (PTH) significantly stimulate bone formation in osteoporotic patients. An oral agent able to stimulate the endogenous secretion of PTH would provide a convenient alternative. Animal experimentation showed that pentoxifylline, a methylxantine derivative with phosphodiesterase inhibitory action, can induce PTH secretion bursts. We hypothesized that similar effects could be observed in humans. The pharmacokinetics and the effects of an oral solution of pentoxifylline on PTH activity and calcium metabolism were investigated in 6 healthy young volunteers (mean ± SD: age=29±8 years). Each subject received four doses of pentoxifylline (50 mg, 100 mg, 200 mg and 400 mg), one oral placebo and one intravenous infusion of EDTA as verum (50 mg/kg over 2 h) in a partly randomised, cross-over, 6-period study, under standardized diet. All oral doses were absorbed rapidly (Tmax= 0.4, 0.3, 0.3 and 0.2 h, Cmax= 243, 746, 1731 and 4211 ug/L after 50, 100, 200 and 400 mg respectively). The average terminal half-life, apparent distribution volume and systemic clearance were 1.2 h, 277 L and 189 L/h respectively. Pentoxifylline induced no change either in PTH plasma levels, or in urinary cyclic AMP excretion, or in phospho-calcic metabolism, compared to placebo. Conversely, the EDTA infusion induced a marked increase in PTH levels and in calcium excretion rate, as well as a profound decrease in total and ionised serum calcium concentrations, lasting for at least 6 h. In conclusion, pentoxifylline does not appear to stimulate PTH secretion.

## P - 138

Effects of Paracetamol on Antioxidant Enzymes in Erythrocytes in Febrile Children Bajcetic M., Mitrovic J., Divac N., Samardzic R.
Faculty of Medicine, Dept. Of Clinical Pharmacology. University Children Hospital, Biochemistry Laboratory, Belgrade, Serbia and Montenegro

Paracetamol has been used for years as a safe antipyretic drug at therapeutic doses for children. However severe hepatotoxicity associated with oxidative stress and gluthatione depletion has been observed in paracetamol intoxication. However strong doubts on optimum dosage and dosing interval of paracetamol in children still remain. The objective of this study was to determine changes in antioxidant enzymes in erythrocytes of febrile children receiving paracetamol in recommended therapeutic doses and intervals. Children aged from 2 months to 12 years were divided in two groups(G).G1: afebrile children (n=21) who did not receive paracetamol. G2: children (n=19) who had fever above 38°C lasting more then 24 h and received paracetamol in the recommended therapeutic dose and intervals. Blood samples were taken for glutathione (GSH),glutathion reductase (GR), glutathion peroxidase (GPx), glutation S transferase (GST),superoxid dismutase (SOD) and liver transaminases. The activities of GR ($p<0.001$), GSH ($p<0.05$) and SOD ($p<0.05$) were significantly reduced in group 2 as compared with group 1, while liver transaminase (AST) level was slightly increased. Paracetamol applied in febrile children in recommended therapeutic doses and intervals significantly reduced erythrocyte antioxidant enzymes levels, which may predict an increased risk of hepatotoxity.

## P - 139

Newer Hypnotic Drugs for Short-Term Pharmacotherapy for Insomnia: a Systematic Review

[1]Dundar Y., [1]Boland A., [1]Dickson R., [1]Haycox A., [1]Strobl J., [1]Walley T.
[1]Liverpool Reviews and Implementation Group, Department of Pharmacology and Therapeutics, University of Liverpool, UK

Background: Insomnia is a common problem (population prevalence 10-38%) and drugs, especially benzodiazepines, are often prescribed (in the second quarter of 2002, UK Prescription Pricing Authority recorded over 1.5 million items of benzodizepines having been prescribed). Non-benzodiazepine hypnotics (zaleplon, zolpidem and zopiclone) may overcome some of the adverse effects associated with benzodiazepines including tolerance, dependency and withdrawal symptoms.
Objective: To assess the clinical effectiveness of newer hypnotic drugs (zaleplon, zolpidem and zopiclone) compared to benzodiazepines licensed and approved for use in the UK for short-term management of insomnia (nitrazepam, loprazolam, lormetazepam and temazepam).
Methods: We conducted a systematic review, using bibliographic databases, The Cochrane Library and handsearches of key articles to identify randomised controlled trials that compared either benzodiazepines to the new drugs or any two of the new drugs in patients with non-organic insomnia requiring short-term pharmacotherapy as well as volunteers. Outcome measures included: sleep latency, sleep duration, number of awakenings, sleep quality, quality of life and adverse effects. A meta-analysis will be carried out; for binary outcomes relative treatment effects will be presented in the form of odds ratios, for continuous outcomes, mean differences will be calculated.
Results: The review is in progress and will be completed for conference presentation, which will include an outline of the review results.

## P - 140

Sustained Hemodynamic Effects of Intravenous Levosimendan

[1]Lehtonen L.A., [2]Kivikko M., [3]Colucci W.S.
[1]Helsinki University Central Hospital, Laboratory Services, Helsinki, Finland; [2]Orion Pharma, Clinical Research, Espoo Finland; [3]Boston University Medical Centre, Boston, MA, USA

The short term infusion of the calcium sensitser drug levosimendan (LS) improves hemodynamic function in patients with decompensated heart failure. LS has metabolites with long-elimination half-life. The goal of this study was to determine whether the hemodynamic effects of LS last beyond the discontinuation of the drug infusion. The study was the continuation phase of a double-blind, placebo-controlled study in patients with decompensated heart failure (cardiac index below 2.5 l/min/m2, pulmonary capillary wedge pressure over 15 mmHg) who received escalating infusion rates (0.1-0.4 mcg/kg/min) of intravenous LS (n = 98) or placebo (n = 48) for 6 hr. At the end of 6 hr infusion, 85 of LS-treated patients were continued on open-label drug (0.1-0.2 mcg/kg/min) for a total of 24 hr, and constitute the study population in this report. After 24 hours infusion patients were again randomized in a 1:1 ratio to an additional 24 hr of LS (n = 43) or placebo(n = 42). Hemodynamics and plasma concentration of LS and its major metabolites OR-1855 and OR-1896 were measured before and 1, 2, 4, 6 and 24 hours after randomised drug withdrawal. The increase in cardiac index and reduction in pulmonary capillary wedge pressure observed at 24 hr were maintained in both the LS continuation and withdrawal groups despite a fall in LS plasma levels. The levels of the active metabolites increased for at least 24 hours after the cessation of the drug infusion. The accumulation of active metabolites of LS results in prolonged hemodynamic effects that may be of therapeutic value in patients who are hospitalised for decompensated heart failure.

## P - 141

The three-arm Trial: Report of a Practical Case Illustrating the Utility of This Approach to Assess the Assay Sensitivity

[1]Videla S., [1]Sust M., [2]Villoria J., [1]Abadías M., [1]Fresquet A., [1]Costa A., [1]Bartlett A.

[1]Laboratorios Dr. Esteve, S. A. Av. Mare de Deu de Montserrat, 221 Barcelona 08041; Spain. [2]PRA International

Introduction: a three-arm trial, including both placebo and a known active treatment can readily assess whether failure to distinguish test treatment from placebo implies ineffectiveness of test treatment or simply the result of a trial lacking the ability to identify an active drug. Here, we provide an example of the usefulness of such a trial.
Methods: 161 patients with a psychiatric disorder were randomized to either placebo, an established treatment (reference, active control), or test treatment in parallel design. Efficacy was evaluated with a validated quantitative scale. Changes from baseline were compared among treatments. An effect size of 2 points was considered clinically relevant.
Results: intra-group mean reductions were 5.6 points (placebo), 5.9 (reference) and 5.7 (test). Between-group differences (mean, lower and upper limits 95% confidence interval) were: test-pla: 0.1 (-1.84, 2.04); ref-test: 0.2 (-1.54, 1.94); ref-pla: 0.3 (-1.51, 2.11).
Discussion: a two-group trial with test and placebo would not have concluded in favour of efficacy of test drug, while such trial with test and active control would have concluded efficacy of test drug (non-inferiority). Inclusion of both controls has provided evidence of the lack of assay sensitivity of the study which precludes obtaining conclusions in one or other way.

## P - 142

Food Effect on the Double Peak Phenomenon Occurrence in Famotidine Bioequivalence Studies

Kopecky J., Zoulova J., Filipova K., Pastera J., Chladek J., Svoboda D., [1]Macek K., Kvetina J.

Institute of Experimental Biopharmaceutics, Joint Research Center of PRO.MED.CS Praha a.s. & the Academy of Sciences of the Czech Republic, Hradec Kralove, [1]Faculty Hospital, Hradec Kralove, Czech Republic

Characteristic pharmacokinetic feature of orally administered H2-blockers, including famotidine, is occurrence of the double peak in the plasma concentration-time profile, explained by site-dependent intestinal absorption. It complicates the evaluation of bioequivalence (particularly in parameters cmax and tmax). We attempted to influence this phenomenon by food. Two bioequivalence (randomized, cross-over, single dose) studies were performed. In both studies, two different famotidine tablet formulations were administered orally (dose 40 mg) to healthy volunteers. The administration was followed by a standardized breakfast 2 hours after famotidine ("fasting" study) or immediately after famotidine ("fed" study). While in "fasting" study the second peak was observed in 46 % of plasma concentration-time profiles, in "fed" study it was only in 6 % of profiles. Thus, food immediately after famotidine administration reduced the double peak occurrence. To explain the mechanism of this reduction, one can speculate about the changes in intestinal transit rates and intestinal water fluxes induced by food.

## P - 143

The Relationship of in Vitro Dissolution and Human Bioavailability on the Model of Two Oral Isosorbide-5-Mononitrate (Is-5-Mn) Formulations

[1]Vyslouzil L., [1]Kopecký J., [1]Pastera J., [2]Macek K., [1]Chládek J., [1]Rezanka V., [1]Kvetina J.

[1]Institute of Experimental Biopharmaceutics, Joint Research Centre of PRO.MED.CS Praha a.s. & Academy of Sciences of the Czech Republic, Hradec Králové; [2]Faculty Hospital, Hradec Králové, Czech Republic

On the model of oral IS-5-MN formulations, we investigated relationship between dissolution rate and bioavailability of substance with high solubility. Two 40 mg IS-5-MN tablet formulations (Monosan, PRO.MED.CS Praha a.s., Czech Republic and Mono Mack, Intercaps Zlín, Czech Republic) were compared in dissolution test (pH 5.8) and in bioequivalence study; it was designed as open, randomised, cross-over. Formulations were administered in a single dose of 40 mg with a wash-out period of 14 days to 24 healthy volunteers (18-53 years). There was no difference in dissolution profile between formulations; ≥90 % of IS-5-MN was released in up to 5 min. Also bioequivalence of the formulations was proven (in all parameters):

| Parameter | | Monosan | Mono Mack | 90% confid. interval |
|---|---|---|---|---|
| $AUC_{0\rightarrow\infty}$ | [ng.h/l] | 7.5±1.5 | 7.6±1.5 | 95-101 % |
| $AUC_{0\rightarrow 32}$ | [ng.h/l] | 7.3±1.6 | 7.5±1.5 | 95-101 % |
| $c_{max}$ | [ng/l] | 1.17±0.30 | 1.12±0.29 | 97-113 % |
| $t_{max}$ | [h] | 0.64±0.40 | 0.59±0.37 | from -0.13 to 0.25 h |
| $k_e$ | [h-1] | 0.130±0.026 | 0.130±0.028 | - |
| $t_{1/2}$ | [h] | 5.6±1.3 | 5.6±1.3 | - |

We conclude that the in vitro dissolution test predicted well in vivo comparative bioavailability of model drug formulations with high water solubility.

## P - 144

The Effect of Food on Bioavailability of Propafenone

[1]Zoulová J., [1]Kopecký J., [2]Perlík F., [1]Anzenbacherová E., [1]Svoboda D., [1]Chládek J., [1]Kvetina J.

[1]Institute of Experimental Biopharmaceutics, Joint Research Center of PRO.MED.CS Praha a.s. and Academy of Sciences of the Czech Republic, Hradec Králové, [2]1st Faculty of Medicine, Charles University, Prague, Czech Republic

The effect of food on pharmacokinetic parameters of propafenone was investigated in two open, randomized, crossover studies involving 12 (fasted state) and 24 (fed state) healthy volunteers. Formulations (Propanorm tab., PRO.MED.CS Praha a.s., Czech Republic vs Rytmonorm tab., Knoll, FRG) were administered in a single oral dose of 300 mg with washout period of 14 days in both studies. Bioequivalence of compared formulations was proven both in the fed and fasted study. Pharmacokinetic parameters AUC and $c_{max}$ were increased when administered with food (Propanorm fasted vs fed: $AUC_{0\rightarrow\infty}$ 883 vs 1310 ng.h/ml, $AUC_{0\rightarrow t}$ 826 vs 1229 ng.h/ml, $c_{max}$ 241 vs 319 ng/ml; Rytmonorm fasted vs fed: $AUC_{0\rightarrow\infty}$ 832 vs 1291 ng.h/ml, $AUC_{0\rightarrow t}$ 767 vs 1226 ng.h/ml, $c_{max}$ 208 vs 314 ng.h/ml). Food had no effect on $t_{max}$. Intrasubject coefficients of variation of pharmacokinetic parameters increased in the fed state (fasted vs fed: $AUC_{0\rightarrow\infty}$ 27.2 vs 42.5 %, $AUC_{0\rightarrow t}$ 31.6 vs 45.3 %, $c_{max}$ 42.8 vs 51.1 %). In conclusion, food increases the bioavailability and variability of propafenone in healthy volunteers after single oral dose.

## P - 145

CYP1A2 Activity in Caucasians - Relationship to Smoking Habits, Use of Oral Contraceptives and 3 SNPs in Intron 1 of the CYP1A2 Gene.

Christensen M., Nordmark A., Aklillu E., Schrey S., Ingelman-Sundberg M., Bertilsson L.
Karolinska Institutet, Clinical Pharmacology, Huddinge University Hospital, SE 141 86 Stockholm, Sweden

Objectives: To determine the influence of mutations in intron 1 and environmental factors on the activity of the drug metabolising enzyme CYP1A2.
Methods: 132 Caucasians were recruited for phenotyping with caffeine using the paraxanthine / caffeine (P/C) ratio in 4 h plasma analyzed by HPLC. Three SNPs in intron 1 at positions -740T®G, -730C®T and -164C®A were analyzed by SNP-specific PCR-RFLP genotyping. The frequency, linkage disquilibrium and genotypes were assessed in relationship to the P/C ratio.
Results: Smoking, use of oral contraceptives and heavy coffee consumption influenced the P/C ratio (P<0.001) shown by ANOVA analysis. None of the 3 SNPs had an effect on the P/C ratio and the effect of -164C®A previously claimed to be associated with CYP1A2 induction by smoking could not be confirmed (1). Four different haplotypes were identified: *1A; *1F; *1J and *1K with the frequency of 25, 72, 2.6 and 0.4%, respectively. Six genotypes were found for different combinations of the 3 SNPs. The -740T®G mutation was always linked to -164C®T whereas -730C®T was always linked to -740T®G, i.e. a subject with -730C®T carries always the other two mutations.
Conclusions: The metabolism of drugs by CYP1A2 is highly influenced by environmental factors. Thus, lower doses of such drugs may be needed when co-administered with oral contraceptives and higher doses are needed in smokers and in heavy coffee consumers. New CYP1A2 genotypes are originated from linked mutations. The different results concerning the -164C®A SNP may be due to different measures of the CYP1A2 phenotype

## P - 146

Paraoxon Induces Apoptosis in EL4 Cells via Activation of Mitochondrial Pathways.

Saleh A.
United Arab Emirates University

The toxicity of organophosphorus compounds, such as paraoxon (POX), is due to their anticholinesterase action. Recently, we have shown that, at non-cholinergic doses (1 to 10 nM), POX (the bioactive metabolite of parathion) causes apoptotic cell death in murine EL4 T-lymphocytic leukemia cell line through activation of caspase-3. In this study, by employing caspase specific inhibitors, we extend our observations to elucidate the sequence of events involved in POX-stimulated apoptosis. Pretreatment of EL4 cells with the caspase-9 specific inhibitor zLEHD-fmk attenuated POX induced apoptosis in a dose-dependent manner, whereas the caspase-8 inhibitor zIETD-fmk had no effect. Furthermore, the activation of caspase-9, -8, and -3 in response to POX treatment was completely inhibited in the presence of zLEHD-fmk, implicating the involvement of caspase 9-dependent mitochondrial pathways in POX stimulated apoptosis. Indeed, under both in vitro and in vivo conditions, POX triggered a dose- and time-dependent translocation of cytochrome C from mitochondria into the cytosol, as assessed by Western blot analysis. Investigation of the mechanism of cytochrome C release revealed that POX disrupted mitochondrial transmembrane potential. Neither this effect nor cytchrome C release was dependent on caspase activation, since the general inhibitor of the caspase family zVAD-fmk did not influence both processes. Finally, POX treatment also resulted in a time-dependent up-regulation and translocation of the pro-apoptotic molecule Bax to mitochondria. Inhibition of this event by zVAD-fmk suggests that the activation and translocation of Bax to mitochondria is subsequent to activation of the caspase cascades.

## P - 147

Fluconazole in Anuric Patients Undergoing Continuous-Veno-Venous-Hemodialysis (CVVHD): Pharmacokinetics and Dosage Simulation

Mueller S.C., Majcher-Peszynska J., Mundkowski R.G., Hickstein H., Drewelow B. Institute for Clinical Pharmacology, University of Rostock, Germany

Background: Invasive candidal infections are a cause of mortality in ICU patients. Efficacy of fluconazole against candida spp. is dose dependent and related to AUC/MIC. To treat patients undergoing CVVHD effectively, therapeutic fluconazole levels have to be secured.
Methods: 10 anuric intensive care patients undergoing standardized CVVHD were included. Blood and dialysate samples were taken before administration and at 11 further timepoints. Pharmacokinetic parameters were calculated and used for simulation of AUC/MIC ratios and trough levels of various dosage schemes.
Results: A saturation coefficient of 0.7 ± 0.2 demonstrated almost unlimited passage of Fluconazol via the dialyzer. Main pharmacokinetic parameters were: t1/2: 23.3 ± 13 h, total body clearance: 25.5 ± 15 ml/min, Cl by CVVHD: 17.3 ± 5 ml/min. Dosage simulation revealed that 400 mg fluconazole/day seem to be sufficient for candida species susceptible (NCCLS), in susceptible-dose-dependent candida species, 800 mg/day seem to be adequate.
Conclusion: CVVHD cleared Fluconazole in anuric patients comparably with healthy individuals. Fluconazol dosage in CVVHD patients should be preferably 800mg/day if candida species with susceptible-dose dependend MIC´s cannot be excluded.

## P - 148

The Effect of Caffeine-Containing Coffee Versus Decaffeinated Coffee on Serum Clozapine Concentrations in Hospitalised Patients

[1]Raaska K., [2]Raitasuo V., [1]Laitila J., [1]Neuvonen P.J.
[1]Department of Clinical Pharmacology, University of Helsinki, Finland; [2]Kellokoski Hospital, Finland

Background: Clozapine and caffeine are metabolised mainly by cytochrome P4501A2 (CYP1A2) enzyme. Previous studies suggest that caffeine in coffee inhibits clozapine metabolism and increases serum clozapine concentrations, but there have been no placebo groups in these studies.
Methods: A randomised placebo-controlled crossover design with two phases, both seven days, was used to study whether coffee in usually consumed amounts has an effect on steady state serum clozapine concentrations. This study comprised twelve hospitalised clozapine-using patients. After a run-in period, either caffeine containing or decaffeinated instant coffee was available ad libitum for seven days. Two patients were dropped out because of non-compliance.
Results: Caffeine-containing coffee increased mean serum clozapine trough concentration by 20% (range -3%- +41%, p= 0.03) and N-desmethylclozapine concentration by 7% (range -10% - +23%; p= 0.02). N-desmethylclozapine/clozapine ratio decreased by 9% (range -26%- +11%; p= 0.06) but the clozapine-N-oxide / clozapine ratio remained essentially unchanged (range -23% - +21, p=0.93). During the decaffeinated coffee phase mean serum caffeine concentration was 5% and paraxanthine concentration 8% of the corresponding concentrations during the caffeine phase.
Conclusions: The regular caffeine-containing instant coffee, in usually consumed amounts, increases only modestly serum clozapine concentration in most patients. The most likely mechanism of this interaction is the inhibition of the CYP1A2 enzyme by caffeine.

ORAL

The Management of Hyperlipidaemia in CAPD Patients

Velickovich- Radovanovich R., Avramovich M., Raicevich R., Mitich B., Kostich S., Djordjevich V.
Institute of Nehrology and Haemodialysis, Clinic Centre Nis Serbia & Montenegro

The high risk of atherosclerosis in continuous ambulatory peritoneal dialysis (CAPD) patients is rather increased by common lipid disorders (hypercholesterolaemia - HC and combined hyperlipidaemia - CHL). High triglycerides (TG) and low HDL- cholesterol levels are typical for CAPD patients, and elevated LDL-C is also common. CAPD patients with CHL (LDL-C> 4,0mmol/l, TG > 2,3mmol/l) and isolated HC (LDL-C> 4,0mmol/l, TG < 2,3mmol/l) participated in a randomised double- blind parallel 24- week comparison between fluvastatin (n=31) and gemfibrozil ( n=29). Fluvastatin was administered 20 mg/dl while gemfibrozil was given 300mg twice daily. Fluvastatin caused decrease a 38,5 - 42% in CHL and HC, while gemfibrozil caused a 15% decrease in H and no change in CHL. Fluvastatin had no effect on TG levels in HC but resulted in a 28% decrease in CHL, and gemfibrozil caused a 52% fall in TG levels in both lipid phenotypes. During treatment no significant side effects were observed and liver and muscle enzymes remained within normal values. Fluvastatin was highly effective in lowering LDL-C in both lipid phenotypes, fluvastatin is consequently preferred treatment of HC and CHL, in CAPD. Gemfibrozil can be used in normocholesterolemic patients high triglyceride levels, in CAPD.

P - 149

Efficacy and Safety Fluvastatın Compared to Simvastatin in Capd Patients

Raicevic R., Velickovic- Radovanovic R., Avramovic M., Kostic S.
Institute of Nephrology and Haemodialysis, Clinic center of Nis Serbia

Dyslipoproteinemia is an important risk factor for cardiovascular disease in uraemic patients on continuous ambulatory peritoneal dialysis (CAPD). This six months study was designed to confirm the efficacy and safety of fluvastatin compared to simvastatin, a marketed agent for low density lipoprotein cholesterol (LDL -C) reduction in hypercholesterolemic patients. After a 6- week placebo baseline phase patients were randomized to receive fluvastatin or simvastatin. We conducted a single blind cross- over study versus placebo, in 46 patients ( mean duration CAPD 28, 23 +/- 14,15 month, age 51,3 =/- 6,7 years) for elevated levels of cholesterol -C (> 6,2mmol/l) and LDL-C (> 3,9mmol/l), to evaluate the efficacy and safety fluvastatin (10mg/ day) and simvastatin (10mg/ day). Fluvastatin significantly lowered LDL-C from baseline by 38,5% compared with 31,5% for simvastatin (p< 0,05). A total of 42 % of fluvastatin patients attained the target level of < 3,4 mmol/l compared to 28% of simvastatin patients. Fluvastatin and simvastatin reduced significantly C and LDL-C in our patients, they are well tolerated and may be useful to reduce LDL-C, indicators of coronary risk. The adverse event profile was similar both treatment groups and neither treatment caused clinically relevant laboratory abnormalities. In conclusion fluvastatin is superior to simvastatin in treating CAPD patients with hypercholesterolemia.

P - 150

HLA Class II Molecules and Drug-Induced Idiosyncratic Liver Disease. A Multicenter Study

[1]Lucena M.I., [2]Andrade R.J., [1]Alonso A., [3]Fernández M.C., [4]Durán J.A., [1]Torres E.L., [1]Seoane J., [1]Verge C., [1]De la Cuesta F.S.
[1]Servicio de farmacología Clínica y [2]Unidad de Hepatología H. Universitario, F Med. Málaga; [3]Servicio de Farmacología Clínica H Torrecárdenas, Almería; [4]S. Ap. Digestivo Hospital H. V. Macarena, Sevilla.

Background: The HLA class II genes of the MHC are central to immune processing of exogenous antigens, and, could be theoretically involved in immunologically-mediated drug-induced idiosyncratic liver disease (DIILD). Recently, an association between amoxicillin-clavulanate induced hepatitis and the haplotype DRB1*1501-DQB1*0602 has been reported. Aims: to investigate if there could exist an association between a particular HLA class II alleles and the propensity to develop DIILD. Methods: 140 patients with probable or definitive DIILD, as assessed by CIOMS scale, in whom a blood sample was obtained, were included in the study. HLA-DRB and -DQB were typed by polimerase chain reaction-sequence specific oligonucleotides (SSO)method genomic DNA (when required PCR-sequence specific primers were used), with 635 volunteer bone marrow and blood donors serving as controls.Results: Frequencies of HLA-DRB and -DQB alleles in patients with DIILD did not differ significantly from the control subjects (Table). Neither the presence of hypersensitivity features nor the type of injury (cholestatic or mixed) or the individual drug co-amoxiclav (n=22) were associated with an specific HLA class II molecule. Conclusions: There is no association between any specific HLA genotype and DIILD considered collectively or when the cohort of patients with co-amoxiclav induced hepatotoxicity was evaluated. ( This study has partly been supported by a grant from FIS nº: 01/1088)

HLA class II phenotypic frequencies in patients with DIILD

| Allele | Patients (n=140) | Controls (n=635) |
|---|---|---|
| DRB1*01 | 23.4% | 20.0% |
| DRB1*15-16 | 35.2% | 22.9% |
| DRB1*03 | 20.0% | 25.2% |
| DRB1*04 | 26.9% | 23.9% |
| DRB1*07 | 23.4% | 35.4% |
| DRB1*13 | 24.1% | 22.9% |
| DRB1*14 | 9.0% | 5.2% |
| DQB1*05 | 42.5% | 36.1% |
| DRB1*06 | 43.8% | 40.8% |

## P - 151

Consumption Trend of Anticonvulsant Agents in Sarajevo Svjetlana

[1]Loga S., [2]Loga S., [1]Mulabegovic N., [3]Skaljic A., [1]Kusturica J., [1]Rakanovic M., [1]Becic F.
[1]Institute of Pharmacology, Faculty of Medicine, University of Sarajevo, Cekalusa 90, 71000 Sarajevo, B&H [2]Neuropsychiatry of University of Sarajevo, Faculty of Medicine Sarajevo [3]Informative Service of Pharmacies of Sarajevo

The goal of this study was to establish anticonvulsant drug consumption in Sarajevo. Sarajevo is a principal and the largest city in Bosnia and Herzegovina (about a half of million citizens). The method of this study was to collect the consumption data of any anticonvulsant agent sold in five biggest pharmacies in Sarajevo. The investigation period was from 01/06/2000 to 31/1/2002 (three years). The most applied anticonvulsant agents in year 2000 were carbamazepine (tbl. a 200 mg) and valproic acid (drag. a 150 mg) with registered significant consumption increase (Yc=201500.00) in comparison to year 2002 (Yc= 152450.00), respectively valproic acid (Yc= 58833.00 versus Yc= 52633.33). The most positive consumption trend had methylphenylbarbitone (tbl. a 30 mg) (Yc=230.00 in year 2000 versus Yc=1250.00 in year 2002), while in the same time, a decreased consumption trend (Yc=10410.00 versus Yc= 4590.00) was registered for valproic acid (sol. 30%). A positive consumption trend was registered for phenobarbitone tablets a 15 mg in year 2001 (Yc= 4380.00). Generally, anticonvulsant agent consumption showed a tendency to decrease during the three years of investigation. However, in year 2002, new anticonvulsants were introduced in therapy protocols, although still in small amounts (lamotrigine and vigabatrin).

## P - 152

Application Dossier for Marketing Authorization in the European Union and Federation of Bosnia and Herzegovina

Todic M., Becic F., Loga-Zec S., Kusturica J.
Institute of Pharmacology and Toxicology, Sarajevo, Bosnia and Herzegovina

The content of the dossier in the European Union is defined in the Common Technical Document agreed in 2000. It consists of five Modules: -
Module 1, Administrative and prescribing information including Summary of Product Characteristics, Labeling and Package Leaflet information, Certificate of authorization in the country of manufacture and information about authorizations in another countries; - Module 2, Quality, Nonclinical and Clinical Summaries; - Module 3, Quality data; - Module 4, Nonclinical studies; - Module 5, Clinical studies. Legislation in the Federation consider following: - Application; - Documentation on clinical, pharmaco-toxicological and laboratory evaluation; - Certificate of authorization in the country of manufacture, Good manufacture practice certificate and List of obtained authorizations in another countries; -
Package Leaflet text; -Safe disposal of expired drug; There is no substantial difference in the content, but considered information in European Union is more defined and extensive. The differences between European and domestic rules for authorization will be discussed, and some propositions that are in our country possibilities have already been adapted.

## P - 153

Diclofenac Systemic Exposure is not Increased When Topical Diclofenac is Applied on Uv-Induced Erythema

[1]Magnette J.L., [1]Kienzler J.L., [1]Sallin D., Ménart C., Nollevaux F., Knops A.
[1]Novartis Consumer Health SA, Nyon, Switzerland

The aim of this trial was to determine if the systemic exposure to diclofenac is enhanced after topical application of diclofenac sodium (new gel formulation) on UV-injured skin. The study was conducted in 18 Caucasian healthy volunteers as a sequential design. Diclofenac sodium was applied twice (total of 25mg) during a single day on 2500 cm2 (about 15% body surface) normal skin and then on the same skin area during the acute phase of an erythema induced by 3 times the UV minimal erythemal dose. In-between, each subject also received 25mg enteric-coated diclofenac sodium given orally 3 times in a single day. The results show that the relative bioavailability of diclofenac when applied on sunburned skin was less than 3% (plasma data, <3% for AUC and <1% for Cmax) to 7 % (urinary excretion over 72 h) of that of oral diclofenac. It was virtually identical to that measured on normal skin with a point estimate of 96% for urinary excretion (90 % CI: 81-114 %). The general safety and local tolerability of the tested diclofenac sodium formulation were very good on both normal and sunburned skin. The local adverse events (erythema, local pain) were related to the UV-exposure.

## P - 154

Information about Drugs Available for our Medical Staff

Beèiæ F., Mulabegoviæ N., Kapiæ E., Kusturica J., Loga-Zec S., Todiæ-Rakanoviæ M. Institute of Pharmacology, Clinical Pharmacology and Toxicology, Faculty of Medicine, University of Sarajevo

National policy of medicines is a very important factor for the progress of any State. Therefore medicine is a priority of any medical system. Safety, effectivity and availability of the medicines with proper quality are basis of the racional pharmacotherapy. Medical worker can find useful information about medicines, their properly and rationaly application in drug register. Different situations demand a necessity of use of medicines with different brand names. Consequently, it is necessary to highlight an application and usage of INN medicines. Unreasonably prescribing of medicines may result with excessive costs of the health care. With regard to a very difficult financial situation in Federation of Bosnia and Herzegovina there is a need for full concerne about rational use of medicines. With a view to costs of health care, objective and better information of the medical staff in Federation of Bosnia and Herzegovina is a necessity. National registers of drugs have been made and four editions have been printed until now. Every new edition was extended by numerous of new registered medicines INN and brand names. The first edition of our register contained 269 INN and 452 brand names. However, fourth edition contained 403 INN and 693 brand names of medicines. The medicines are selected according to anatomical-therapeutically-chemical- classification of medicines (ATC). In addition, the basis data about safety, effectivity, availability and cost of the medicines are stated for every medicine. National register of medicines is very important and reliable source of objective and demonstrated information about medicines for medical staff and patients.

## P - 155

Drugs Available for Treatment of Asthma Bronchale

Beèiæ F., Mulabegoviæ N., Kapiæ E., Kusturica J., Rakanoviæ-Todiæ M., Zec S.L.
Institute of Pharmacology, Clinical Pharmacology and Toxicology, Faculty of Medicine, University of Sarajevo.

Asthma bronchale is a serious global health problem. This chronic airway disorder can be severe and sometimes fatal. The prevalence of asthma is increasing everywhere, especially among children. Asthma is a significant burden, not only in terms of health care costs but also of lost productivity life. Asthma requires continuous medical care to control symptoms, prevent the attacks and make life with asthma trouble free. Our goal is to assess which drugs are available in our country and if the new treatments of asthma are available. We made retrospective literature review of the registered drugs in the Federation of Bosnia-Herzegovina until 2002. Year. WHO Model Formulary stated following drugs for treatment of asthma (Chapter 25.I): salbutamol, beclomethasone dipropionate, theophylline/aminophylline, and sodium cromoglicate/ipratropium bromide. In our National register of drugs, stated drugs for treatment of asthma are: salbutamol, salmeterol, fenoterol/ipratropium, beclomethasone, ipratropium bromide, ipratropium/salbutamol, theophylline, aminophylline, and montelukast. We can conclude that our physicians have suitable medicines for the treatment of acute exacerbation of asthma and chronic obstructive pulmonary disease.

## P - 156

Incorporating Pharmacology Education into an Intergrated Medical Curriculum.

Franson K.
Centre for Human Drug Research, University of Leiden, Netherlands.

Incorporating pharmacology education in an integrated medical curriculum Due to curricular integration in many medical schools, clinical pharmacology is no longer a dedicated course taught by clinical pharmacologists. At Leiden University, the Teaching Resource Centre (TRC) is providing pharmacology education using an ability-based process. First, ability outcomes and corresponding knowledge content were identified. Then two learning strategies by which students could practice and evaluate their performance on the outcomes were introduced throughout the curriculum. 1) TRC Pharmacology Database (TRCP): Using a newly developed graphical language for uniformity, the TRCP contains graphical material, supportive text and charts, and formative feedback questions. TRCP can "teach" a student how a drug's mechanism of action interacts with physiologic or pathophysiologic processes when they follow a tutorial. TRCP also contains a back-end, which reports program utilisation and performance on self-assessment questions. 2) Patient evaluation and Plan (PEP): PEP provides a standardized format for therapeutic decision making and communicating a therapeutic plan. Students are provided multiple opportunities to practice PEP writing via interactive web-based cases. PEP writing fits especially well in the clinical part of the curriculum. After two years, 60% of the curriculum has adopted our methods to consistently present and reiterate pharmacological principles.

## P - 157

Attitudes to Feed-Back with Prescribing Profiles among Prescribers in Rijeka, Croatia and Stockholm, Sweden

Palcevski V.V., Wettermark B., Prpic I., Bergman U.
Karolinska Institute, Huddinge University Hospital, Division of Clinical Pharmacology

Feedback on prescribing is essential for quality assurance. Several drug-related quality indicators have been introduced, focusing on irrational drugs, ratios between treatment alternatives, range of drugs, drug combinations or adherence to guidelines. DU90% - Drug Utilization 90% - focusing on 90% of drug use and adherence to guidelines has been introduced as a simple method for assessing the quality of drug prescribing. As drug-related quality-indicators have been suggested to be of limited value for prescribers to support the decision-making we evaluated the credibility and usefulness of DU90%-method among physicians in Rijeka, Croatia and Stockholm, Sweden. In Rijeka 217 and in Stockholm 215 physicians received DU90%-profiles and a questionnaire. On a VAS-scale of zero to 10 (most positive) the prescribers were asked to what extent the prescribing profiles provided a relevant and clear picture and to what extent they considered that DU90% profiles would increase the quality in drug prescribing and use at their practices. The response-rate was 85% in Rijeka and 77% in Stockholm. The prescribers found the profiles clear and relevant (median 10 and 8) and considered that they would increase the quality in drug prescribing at their practices (median 10 and 8).

## P - 158

Pharmacoeconomic Comparison of Switch and Intravenous Antibiotic Therapy for Lower Respiratory Tract Infections in Elderly Patients

Wawruch M.,Bozekova L.,Krcmery S.,Slobodova Z.,Kozlikova K.,Lassan S.,Kriska M.
Department of Pharmacology, Faculty of Medicine, Comenius University, Slovakia.

Background: As a consequence of the growing cost of antibiotic therapy, the demand for a pharmacoeconomic evaluation is rising. The aim of this essay is to undertake a pharmacoeconomic comparison of switch and intravenous application of antibiotics.
Methods: By analyzing the cost effectiveness, we retrospectively evaluated a group of 96 inpatients with acute lower respiratory tract infection at the Geriatric Clinic LFUK in Bratislava from January 1, 1999 to December 31, 2001. The clinical trial group only included patients in which the first given antibiotic (ATB) had a successful outcome. The resulting parameter of the analysis was represented by the cost effectiveness coefficient (cost/E).
Results: Cost/E (expressed in Slovak Crowns per a symptom free day) of switch administration of ATB was significantly lower in comparison to intravenous administration of ATB: amoxicillin clavulanate 208.8 versus 411.8; ampicillin sulbactame 93.9 versus 168.1; cefuroxime 90.0 versus 123.3; ciprofloxacin 31.7 versus 54.1.
Conclusion: It is possible to reduce the cost of antibiotic therapy by quickly switching from intravenous to oral administration of antibiotics in suitable patients.

## P - 159

Hepatic Toxicity of Benzarone and Benzbromarone

[1]Kaufmann P., [1]Hänni A., [2]Gasser R., [1]Török M., [1]Krähenbühl S.T.
Department of Clinical Pharmacology and Toxicology, University Hospital of [1]Basel and F. Hoffmann-La [2]Roche, Basel, Switzerland

Patients treated with benzarone or benzbromarone can suffer hepatic injury, sometimes with fatal outcome. These drugs show structural elements similar to amiodarone, a well-known mitochondrial toxin. Therefore amiodarone, benzarone, benzbromarone and the analogues benzofuran and 2-butyl-benzofuran were investigated with regard to their effect on mitochondrial function. In rat hepatocytes, benzarone and benzbromarone decreased the mitochondrial membrane potential by 54 and 82%, respectively, at 20mmol/L. Additionally, amiodarone, benzarone and benzbromarone, but not benzofuran, stimulated the glutamate-supported state u respiration. In rat liver mitochondria, amiodarone, benzarone and benzbromarone, but not benzofuran, decreased state 3 glutamate and succinate oxidation and the respiratory control ratio. b-oxidation was decreased by 71, 87 and 58% in the presence of 100mmol/L benzarone, amiodarone or 50mmol/L benzbromarone, but unaffected by benzofuran. 2-Butyl-benzofuran showed a weak inhibition of state 3- and b-oxidation only at the highest concentration (100mmol/L). Acyl-CoA-dehydrogenase and b-kethothiolase were inhibited by amiodarone, benzarone and benzbromarone, but at higher concentrations compared to b-oxidation. The benzofuran structure alone is not responsible for the toxicity of these compounds, but the p-hydroxybenzene structure plays an important role. The sidechain at position 2 enhances the toxicity but does not fully explain it. Bromide is not essential but enhances the mitochondrial toxicity.

## P - 160

Onset of Action of Alfuzosin Once-Daily in Men with Symptomatiic Benigin Prostatic Hyperplasia

[1]Jacobs S., Leonard S.M., City C., CA; Roehrborn C., Gittelman M., Forrest J.
Sanofi-Synthelabo

Early effects of alfuzosin once daily (OD) on maximum urinary flow rate (Qmax) and safety were evaluated in a double-blind, placebo-controlled study in 49 men with symptomatic benign prostatic hyperplasia (BPH) who were proven alpha-blocker responders. After a 14-day placebo washout period, patients were randomized to receive alfuzosin 10 mg OD or placebo for 7 days (days 1–8). This was followed by a 7-day placebo washout period and crossover to the alternate therapy for 7 days (days 15–21). Qmax was measured 8 hours after dosing on days 1, 4, 8, 15, 18, and 21. Response data for each treatment sequence were combined for alfuzosin or placebo (ie, day 1/15, day 4/18, and day 8/21). Excluding early dropouts, the 2 sequence groups (n = 22 for alfuzosin/placebo and n = 23 for placebo/alfuzosin) were respectively matched for age, prostate volume, and predose Qmax. The mean differences in Qmax for patients treated with alfuzosin were 1.4 mL/s on day 1/15 (P <.05) and 1.9 mL/s on day 4/18 (P <.05). Only dizziness (3 patients on alfuzosin and 1 on placebo) was considered drug related. In men with lower urinary tract symptoms, alfuzosin OD exhibits a urodynamically measurable effect on bladder outlet obstruction due to BPH within hours of administration of the first dose.

## P - 161

Veno-Occlusive Disease (VOD) in a Patient Treated with Cyclophosphamide (CPA) and Roxithromycin (ROX)

Kaufmann P., Beltinger J., Wenk M., Bogman K., Török M., Krähenbühl St.
[1]Department of Clinical Pharmacology and Toxicology, University Hospital of Basel

High doses of CPA are known to cause VOD. At immunosuppressive doses, this adverse effect has not been reported. We observed a patient treated with immunosuppressive doses of CPA and ROX, who developed VOD. ROX inhibits cytochrome P450 (CYP) 3A4, an isoenzyme involved in the CPA-metabolism.Therefore, the patient's liver may have been exposed to higher levels of toxic metabolites than expected. The relative distribution of the metabolic pathways of CPA was studied in vitro. The toxic effect of CPA, ROX and the CPA/ROX-combination was tested. Furthermore, the impact on p-glycoprotein (pgp) was assessed and the mechanism of toxicity investigated. ROX did not favour the generation of toxic CPA-metabolites, but led to accumulation of CPA due to inhibiton of both metabolic pathways (CYP 3A4 and 2B6). While CPA and ROX showed no or minor toxicity on endothelial cells, the CPA/ROX-combination was highly toxic. ROX is a pgp-inhibitor, but the increase in toxicity of CPA by ROX could not be demonstrated with other pgp-inhibitors. Only the CPA/ROX-combination but not the single compounds led to chromatin condensation and was toxic to endothelial cells. In conclusion, the combination roxithrothmycin/cyclophosphamide induces apoptosis and is more toxic than the single compounds.

## P - 162

'Selective' Switching from Non-Selective to Selective Non-Steroidal Anti-Inflammatory Drugs (NSAIDs).

Bennett K., Teeling M., Feely J.
Department of Pharmacology and Therapeutics, Trinity Centre for Health Sciences, St James's Hospital, Dublin 8.

Non-steroidal anti-inflammatory drugs (NSAIDs) account for almost 25% of all adverse drug reactions, primarily gastro-intestinal (GI) toxicity. Selective COX 2 inhibitors have been shown to preferentially inhibit activity of the cyclo-oxygenase-2 enzyme, but with reduced GI toxicity. Objective: To determine the degree of switching from non-selective NSAIDS to COX-2 inhibitors and associated factors. Methods: The General Medical Services Scheme prescription database (~1.2 million) was examined for NSAID prescriptions during December 1999-November 2001. All those receiving non-selective NSAIDs and those switching to selective COX-2 inhibitors after at least one month on a non-selective NSAID were identified. Results: A total of 81,538 of the 480,573 patients (17%), initially prescribed non-selective NSAIDs were switched to COX-2 inhibitors during the study. The elderly (aged ³ 65 years) were more likely to have their NSAID switched (OR=1.81, 95% CI 1.79-1.84), as were women (OR=1.25, 95% CI 1.23-1.27), those on >15 DDDs of non-selective NSAID (OR=1.83, 95% CI 1.80-1.86), and those previously prescribed anti-peptic ulcer drugs (OR=5.24, 95% CI 5.14-5.34). Conclusions: Prescribers are more likely to switch older female patients, on a previously high dose of non-selective NSAID, and with past history of peptic ulcer disease. This suggests that doctors do take risk factors into consideration when prescribing NSAIDs.

## P - 163

A Role for Aldosterone in Essential Hypertension

Mahmud A.
Trinity College, Dublin

Objective: As aldosterone increases stiffness in large vessels it is suggested that decreased arterial compliance is one mechanism for hypertension in hyperaldosteronism. To determine whether aldosterone contributes to essential hypertension we compared aldosterone antagonism with spironolactone (Spir 50 mg) to a diuretic antihypertensive (bendrofluazide Bend 2.5 mg).
Design and Methods: Twenty untreated patients (mean age 53±3, 9 female) with essential hypertension were randomised in a cross-over design for 4 weeks therapy with an intervening one month washout period. Blood pressure (BP mmHg, Omron Model 705), arterial wave reflection in the aorta (AIx, height of the late systolic peak/pulse pressure by Sphygmocor) and carotid-femoral pulse wave velocity, (PWV, Complior) were measured. Statistical analysis was performed by the Student's t test and regression analysis.
Results: Both therapies reduced BP but Spir produced a significantly greater fall in BP than Bend (19±3/11±7 vs 9±2/5±2). Only Spir reduced PWV and AIx (*p<0.01). The reduction in PWV and AIx with Spir compared to Bend remains significant (p<0.01) when adjusted for the baseline values as well as the greater fall in mean BP.
Conclusion: The significant reduction in PWV and AIx with Spir, but not with Bend, suggests that aldosterone antagonism has BP independent effects on arterial stiffness. Also its antihypertensive effects is greater than expected from a diuretic. Aldosterone may contribute to blood pressure in essential hypertension.

## P - 164

Chronopharmacologic Study of the Local Anaesthetic Activity of Mepivacaïne in Children Dental Care

[1]Boughattas N.A., [2]Amor S.H., [3]Attia M.B., [1]Letaief M., [2]Maatoug F., [4]Bouzouita K..
[1]Faculté de Médecine, 5019 Monastir, Tunisia; [2]Faculté de Médecine Dentaire, 5019 Monastir, Tunisia; [3]Faculté des Sciences de Bizerte, 7021 Zarzouna, Tunisia; [4]Faculté de Médecine, 1006 Tunis, Tunisia.

The present study aims to investigate whether the duration of local anaesthesia (L.A.) varied according to the day-time of mepivacaïne (Scandicaïne®) injection. A total of 36 children aged between 10 and 15 years and synchronized with a normal sleep-wake rhythm was included in the study for various dental care (on one root teeth). Six 2 h-intervals (from 7 a.m. to 7 p.m.) were selected for drug injection. All children (6 patients/interval-time) received the same dose of mepivacaïne (1.8 ml at 2%). The duration of L.A. was determined at the appearance of the first sensations revealed by a mechanic-test (with a probe) associated to a cold-test (with ethyl chloride). The data were analyzed by the cosinor procedure. The duration of L.A. varied significantly according to the dosing-time (p < 0.001). The lowest and the highest values of such variation were 13 min and 39 min respectively. The cosinor analysis revealed a diurnal rhythm in L.A. with an acrophase (peak-time) localized at around 2 p.m. Such diurnal variation in L.A. could not be related to the plasma bioavailability since the drug was locally injected. The mechanism should result from circadian changes in membrane permeability to ions.

## P - 165

The Improvement of Digoxin Therapy after Implementation of Pharmacokinetic Interpretation

Grundmann M., Kacirova I., Koristkova B., Brozmanova H.
Dept. of Clinical Pharmacology University Hospital and Medico Social Faculty, University of Ostrava, Ostrava, Czech Republic

The therapeutic drug monitoring (TDM) of digoxin started in our department in 1997. The information about body weight, serum creatinine level, dosage of digoxin and concomitant therapy has been required. The pharmacokinetic modeling and interpretation has been provided. The outcomes in 1997 and 2001 were compared. 777 samples from 553 geriatric patients (60% females, age 76±7 years, no more information available) analyzed in 1997 and 402 samples from 347 patients (66% females, age 76±7 years, body weight 72±13 kg, serum creatinine 119±72 umol/) analyzed in 2001 were included. There was no information about dosage in 1997. In 2001 mean dose was 0.170±0.100 mg, the dose related to body weight 2,5±1,4 ug/kg. In 1997 mean plasma level was 1,13±0,70 ng/ml, while 0,93±0,51 in 2001. Frequency of toxic levels dropped from 12% to 5%, while the amount of therapeutic levels remained the same (58%, 59% resp.). The providing of pharmacokinetic service decreased significantly adverse drug reactions about 58 %.

## P - 166

A Novel in-vivo PK/ in-vitro PD Model for the Combined Simulation of Bacterial Killing of Two Antimicrobial Agents: A case Study on Fosfomycin and Cefpirome

Zeitlinger M., Müller M., Joukhadar C.
Department of Clinical Pharmacology, Division of Clinical Pharmacokinetics University of Vienna Medical School, Vienna; Austria

Objective: Static microbiologic models seem insufficient to simulate the dynamically changing conditions in the human body. Using an in-vivo pharmacokinetic (PK)/ in vitro pharmacodynamic (PD) approach allows for the investigation of target site effect of anti-infective agents in select tissues. In the present study we set out to compare the PDs of cefpirome and fosfomycin, a commonly administered drug combination in intensive care treatment. Methods: The time-concentrations profiles of cefpirome and fosfomycin in serum and muscle tissue of intensive care patients were obtained by microdialysis (MD), in order to measure unbound concentrations. Based on this data we developed an in-vitro model to determine bacterial killing of cefpirome and fosfomycin on select strains of Staphylococcus aureus and Pseudomonas aeruginosa. Results: CFU/ml of Staphylococcus aureus (ATCC 29213) and Pseudomonas aeruginosa (clinical isolate) decreased by approximately 2-log10 for plasma and muscle tissue six hours after cefpirome and fosfomycin administration compared with baseline, respectively. The simulation of plasma and tissue PKs for the combined administration of these antibiotics resulted in complete eradication of S. aureus within five hours after drug exposure. No bacterial re-growth could be observed in any of the simulations within six hours. Conclusion: Both antibiotics seem suitable for the therapy of tissue infections caused by S. aureus in intensive care patients. However, the PK/PD simulation has shown that the combined administration of both antimicrobial agents results in more pronounced bacterial killing of S. aureus and P. aeruginosa strains than compared with monotherapy.

## P - 167

An Exploration of the Therapeutic Arsenals of Antibiotics in European Countries Using the Drug Utilisation 90% Method

Ferech M., Stichele R.V., Elseviers M., Goossens H.
ESAC Management Team, University of Antwerp, Belgium

ESAC (European Surveillance of Antibiotic Consumption, granted by DG SANCO of the EC) is an international network of national surveillance systems, aiming to collect comparable antibiotic consumption data in Europe. Within the project, the aim of this study was to investigate the number and nature of commonly used antibiotics in different countries, using the DU90 Methods. We collected data from ambulatory care (AC) in 31 countries, using the Anatomic Therapeutic Clinical Classification (ATC-WHO, version 2002), and expressing results in Defined Daily Doses (DDD) for the period 1997-2001. For each of the 206 antibiotics (including combinations), currently listed in the ATC J01 group (Antiinfectives for systemic use), the volume of use in terms of DDD was determined in each country, and ranked in a Lorenz curve distribution, with a cut off at 90% of the total consumption. Results The ESAC team succeeded in collecting acceptable AC data for 1997-2001 from 16 European countries. Of the 206 available ATC codes, no consumption whatsoever was recorded in any country for 67 ATC codes; 24 ATC codes were used in only one country; 115 ATC codes were used in at least two countries. The median number per country of ATC codes with some tracable consumption was 60 (P25-P75 48-66), with Norway at the extreme low range (32) and Spain at the extreme upper range (75). Conclusions. Remarkable differences between the therapeutic arsenals of antibiotics were identified within a representative sample of European countries. This variability may reflect differences in quality of care and explain the diverging patterns of emergence of antibiotic resistance in Europe.

## P - 168

Pattern of Use of Benzodiazepines (BDZ) in Hypertensive Patients in General Practice (GP) in Serbia

[1]Divac N., [2]Veljkovic S., [1]Bajcetic M., [1]Samardzic R.
[1]Institute of Clinical Pharmacology, School of Medicine, Belgrade, [2]Institute of Physiology, Faculty of Medicine, Nis

It has been established that benzodiazepines (BDZ) are the most frequently prescribed drugs in Serbia. In previous studies it has been noted that hypertension is the second most frequent indication for benzodiazepines (after anxiety) in GP in Serbia. This study is aimed to investigate the pattern of use of BDZ in hypertensive patients in GP. 136 patients with hypertension (mean age 50.6±7.9 years, 53.7% male) completed questionnaires: 42.6% were taking BDZ. BDZ (in average daily dose equivalent to 5mg/day of diazepam) were prescribed for anxiety in 62.1%, hypertension in 20.7% and insomnia in 17.2% of cases. BDZ were regularly used in 44,8% and "as needed" in 55,2% of patients, over a period of several months (74,1%) or of several years (25,9%). Risk of dependence was known to 55,2%. No differences between hypertensive patients who used BDZ and those who did not were noted in terms of blood pressure (160.0±3.9/100.0±2.7 vs. 163.5±5.1/101.5±1.4 mmHg ), smoking habits, education level, age and sex. There are significantly more ($X^2_{0.01;1}=9$) obese patients (with body mass index>30) in the group of BDZ users than in the group of non-users. No difference has been found between antihypertensive therapy of these two groups of patients. It is concluded that the use of BDZ in hypertensive patient is frequent, but inadequate in terms of indications and dosage, and no predictors, except body mass index, of BDZ use could be detected in this study.

## P - 169

Pharmacoeconomical Evaluation of Antimicrobial Treatment Patients with Antibiotic-Resistant Pseudomonas Aeruginosa Pneumonia in Intensive Care Units

Kadusevicius E., Zmuidaite V., Stankeviciene I., Zaliaduonyte D.
Kaunas Medical Univesity Hospital, Department of Clinical Pharmacology, Eiveniu str.2, Kaunas 3000, Lithuania

Objective: to evaluate clinical and pharmacoeconomical results of antibimicrobial treatment patients (pts) with antibiotic-resistant Pseudomonas aeruginosa pneumonia. Methods: data were analysed from histories of 102 (pts) with positive clinical cultures for P.aeruginosa who were treated in Intensive care units (ICU) of Kaunas Medical University Hospital. In-hospital mortality and length of stay were examined in 66 pts. who had P.aeruginosa resistant to Imipenem, Meropenem, Ceftazidime or Amikacine and compared to the rest of 36 pts. that had P.aeruginosa susceptible to the earlier mentioned antibiotics. The overall in-hospital mortality in ICU during 2000 year was 15.47 %, the mortality in pts. with susceptible P.aeruginosa was 38.88 % vs. to 63.63 % of pts. from whom resistant P.aeruginosa was isolated (relative risk [RR], 1.64; 95% confidence interval [CI], 1.087-2.645). The duration of hospital stay for pts. with a susceptible P.aeruginosa was 9 (8,6+/-1,2) days vs. 19 (19,4+/-2,3) days for pts. who had resistant P.aeruginosa isolated (p<0.001). In pts. group with resistant P.aeruginosa (n=66) rational treatment with main antipseudomonal antibiotics (I, M, CF and A) was more effective than that with other antibiotics (mortality 53.3 % vs. 85.7 %, p<0.05). Descending (strong - weak) empiric treatment was more effective than ascending (mortality 30 % vs. 52.43 %, p=0.08), RRR - 0,428; 95% [CI] (-0,042-0,729), NNT to prevent one death - 4,457; 95% [CI] (2,383-infinity), ICER per death avoided – 1194.05 €.
Conclusion: Treatment with I, M, CF and A was cost effective.

## P - 170

Effect of St. Johns Wort (Hypericum Perforatum, SJW) on Human CYPs

Wenk M., Todesco L., Krähenbühl S.
Division of Clinical Pharmacology and Toxicology, University Hospital, Basel, Switzerland

St. John's wort is a popular over-the-counter herbal antidepressant. While induction of CYP3A4 by SJW has been demonstrated, the results for other CYPs are less clear. We investigated CYP induction by SJW in 16 healthy volunteers (8 males and females). Subjects were treated with Jarsin® (3 x 300 mg/day) for 14 days. Before and at the end of treatment, subjects were phenotyped with oral caffeine (1A2), dextromethorphan (DMO) (2D6 or 3A4), and the cortisol (C) to 6-OH-cortisol (6OHC) ratio in urine. The caffeine metabolic ratio for CYP1A2 in saliva and urine did not change after SJW in males, but increased significantly in females (p<0.025). The 1A2 polymorphisms -3858G->A (CYP1A2*1C) and -164A->C (CYP1A2*1F) were not predictive for induction. For CYP3A4, the metabolic ratio 6OHC/C in urine was increased in both sexes (p<0.01), whereas the metabolic ratio obtained with DMO was elevated only in females (p<0.01). No influence of SJW could be observed on the activity of CYP2D6. Our study suggests that induction of CYP1A2 by SJW is gender-dependent and not predicted by known 1A2 polymorphisms. Regarding CYP3A4, the known induction by SJW could be confirmed. DMO may not be as reliable as the urinary 6OHC/C ratio to determine CYP3A4 induction.

## P - 171

Interactions Between Herbal Drugs and Warfarin

Dobric S., Dragojevic-Simic V., Kilibarda V., Bokonjic D.
National Poison Control Centre, Military Medical Academy, Crnotravska 17, 11000 Belgrade, Serbia and Montenegro

Increase in herbal products use worldwide has made information about potential herb and drug interactions very important, especially for drugs with a narrow therapeutic index such as warfarin. The aim of this study was to revealed potential and documented herb-warfarin interactions. Searches of the computerized databese MEDLINE (1995-2002) and current editions of leading tertiary references on dietary supplements and drug interaction (e.g. Natural Medicines Comprehesive Database, German Commission E Monographs, Drug Interactions Facts, etc.) were conducted. Herbal medicines that have been associated with documented reports of interactions with warfarin include danshen (Salvia miltiorrhiza), devil's claw (Harpagophytum procumbens), dong quai (Angelica sinensis) and papain (increase in warfarin's effects) as well as coenzyme $Q_{10}$, ginseng and green tea (decrease in warfarin's effects). However, much more herbal products may have the potential to interfere with warfarin therapy. Among them are several of the most used herbal drugs such as angelica root, arnica flower, anise, feverfew, garlic, ginger, ginkgo, horse chestnut, etc. Continued efforts by health care professionals to recognize and report suspected interactions between prescription medications and herbal drugs should ultimately increase knowledge and awareness of interactions and improve the quality of patient care.

## P - 172

Influence of Glyceryl Trinitrate on Anti-Inflammatory and Ulcerogenic Actions of Indomethacin in Rats

[1]Dobric S., [2]Velev R., [3]Cupic V., [1]Milovanovic Z., [1]Jacevic V., [1]Bokonjic D.
[1]National Poison Control Centre, Military Medical Academy, Belgrade, Serbia and Montenegro [2]Faculty of Veterinary Medicine, Skopje, FYR Macedonia [3]Faculty of Veterinary Medicine, Belgrade, Serbia and Montenegro

It has been demonstrated that nitric oxide (NO) may play an important role in gastric mucosal defense and that NO-donors may protect against experimentally induced gastric lesions. The aim of this study was to evaluate the influence of glyceryl trinitrate (GTN), NO-generating compound, on anti-inflammatory and ulcerogenic actions of indomethacin (IND), a strong nonsteroidal anti-inflammatory drug (NSAID) in rats. Adult male Wistar rats starving for 16-20 hours before the experiment were used. GTN (1, 3 and 6 mg/kg po) was given 60 minutes before or immediately after IND (25 mg/kg po). For estimating anti-inflammatory activity of IND the carrageenan-induced rat paw oedema test was used. Its ulcerogenic action was evaluated by determining the length, area and intensity of gastric lesions as well as by the pathomorphological examination of the stomach of treated animals. It was shown that GTN, given either 60 minutes before or immediately after IND, dose-dependently and significantly reduced all parameters of ulcerogenic activity of the NSAID without changing its anti-inflammatory action. Efficacy of GTN was more pronounced when the drug had been given immediately after IND. These results confirm the potential use of NO-donors as gastroprotective drugs in patients treated with highly ulcerogenic NSAIDs like IND.

## P - 173

The Organization and Teaching of Clinical Pharmacology in Serbia and Montenegro Army

Dragojevic-Simic V., Dobric S., Jandric D., Stojiljkovic M.P., Jovanovic D., Bokonjic D.
Military Medical Academy, Belgrade, Serbia and Montenegro

Army clinical pharmacology was closely connected and derived from civil one, which was established as an independent medical speciality in Serbia and Montenegro since 1981. However, many clinical pharmacology services were provided in Military Medical Academy (MMA), the largest army hospital in former Yugoslavia, before this formal date. Its clinical specialists e.g. were permitted to carry out drug clinical trials by Republic Secretariat of Health and Social Politics from 1973. Detailed direction on the organization of these trials, as well as standing orders of MMA board of commissioners entrusted with drugs was established. First clinical pharmacologists completed their speciality at the Medical School in Belgrade, and it was decided that the Yugoslav Army should has one such training program located in MMA. It consists of the following: 7.5 months at an Institute of Basic Toxicology and Pharmacology, 10.5 months of formal lectures and 15 months of clinical training. Special attention is devoted to drug development programs which include drugs for defense against chemical and nuclear weapons of mass destruction.

## P - 174

Dose Selection of Cytoprotector Amifostine for Chronic Rat Study of Doxorubicin Toxicity

Dragojevic-Simic V., Dobric S., Bokonjic D.
Military Medical Academy, Belgrade, Serbia and Montenegro

Cytoprotector amifostine (AMI) provides protection of normal tissue against many antineoplastic drugs. Dose-limiting toxicities of doxorubicin (DOX) prevent its application in appropriate therapeutic dose. The aim of this study was to determine the AMI dose which reduce the mortality as well as whole-body toxicity of multiple application of DOX in rats. Firstly, maximum tolerated dose of AMI in chronic use was determined. For this purpose the animals were treated with increasing doses of AMI (75, 150 and 300 mg/kg ip) 4 times a week for 4 weeks. According to mortality, behavior and body weight reduction of rats the AMI dose of 75 mg/kg ip was selected. It was given 20 min. before DOX (1.25 mg/kg ip 4 times a week for 4 weeks) and the rats were observed for another 4 weeks. Pretreatment with AMI significantly reduced rat mortality (90 vs. 63.5 %), as well as body weight reduction and gross anatomic changes caused by DOX-induced toxicity. Selected dose of 75 mg/kg was 1/4 of that used for protection from DOX single-dose toxicity in our previous experiments, according to its use in clinical settings.

## P - 175

Retrospective Prospective Analysis of Pilot Study of Pharmaco-Economy at the Model of Application of Antibiotics in Surgical and Internal Medicine Department Through the Analysis of ATC/DDD and ABC.

[1]Begovic B., [2]Zulic I., [3]Hadzovic S.
[1]Institute of Clinical Pharmacology, Clinical center University of Sarajevo, Bolnicka 25, Bosnia and Herzegovina [2]Institute of pharmacology, clinical pharmacology and toxicology, Cekalusa 90/II, Sarajevo, Bosnia and Herzegovina [3]Faculty of Pharmacy, Cekalusa 90, Sarajevo, Bosnia and Herzegovina

Objectives: To examine relations between effectiveness and cost (CEA) in retrospective-prospective pilot study of pharmaco-economy in surgical and internal medicine departments. To make conclusions on variability of this model in the coming period, based on ATC/DDD and ABC analysis.
Method: The study consists of two sections: retrospective one and prospective one. During one year period of time, based on engaging criteria, we have selected 120 patients who were treated at internal medicine and surgical departments, analized drugs applied (the average daily dose) and calculated the consumption of drugs on the basis of defined daily dose as well as total cost of therapy applied.
Results: Prospective part of the study witnessed decrease of the average cost of treatment. Adequate application of antibiotics (cheaper antibiotics were applied in appropriate indications and were individually dosed) and shortening of the period of time of treatment by antibiotics did lower the total price of treatment of patients at this department.
Discussion: This method of drug application with continuous analysis of application may lead us toward significant saving in treatment of patients. It is necessary to apply appropriate therapeutical guides that limit treatment freedom when applying particular therapy, to some extent, but, at the same time, sustain significant saving of funds necessary for treatment of patients.

## ORAL

Population Pharmacokinetics of Rac-, (R)- and (S)-Methadone in Methadone Maintenance Subjects

Somogyi A.A., Foster D.J.R, Bochner F., White J.
Department of Clinical and Experimental Pharmacology, University of Adelaide, Adelaide, Australia

Variability in the pharmacokinetics of racemic methadone influences withdrawal symptoms and therapeutic success in maintenance treatment. We developed a population pharmacokinetic model for rac-, (R)- and (S)-methadone using P-Pharm software. The model-building data comprised 38 patients (39% females; mean±s.d.; 74±15 kg; 36±8 years), on 7.5-150 mg/day (463 plasma concentration-time points). The data were best modelled by a two compartment open model with first-order input and a lag phase, and assumed log-normal parameter distribution. The model was validated with data from 21 patients (48% females; 69±12 kg; 32±7 years on 20-160 mg/day; 262 plasma concentration-time points). The model development and validation data sets were combined and used to refine the population models and identify explanatory covariables. The apparent volume of the central compartment was found to increase with decreasing plasma a1-acid glycoprotein concentration and was higher in males, while the delay in absorption was longer at higher doses. No covariates were identified for oral clearance (CL/F), which ranged approximately 7-fold for all analytes. There was marked stereoselectivity for all pharmacokinetic parameters except CL/F. Using MAP Bayesian prediction, the population pharmacokinetic models were able to accurately predict CL/F values from limited (1 or 2 samples) blood sampling protocols.

## P - 176

Clinical Research of Efficiency, Tolerability and Safety Using Repaglinide in Treatment of Patients with Diabetes Mellitus Type 2

[1]Begovic B., [2]Zulic I., [3]Grujic M., [3]Stevanovic D., [5]Babic D., [4]Ler Z., E.S. [5]Waltonand, [4]Kanc K.
[1]Institute of clinical pharmacology, Clinical center University of Sarajevo, Bolnicka 25, Bosnia and Herzegovina [2]Institute of pharmacology, clinical pharmacology and toxicology, Cekalusa 90/II, Sarajevo Bosnia and Herzegovina [3]General Hospital, Kranjceviceva 12, Sarajevo, Bosnia and Herzegovina [4]Novo Nordisk A/S, ROSEE, Zelezna 18, Ljubljana, Slovenia [5]Novo Nordisk A/S, Repr. Office Sarajevo, Bosnia and Herzegovina

Introduction: Repaglinide is novel fast acting oral antidiabetic agent. In this study we investigated efficacy and safety of repaglinide in treatment of type 2 diabetc patients.
Materials and methods: 17 type 2 diabetic patients: 8 treatments naive and 9 previously sulphonylurea-treated patients, with moderate to poor glycemic control (pre-prandial glucose levels 7.8-12.0 mmol/L) were treated with repaglinide in optimally titrated dose (dose range 1.5 to 9.0 mg/day), for 14 weeks. Serum glucose was measured pre-prandially at each visit according to the protocol (8-times). BMI was calculated at baseline, when repaglinide was intoduced (after «wash-out» period ) and at final patient visit.
Results: at baseline, the mean pre-prandial serum glucosa level was 9.67 (SD 2.02) mmol/L. At final visit the mean pre-prandial serum glucose level was 8.34 (SD 1.84) mmol/L, ($p<0.02$). At baseline the mean BMI was 29,69 kg/m2 (SD 3.57) and at final visit 29.09 kg/m2 (SD 3.68), ($p = 0.05$). All 17 patients tolerated the drug very well. There were no hypoglycaemic episodes registered. There were no repaglinide related adverse events.
Conclusion: Repaglinide is very effective in improvement of glycaemic control. No weight gain has been observed. Moreover there was a significant trend towards weight loss, what is consistent with findings in other studies. The drug was well-tolerated and no drug-related adverse events were observed.

## P - 177

Grapefruit Juice even in Small Amounts Increases Considerably Plasma Concentrations of Simvastatin and Simvastatin Acid

Lilja J.J., Neuvonen M., Neuvonen P.J.
Department of Clinical Pharmacology, University of Helsinki, FIN-00290 Helsinki, Finland

Background: Simvastatin is an HMG-CoA-reductase inhibitor extensively metabolised by CYP3A4 and carboxyesterases. High plasma concentrations of simvastatin acid increase the risk of musculosceletal adverse effects of simvastatin. We wanted to study the effect of a small amount of grapefruit juice on the pharmacokinetics of simvastatin.
Methods: Ten healthy volunteers drank in a randomized, two-phase crossover study either 200 ml normal-strength grapefruit juice or water on two consecutive mornings (in addition to normal diet). On day 3, a single 40 mg dose of simvastatin was taken with 200 ml grapefruit juice or water. Plasma concentrations of simvastatin and simvastatin acid were measured by LC-MS-MS up to 24 hours.
Results: Grapefruit juice increased the AUC(0-33) of simvastatin 3.6-fold (range, 1.8-fold to 6.0-fold; $P < 0.001$) and Cmax 3.9-fold ($P < 0.001$). The AUC(0-33) of simvastatin acid was increased 3.3-fold (range 2.1-fold to 5.6-fold; $P < 0.001$) and Cmax 4.3-fold ($P < 0.001$) by grapefruit juice.
Conclusions: Even a small amount of grapefruit juice ingested daily with simvastatin increases considerably plasma concentrations of both simvastatin and its active metabolite, simvastatin acid. This interaction, caused by the inhibition of CYP3A4-mediated first-pass metabolism in the intestinal wall, can increase the cholesterol lowering effect and the risk of concentration-dependent muscle adverse effects of simvastatin.

## P - 178

Input and Elimination of Resistant Bacteria in Sewage Treatment Plants

Kümmerer K., Unger J., Wiethan J., Tietze A.B.
Institute of Environmental Medicine and Hospital Epidemiology University of Freiburg,Germany.

With respect to the causes of resistance, the focus is on the use of antimicrobials in hospitals, by medical practitioners and in animal husbandry. In order to minimize the associated risk a significant reduction of pathogens is necessary during sewage treatment process. We investigated the input and elimination of resistant pathogenic bacteria in three different municipal sewage treatment plants. Elimination rates were 95%-99% for E.coli, Pseudomonas spp. and Enterococcus spp. For resistant bacteria the elimination was 93.5% - 100%.Therefore it is questionable whether advanced treatment of STP effluent is necessary. There was no difference between resistant and not resistant bacteria. We found that the number of multi resistant bacteria correlated with the size and the number of hospitals connected to a STP. The numbers of resistant bacteria found in the effluent of an ICU of a hospital with maximum medical service spectrum were in the same range as found fort the influent of municipal STP despite the fact that hospital waste water is diluted at least by a factor of 100 by municipal sewage. Therefore, the community and not the hospitals are the main source of resistant bacteria in sewage. With respect to the elimination rates the question is, whether advanced technologies such as waste water disinfection are necessary. The work presented here was supported by the German ministry of Research and Education (BMB+F), Grant No. 02WU9871/2

## ORAL

Chemotherapy for Lung Cancer: Rationalization of Costs

Cervellino J.C., Araujo C.E., Fligman M.D., Pires E.A.
Chair of Pharmacology, School of Medicine, University of Buenos Aires (Argentina).

The development of new drugs for non-small cell lung cancer could be a big success in the treatment of this disease, improving objective response rate and quality of life. To cope with this formidable challenge, interest seems to be focused exclusively in the development of new molecules. But, what about the well-known old agents combinations? Are they not useful anymore? Generally speaking, modern cancer chemotherapy includes combination of new drugs exclusively. However, recent results are often quite similar to those achieved in the past at low cost and with mild toxicity. Comparison with the national history of the disease could shed some light to the actual value of trials' result. According to P. Bunn (ESO Monograph, 1991), median survival (MST) for non-small cell lung cancer was 27 weeks, which is quite similar to most data reported in the last 20 years (Table). If the therapeutic benefit over old treatments is null, is the benefit obtained from an economic analysis? Again, the answer is negative (Table), Considering the higher cost of new drugs and their severe toxicity, the cost-benefit relationship does not seem to be better.

| Chemotherapy | OR (%) | MST (mo) | Six cycles cost (US$) |
|---|---|---|---|
| Gemcitabine + DDP | 30 | 9.8 | 30,006 |
| Paclitaxel + carboplatin | 32 | 9.9 | 40,200 |
| Ifosfamide + epirubicine | 51 | 12.0 | 16,938 |
| Cyclophospamide | 38 | 9 | 504 |

Probably a smarter approach could be to combine both old and new agents, in order to achieve better results when analyzed from the patient's point of view.

## P - 179

Patterns of Systemic Antibiotic Use in a Tertiary Hospital in Israel in the Years 1998-2000

Kitzes-Cohen R., Coos D., Levy M.
Carmel Medical Center and Hadassh University Hospital, Israel

Objectives: To investigate the pattern of antibiotic use in the hospital over a three years period according to individual drugs and hospital departments. The data base should allow comparison of utilisation patterns of antibiotics in Europe according to the EuroDURG (European Drug Utilisation Research Group) and ESAC (European Surveillance of Antimicrobial Consumption) initiatives.

Setting: Three hundred thirty five adult beds of a tertiary hospital in Northern Israel during the years 1998-2000. An antibiotic control policy restricts the use of the most expensive antibiotics and those with broad spectrum of activity and a major impact on bacterial resistance.

Methods: The ATC/DDD and DU 90% methodologies were used. The use of antibiotics was expressed as the number of defined daily doses (DDD) per 100 bed-days.

Results: The total antibiotic use varied during the study period from 93.7 to 101.0 DDD/100 bed-days ($p<0.1$). Thirteen drugs accounted for 90% of the total volume. The use of broad-spectrum penicillins was the highest of all drugs followed by cephalosporins and oral quinolones. The highest rates of antibiotic use were found in the departments of ENT, urology, gynecology and orthopedics and in the intensive care unit (ICU). The total restricted antibiotics use was 7.2 DDD/100 bed - days and was the highest in the ICU.

Conclusions: The ATC/DDD methodology provided deliniation and interpretation of antibiotic usage patterns in the hospital. Although the overall use is higher then that found in several reports from European hospitals, stratification by individual drugs and by hospital department yielded similar trends.

## P - 180

Association Angiotensin Converting Enzyme Inhibitor-Antagonists of Angiotensin II Receptors to Reduce Renal Risk in Diabetic Patients Study Among 25 Patients

Ory J.P., Combes J.
CHIC Hte Saône Site de Vesoul Service de Médecine Interne 41, avenue A. Briand Vesoul Cedex, France.

Micro Hope study has shown the great interest to use ACEI when exists diabetes for renal protection, and LIFE study has shown the reduction of cardiovascular morbidity and mortality by AAIIR intervention. At the beginning, the association ACEI - AAIIR was contra-indicated. At present, that is just non indicated. The association permits to act on two different sites to block renin-angiotensin system. 25 patients (8 males - 17 females), 61 old years (42 to 74), presenting type 2 diabetes with proteinuria at 450 mg/24 hours (range : 250 to 1 150) were treated for more two years by Quinapril 20 mg/day. Creatinine clearance was measured : 72 ml/mn (55 to 88). Blood pressure was 138/82. In addition, they were treated by 300 mg/d of Irbesartan. 3 days later : stability of kaliemia : 4.7 meq/l (3.8 to 5.2) and creatinine clearance. 3 months later : blood pressure : 129/78, proteinuria : 280 mg/24 h (95 to 1 180 mg). Natremia, kaliemia and clearance stayed stable. Association needs strict supervision but seems interesting for renal protection with 4.5 years of observation.

## P - 181

Investigation of the Functional Responses of Corpus Cavernosum Smooth Muscle in Secondhand Smoked Rabbits

[1]Göçmez S.S., [1]Utkan T., [2]Duman C., [1]Yıldız F., [1]Gacar M.N., [1]Ulak G., [1]Erden F.
[1]Kocaeli University Medical School, Department of Pharmacology, Kocaeli, Turkey, 41900 [2]Kocaeli University Medical School, Depatment of Biochemistry, Kocaeli, Turkey, 41900

Impaired relaxation mechanisms of corpus cavernosum smooth muscle (CCSM) may lead to erectile dysfunction (ED). Smoking has been reported to cause ED. However underlying mechanism(s) is unclear. Therefore, we aimed in vitro to investigate the effects of passive smoking on neurogenic and endothelium-dependent relaxant responses of CCSM in rabbit. Twenty-seven New Zealand male rabbits were divided into three groups. Group 1: Control group (n=9), Group 2: Rabbits exposed to smoke for 10 weeks (n=9), Group 3: Rabbits exposed to smoke and received orally L-arginine (1mg/ml). Endothelial and neurogenic relaxation of the CCSM significantly decreased in the smoking group compared to the control ($p<0.05$). However endothelial and neurogenic relaxant responses were improved in the L-arginine treated group. There was no significant differences in KCl, sodium nitroprusside and papaverine induced relaxant responses in all groups. Phenylephrine-induced contractile responses of smoking and treatment group were significantly decreased compared to the controls ($p<0.05$). Our study showed that smoking impaired neurogenic and endothelium-dependent relaxant responses in the isolated rabbit CCSM. These relaxant responses improved with L-arginine treatment. In the light of these findings L-arginine may be effective in the treatment of smoking-induced ED. But further work is needed to determine these evidence.

Index Words: Smoking, L-arginine, Nitric oxide, Erectile dysfunction, Corpus cavernosum.

## P - 182

Risk Factors for Extrapyramidal Symptoms (EPS) During Treatment with Selective Serotonin Reuptake Inhibitors (SSRI's)

[1]Hedenmalm K., [1]Yue Q.Y., [2]Dahl M.L., [3]Spigset O.
[1]Drug Epidemiology Unit, Medical Products Agency, Uppsala, Sweden, [2]Department of Medical Sciences, Clinical Pharmacology, University Hospital, Uppsala, Sweden, [3]Department of Clinical Pharmacology, St Olav's University Hospital, Trondheim, Norway

This study of risk factors for EPS with SSRI's included all reports on SSRI's coded as EPS submitted to the Swedish Adverse Drug Reactions Advisory Committee until end of 1999 (n=61). Reporting physicians received a form for collection of information on use of SSRI's and antipsychotics, alcohol or substance abuse, central nervous system (CNS) damage, a history of epilepsy or EPS, and family history of Parkinson's disease. Physicians were asked to contact patients for blood sample collection for genotyping of the cytochrome P-450 enzymes CYP2D6, CYP2C9 and CYP2C19. Twenty-eight forms (46%) were returned; 20 blood samples were obtained. Drugs included citalopram (n=24 total; n=13 forms; n=8 samples), paroxetine (n=22 total; n=9 forms; n=6 samples), sertraline (n=7 total; n=2 forms; n=2 samples), fluoxetine (n=5 total; n=2 forms; n=2 samples) and fluvoxamine (n=5; n=2 forms; n=2 samples). One report concerned two SSRIs. Reactions included involuntary muscle movements (23%), parkinsonism, akathisia, bruxism, rigidity (each 13%), acute dystonia (10%), hyperkinesia, myoclonus (each 5%), tremor (3%), and tardive dyskinesia (2%). The CYP2D6, CYP2C9 and CYP2C19 genotypes did not cosegregate with EPS during SSRI treatment. Potential risk factors included present (21%; 6/28) or past (32%; 9/28) antipsychotic treatment, CNS damage (25%; 7/28), alcohol/substance abuse (21%; 6/28), and previous EPS (21%; 6/28).

## P - 183

Concentrations of Ciprofloxacin and Ceftazidime in Surface Waters.

Wiethan J., Al-Ahmad A., Henninger A., Kümmerer K.
Institute of Environmental Medicine and Hospital Epidemiology, University of Freiburg,Germany.

Simulation of the selection pressure of the antibiotics ciprofloxacin and ceftazidime in surface waters by means of classical methods. Due to the frequent detection of antibiotics in the aquatic environment it has been investigated, whether a selection pressure can be stimulated by these substances in surface water within the microbial flora. The fate of two antibiotics, ciprofloxacin and ceftazidime, was investigated on the base of the closed bottle test, as a simple model for surface water, by means of HPLC in two concentrations respectively. Their effects on the inoculum were investigated by classic microbiological procedures. In high concentration ciprofloxacin proved as persistent and caused growth inhibition as well as strong shifts in the germ spectrum while it remained unobtrusive in low concentration within the scope of the test selection. Ceftazidim was eliminated approximately by half within 28 days, at which a large part was caused by non-biotic elimination. The effects on the inoculum remained restricted in both concentrations to a test internal selection, which had to be attributed to the experimental conditions. A well-founded assumption exists, that the actually available average concentrations of ciprofloxacin and ceftazidme in surface water will be clearly below the low test concentrations, which caused no influence. Under this condition it seems to be improbable, that selective effects on bacterial communities are caused by these substances in surface waters. However, some methodical restrictions have to be taken into account.

The work presented here was supported by the German ministry of Research and Education (BMB+F), Grant No. 02WU9871/2

## P - 184

Effects of Combined Hypolipemic Diet on Serum Lipids

Krehic J., Cabaravdic A., Begovic B., Veletovac-Causevic V.
Institute for Clinical Pharmacology, University Clinical Centre Sarajevo, Bosnia and Herzegovina

Introduction: Until these time there are different kinds of hypolipemic diet, but the most patients are following advises from Step I and Step II diet of American NCEP. Alternative strategy is "Mediterranean diet". We evaluated the effects of short term combined diet (Step I, II and Mediterranean) reach in antioxidants. Methodology: Twenty patients with dyslipidemia Fredrickson's Tip IIa and IIb were included for a period of 4 weeks. Laboratory tests were performed before and after this period.
Results: TC; Tg; HDLC; VLDLC; LDLC; ApoB; ApoA1; C/HDLC; phospholipids; alpha; pre-beta1; beta; index beta/alpha; lipemia degree and atherogenic index were changed after 4 weeks of diet by -9,7%; -15,5%; -15,5%; -9%; -4,7%; -11,8%; -5,9%; -3,9%; -10,3%; +2,5%; -12,5%; +5,4%; -6,4%; -10,1% and -3,4% respectively. TC, ApoB, ApoA1, phospholipids and lipemia degree changes were statisticaly significant.
Conclusion: Comparing to the results from other studies conducted throughout longer diet period, results from our study are comparabile even for shorter period, with combined diet and without any adverse catabolic reactions. Key words: diet, lipids

## P - 185

### Pharmacokinetics of Ciprofloxacin and Levofloxacin in Patients with Liver Cirrhosis: Influence of Albumin Dialysis

Majcher-Peszynska J., Klammt S., Mundkowski .R, Berg A., Mueller S.C., Peszynski P., Mitzner S.R., Drewelow B.
Institute for Clinical Pharmacology, University of Rostock, Germany

Fluoroquinolones are frequently used in patients with liver cirrhosis. Albumin dialysis by Molecular Adsorbent Recirculating System (MARS) is a new extracorporeal detoxification method with growing clinical acceptance for the therapy of liver failure. The aim of this clinical investigation was to determine the pharmacokinetics of ciprofloxacin and levofloxacin in patients with end-stage liver disease during albumin dialysis. During 11 clinical MARS treatments the elimination of ciprofloxacin (n= 6) and levofloxacin (n=5) were evaluated. PK parameters (mean ± SD):

| | $t_{1/2}$ [h] | AUC [mg*h/l] | $Cl_{total}$ [ml/min] | $Cl_{MARS}$ [ml/min] | $Cl_{MARS}/Cl_{total}$ [%] |
|---|---|---|---|---|---|
| Ciprofloxacin | 7,1 ± 2,5 | 12,5 ± 5,5 | 264,2 ± 90,4 | 86,8 ± 15 | 4,9 ± 10,8 |
| Levofloxacin | 14,6 ± 3,8 | 81,8 ± 13,5 | 89,1 ± 17,3 | 65,3 ± 13,8 | 73,8 ± 15,3 |

Elimination was found to be decreased in decompensated liver disease (Child C). Although during the entire MARS treatment period both fluoroquinolones were removed to a significant degree, no negative impact on antimicrobiological therapy could be assumed with respect to PK/PD relationship. The impaired endogenous clearance might be compensated in part by extracorporeal clearance. Therefore, no dosage adjustment of ciprofloxacin and levofloxacin seems to be necessary for patients with end stage liver disease during albumin dialysis.

## P - 187

### Monitoring Digoxin Serum Concentrations

Donado E., García M., Tato F., Tarragó J., Velasco M., Durán C.
Department of Clinical Pharmacology, Santiago de Compostela and Primary Health Care Service, Lalín (Spain)

Background: A large number of uncontrolled patients could result from the habitual prevention in avoiding the digoxin toxicity
Objective: To determine the frequency of out of the range serum digoxin concentration (SDCs) on the basis of our population data.
Methods: The SDCs, that asked for our service during a 14-year period, have been classified into three groups: low therapeutic range, high therapeutic range and exact therapeutic range. The following variables have been analyzed: age, gender, source, dose and dosage interval.
Results: Data were collected on 1185 patients. 51% of them had low SDCs, 10% had elevated SDCs and 40% were within the therapeutic range (0,8 - 2 ng/ml). The distribution of the variables in the three groups shows that women present high therapeutic levels most frequently, people who are aged 75 or older usually have lower levels and that in primary health care are more frequent to find low therapeutic levels that in hospital services.
Conclusions: 1) A large number of patients have an inadequate level. 2) Some of the analyzed variables are associated with out of the range SDCs (age, gender, source). 3) We propose educative measures to improve this problem.

## P - 186

### Adverse Events in Healthy Volunteers: a Phase I 5-years Survey

Lutfullin A., Kuhlmann J., Wensing G.
Institute of Clinical Pharmacology, Bayer AG, Wuppertal, Germany

This study analysis all adverse events (AEs) in healthy volunteers which occurred in a phase I center over a 5-years period. It includes 142 phase I studies with 1559 participants, 2955 treatments and 29664 follow up days. The incidence of AEs was defined as the ratio between the number of AEs and follow-up days. Incidences were compared using the Chi-squared test. There were a total of 2604 AEs of 291 types (overall incidence 8,78%) with headache and diarrhoea as the most frequent. Almost half of all AEs were drug related (ADR). Only 11 AEs were serious, all resolved completely. AEs occurred 3- (all AEs) and 6-fold (ADRs) more frequent in multiple dose than in single dose trials. Within placebo-controlled studies there was a significant difference between active drug and placebo (all AEs :14,15% vs. 8,96%; ADRs: 7,4% vs. 1,4%). This difference resulted from multiple dose studies only. Other determinants for higher AE-incidences were: first period, first study day, elderly, females, high body weight. In conclusion, multiple dose studies are necessary to define a substance-specific AE-profile.

## P - 188

### Dynamics of a Level of Endothelin-1 and Parameters of an Immunological Homeostasis in Patients with Myocardial Infarction Under Influence of Thrombolytic Therapy

Pivovar S., Rudyk Y., Gorb Y.
Research Institute of Therapy of Academy of Medical Science of Ukraine, Kharkov, Ukraine.

This research is devoted to study of changes of level of endothelin-1 and parameters of an immune reactivity in patients with myocardial infarction after the thrombolytic therapy by kabikinase (streptokinase) . The study of level of endothelin-1 (by radioimmunological method) and parameters of immunity reactivity were performed in 144 patients with Q-myocardial infarction (day 1, 7, 14). In 66 patients the thrombolytic therapy was carried out. It is established, the level of endothelin-1 increases (on 34.3 %) per the first day after thrombolytic therapy. Under influence streptokinase by the end of the first day increase content of granulocyte (on 85.7%), decrease their cytophagous activity (on 23.8%) and content of eosinophyle (on 71.9%), increase complement of activity (by 21.7%) and content of CD8+ lymphocyte (on 18.5%). For 5-7 days after thrombolytic therapy decrease content of leukocytes (on 20.2%), granulocyte (on 10.1%) increase account of eosinophyle (on 65.0%), lymphocytes (on 32.0%), and cytophagous activity of granulocytes (by 16.8%). On 12-14 day raise contents of leukocytes (on 43.9%) and CD4+ lymphocytes (on 11.1%).
Conclusions: The application of streptokinase in patients with myocardial infarction conducts to rising of level of endothelin-1 per first day, increasing of postnecrosis inflammation activiti. Key words: myocardial infarction, endothelin-1, immune system.

## P – 189

**Lack of Influence of Glutathione S-transferase (GSTM1) and (GSTT1) Null Genotypes and T-allele Frequency at the MDR-1 Gene on Susceptibility to Parkinson's Disease**

Bernal L.
University of Zaragoza

Both environmental and genetic factors are involved in the development of Parkinson's disease (PD). Biotransformation of exogenous and endogenous compounds may play a role in the inter-individual susceptibility. Glutahione S-transferases (GSTs) protect cellular damage and P-glycoprotein (P-gp), codified by the MDR1 gene, prevents xenobiotics penetration into the brain. The objective of this work was to determine the association between the risk of developing PD and the polymorphic traits GSTM1*0, GSTT1*0 or MDR1 C3435T. The sample consisted of 99 PD patients and 100 healthy controls. GSTM1 and GSTT1 genotypes were assayed by a multiplex PCR and P-gp polymorphisms by a PCR-RFLP assay. The results showed no statistically significant differences between patients and controls regarding the frequencies of homozygous delection of GSTM1 (GSTM1*0) (OR: 0.831; 95% CI: 0.475 to 1.454; $p > 0.05$) or GSTT1 (GSTT1*0) (OR: 1.441; 95% CI: 0.716 to 2.901; $p > 0.05$). MDR-1 allele frequencies (C vs T) were also similar in both groups (OR: 0.961; 95% CI: 0.551 to 1.676; $p > 0.05$). The data do not suggest a substantial interaction effect between genotypes GSTM1 null, GSTT1 null, or MDR1 T/T and risk of developing Parkinson´s disease .

## P – 190

**GH Deficiency and rhGH Treatment Alter CYP3A Activity in Children: Influence of: Gender and Pubertal Status**

Sinues B.
University of Zaragoza

Growth Hormone (GH) seems to exert an essential role in the interphase pharmacogenetic-development by modulating the expression of genes encoding metabolising enzymes. In this work, 34 GH-deficient children, 15 boys and 19 girls, were studied before and 4 weeks after starting therapy with rhGH (dose:0.166 mg/Kg/week).There were 11 boys and 12 girls in prepubertal status. The control group consisted of 34 healthy children matched for age and sex with patients. The biomarker of CYP3A activity was the ratio beta-hydroxycortisol/ free cortisol in overnight urine. A significant higher CYP3A activity was observed in GH deficient children before treatment ($p=0.0001$) in the total group; independently to de sex ($p= 0.014$ in boys and $p= 0.02$ in girls), but observed only in those in prepubertal status. By contrast, GH treatment derived in a gender dependent effect consisting in a decreased activity only in prepubertal boys ($p= 0.008$), with a non significant increase in girls ($p> 0.05$). By comparing CYP3A activity between controls and children after 1 month on GH treatment, a superior activity was detected in girls ($p=0.001$) without differences in boys. This effect was only seen in prepubertal girls. These results are the first observations in humans beings and are consistent with most data previously reported in rodents.

## P – 191

**Polypharmacy and Adverse Drug Reactions in Patients of Different Age**

Đaković-Švajcer K., Vujisić A.
Dept of Pharmacology, Toxicology and Clinical Pharmacology, Faculty of Medicine, Novi Sad, Serbia & Montenegro

The review of medical documentation from 1989, 1994 and 2000 has been used in order to evaluate drug utilization and accompanying adverse drug reactions (ADRs) in the territory of one local primary care unit. Examined groups of patients were related to children (aged 3-5), adults (aged 30-35) and to the elderly (aged over 65). The patients were chosen by chance (40 of each group and of each year, as well). The number of prescripted medicines per visit was approximately the same at children and elderly group (1,73 and 1,84, respectively). The number of prescripted medicines was significantly increased at elderly patients prevailing in chronic diseases (3.16). ADRs were notified at 8,3% of treated children, 9,1% of treated adults and 43,3% of elderly patients. Two ADRs were recorded at 12,5% of patients over 65 years of age. The number of recorded ADRs was in exponential accordance to the concomitantly used drugs (10 cases in children group, 11 in adults and 67 in elderly). This increase of ADRs is likely to be the consequence of interaction of concomitantly used drugs.

## P – 192

**Experience with Transdermal Fentanyl in Hospitalised Chronic Pain Patients**

Girardin F., Piguet V., Desmeules J., Escher M., Vernaz N., Offner J.M., Dayer P.
Multidisciplinary Pain Centre, Division of Clinical Pharmacology and Toxicology, Geneva University Hospital, CH-1205 Geneva, Switzerland

Since 1997, transdermal fentanyl has been available in Switzerland. We retrospectively analysed the use of transdermal fentanyl in 1683 pain inpatients, consecutively referred to a pain centre in Geneva between 1998 and 2003. At the first consultation, 101 patients were already treated with transdermal fentanyl. During the follow-up period, transdermal fentanyl was introduced in 72 inpatients, so that in all 173 were exposed (67% of them are cancer patients). The main reasons for introducing transdermal fentanyl were poor compliance with oral opioids and stable pain intensity. Controlled pain (decreased intensity more than 50%) was obtained in 77 (45%) patients receiving transdermal fentanyl. In 46 patients (27%), transdermal fentanyl was interrupted, mainly because of poor pain control and adverse effects. Transdermal fentanyl remains an alternative analgesic treatment in a limited number of inpatients referred to our pain centre, due to the fact that the pain conditions dealt with are not stable and undergo major fluctuations. Nevertheless, total oral and transdermal inhospital opioid consumption during this period constantly increased.

## P - 193

Lumiracoxib does not Affect the Pharmacokinetics of Methotrexate in Patients with Stable Rheumatoid Arthritis

[1]Hartmann S., [2]Scott G., [1]Rordorf C., [3]Milosavljev S., [1]Branson J., [4]Chales G., [5]Juvin R., [6]Lafforgue P., [7]Le Parc J.M., [8]Tavernier C., [9]Meyer O.
[1]Novartis Pharma AG, Basel, Switzerland, [2]Novartis Pharmaceuticals, Horsham, UK, [3]Novartis Pharmaceuticals Corporation, East Hanover, NJ, USA, [4]Hôpital Sud Rennes, France, [5]Hôpital Michallon Grenoble, France, [6]Hôpital - la Conception Marseille, France, [7]Hôpital Ambroise Paré Boulogne Billancourt, [8]CHRU Dijon, France, [9]Hôpital Bichat-Claude Bernard, Paris, France

Lumiracoxib (Prexige®) is a cyclooxygenase-2 selective inhibitor under investigation for treatment of osteoarthritis, rheumatoid arthritis (RA) and acute pain. The safety, tolerability and effect of lumiracoxib (400 mg od, orally for 7 days) on methotrexate pharmacokinetics (7.5–15 mg orally once a week), was evaluated in 18 patients with RA in a multicentre, randomized, double-blind, placebo-controlled, two-way crossover study. Serial blood and urine were collected for 24 hours post methotrexate dose on Day 1 (methotrexate alone), Day 8 and 15 (co-administration phase with either lumiracoxib or placebo) for the determination of methotrexate and 7-hydroxymethotrexate levels (HPLC-UV) and methotrexate-protein binding. Patients (15 female, 3 male) were of mean age 49 years and mean weight 67 kg. Plasma methotrexate levels ($AUC_{0-t}$ [ngΣh/mL], $C_{max}$ [ng/mL], $T_{max}$ [hours]) and methotrexate protein binding (%) were similar for methotrexate alone (108.0, 26.7, 1.5 and 57.1, respectively), methotrexate/lumiracoxib (110.2, 27.5, 1.0 and 53.7, respectively) and methotrexate/placebo (101.8, 22.6, 1.0 and 57.0, respectively). Similarly, no difference was found in plasma 7-hydroxymethotrexate levels, or urinary excretion of methotrexate and 7-hydroxymethotrexate. In conclusion, lumiracoxib was well tolerated with no significant effect on the pharmacokinetics, protein binding or urinary excretion of co-administered methotrexate in patients with RA.

## P - 194

Fluconazole does not Affect Lumiracoxib Pharmacokinetics in Healthy Subjects: a two-stage, open-label, randomized, crossover study

[1]Yih L., [2]Scott G., [1]Yeh C.M., [1]Milosavljev S., [3]Laurent A., [4]Rordorf C.
[1]Novartis Pharmaceuticals Corporation, East Hanover, NJ, USA, [2]Novartis Pharmaceuticals, Horsham, UK, [3]PPD, Austin, TX, USA, [4]Novartis Pharma AG, Basel, Switzerland

As lumiracoxib (Prexige®), a cyclooxygenase-2 selective inhibitor, is metabolized by cytochrome P450 (CYP) 2C9, the effect of fluconazole (a CYP2C9 inhibitor) on lumiracoxib pharmacokinetics was investigated. Healthy volunteers (n=13; 4 male, 9 female) received fluconazole (400 mg od on Day 1 and 200 mg od on Days 2–4) with a concomitant single-dose of lumiracoxib 400 mg on Day 4 or no treatment (Days 1–3) and single-dose lumiracoxib 400 mg on Day 4 in an open-label, randomized, crossover design. Plasma lumiracoxib profiles were obtained on Day 4 of each sequence. Thromboxane $B_2$ ($TXB_2$) was measured pre dose and 2 hours post dose (Day 4) to assess cyclooxygenase selectivity. Plasma lumiracoxib was measured by HPLC-MS and $TXB_2$ by immunoassay. Subjects were of mean age 41.5 years and mean weight 66.1 kg. Fluconazole increased lumiracoxib $AUC_{0-t}$ and $AUC_{0-\infty}$ by 18% ($p<0.001$) and $C_{max}$ by 12% (ns). $T_{max}$ for each treatment was similar while $t_{1/2}$ was modestly increased with fluconazole (7.28 vs 6.19 hours). $TXB_2$ inhibition was similar ± fluconazole (ns). None of the pharmacokinetic changes observed are considered to be clinically relevant. In conclusion, lumiracoxib dose adjustment appears unnecessary when co-administered with CYP2C9 inhibitors.

## P - 195

Pharmacokinetics of Lumiracoxib in Synovial Fluid and Plasma of Patients with Rheumatoid Arthritis

[1]Reynolds C., [2]Scott G., [3]Looby M., [1]Milosavljev S., [4]Huff J.P., [5]Ruff D.A., [3]Rordorf C.
[1]Novartis Pharmaceuticals Corporation, East Hanover, NJ, USA, [2]Novartis Pharmaceuticals, Horsham, UK, [3]Novartis Pharma AG, Basel, Switzerland, [4]Arthritis Center, South TX, USA and [5]Healthcare Discoveries, San Antonio TX, USA

Lumiracoxib (Prexige®) is a cyclooxygenase-2 selective inhibitor developed for management of rheumatoid arthritis (RA), osteoarthritis and acute pain. This open-label, multiple-dose study investigated lumiracoxib pharmacokinetics in synovial fluid (SF) and plasma from 22 patients (17 female, 5 male) with RA. Each patient received lumiracoxib 400 mg od for 7 days. On Day 7, following an overnight fast, a final dose of lumiracoxib was administered and serial blood samples and sparse SF samples were collected for up to 28 hours post dose. Lumiracoxib and metabolites were measured using LC/MS. Plasma and SF data were analysed using a population model. Patients were of mean age 51 years and mean weight 76.7 kg. Lumiracoxib was rapidly absorbed ($T_{max}$ 2 hours) and the plasma terminal half-life was short (6 hours). Plasma concentrations were low in the latter part of the dose interval. In contrast, concentrations of lumiracoxib in SF remained substantially higher than in plasma at the end of the dose interval; $AUC_{12-24}$ for SF was 2.6 fold higher than for plasma. Metabolite concentrations remained low in plasma and SF throughout. The pharmacokinetics of lumiracoxib are characterised by rapid absorption, a short plasma half-life but with sustained higher concentrations in SF.

## P - 196

Lumiracoxib Shows Similar Bioavailability at Different Sites in the Gastrointestinal Tract

[1]Wilding I.R., [1]Connor A.L., [2]Carpenter P., [3]Rordorf C., [3]Branson J., [4]Milosavljev S., [2]Scott G.
[1]Pharmaceutical Profiles Ltd, Nottingham, UK, [2]Novartis Pharmaceuticals, Horsham, UK, [3]Novartis Pharma AG, Basel, Switzerland, [4]Novartis Pharmaceuticals Corporation, East Hanover, NJ, USA

This study compared the absorption and pharmacokinetic profile of lumiracoxib (Prexige®), a cyclooxygenase-2 selective inhibitor, at four sites in the gastrointestinal (GI) tract. Eleven healthy male subjects were randomised, in a 4-way crossover study, to receive single dose lumiracoxib 100 mg delivered to either the stomach (reference), proximal small bowel (PSB), distal small bowel (DSB) or ascending colon (AC), with inter-treatment wash out ≥4 days. Site specific drug delivery in the gut was achieved by remote controlled capsules. Location of the capsule in the intestine prior to drug release was tracked by g-scintigraphy. 24-hour plasma lumiracoxib pharmacokinetic profiles were obtained following each dose at each site. Ratios for $AUC_{0-\infty}$, $AUC_{0-t}$ and $C_{max}$, relative to the stomach, were close to unity for the PSB (1.04, 1.01 and 1.08, respectively), DSB (1.10, 1.09 and 1.52, respectively) and AC (0.85, 0.82 and 0.82, respectively). Median $T_{max}$ following release in the stomach was 2.0 hours compared with 1.0 hour for all other sites. In conclusion, lumiracoxib was rapidly and efficiently absorbed throughout the GI tract. There were no major differences in the bioavailability of lumiracoxib following absorption at different sites along the GI tract.

## P - 197

Multiple-dose Lumiracoxib Shows Rapid Absorption and COX-2 Selectivity without Accumulation in Patients with Rheumatoid Arthritis

[1]Scott G., [2]Rordorf C., [3]Milosavljev S., [4]Chase W., [5]Fleischmann R., [6]Kivitz A.
[1]Novartis Pharmaceuticals, Horsham, UK, [2]Novartis Pharma AG, Basel, Switzerland, [3]Novartis Pharmaceuticals Corporation, East Hanover, NJ, USA, [4]Seton Medical Park Tower, Austin, TX, USA, [5]University of TX Southwestern Medical Center, Dallas, TX, USA, [6]Altoona Center for Clinical Research, Duncansville, PA, USA

The pharmacokinetic profile and selectivity of supratherapeutic doses of the cyclooxygenase-2 (COX-2) selective inhibitor lumiracoxib (Prexige®) was assessed in patients with rheumatoid arthritis (RA) participating in a 4-week multicentre, randomized, parallel-group study of lumiracoxib 800 mg od, lumiracoxib 1200 mg od and naproxen 500 mg bid. Lumiracoxib pharmacokinetic data were collected from a subset of 25 patients (12 in 800 mg and 13 in 1200 mg group) on Days 0, 14 and 28. On the same days, platelet aggregation data were collected from 33 patients (11 in lumiracoxib 800 mg, 10 in lumiracoxib 1200 mg and 12 in naproxen group). Patients (17 female, 8 male) who provided pharmacokinetic samples were of mean age 47.6 years and mean weight 72.8 kg. Within each group, lumiracoxib plasma concentration profiles and pharmacokinetic parameters ($AUC_{0-12h}$, $C_{max}$, AUCt and apparent clearance) were similar on Days 0, 14 and 28. Plasma levels rose rapidly with median $T_{max}$ of 2.0 hours in both lumiracoxib groups. An under-proportional dose-dependent increase in $C_{max}$ and AUC was observed. Naproxen, unlike lumiracoxib, inhibited arachidonate-induced platelet aggregation. Lumiracoxib was quickly absorbed and plasma levels rapidly reached steady-state without accumulation. COX-2 selectivity of lumiracoxib was maintained at a dose of 1200 mg/day.

## P - 198

Lumiracoxib does not Alter the Pharmacokinetic Profile or Efficacy of the Triphasic Oral Contraceptive Triphasil®-28

[1]Kalbag J., [2] Rordorf C., [1]Wang Y., [3]Caldwell J., [4]Leese P., [5]Scott G.
[1]Novartis Pharmaceuticals Corporation, East Hanover, NJ, USA, [2]Novartis Pharma AG, Basel, Switzerland, [3]Radiant Research, Daytona Beach, Florida, USA, [4]Quintiles, Lenexa, Kansas, USA, [5]Novartis Pharmaceuticals, Horsham, UK

This study evaluated whether co-administration of lumiracoxib (Prexige®), a cyclooxygenase-2 selective inhibitor, alters the pharmacokinetics or contraceptive efficacy of ethinyl oestradiol (EO) and levonorgestrel (LN) (Triphasil®-28). Healthy women (n=35, mean age 25.2 years and mean weight 64.5 kg) taking Triphasil®-28 were enrolled in this three treatment period, placebo-controlled study. In treatment period one, women received Triphasil®-28 alone and in periods two and three they received either Triphasil®-28/lumiracoxib 400 mg od or Triphasil®-28/placebo for 28 days in a randomized, double-blind, crossover design. Plasma pharmacokinetic profiles for EO and LN were assessed on Day 21 of periods two and three. During each period, serum progesterone (concentration >3 ng/mL being considered as hormonal evidence of ovulation) and sex hormone-binding globulins (SHBG) were measured pre dose and 2 hours post dose on Day 21. Mean ratios for $AUC_{0-12h}$, $AUC_{0-24h}$, $C_{max}$, and $C_{min}$ of EO and LN between the lumiracoxib and placebo treatment periods were generally close to unity (range 0.94–1.13) demonstrating that lumiracoxib did not alter the pharmacokinetics of either EO or LN. Moreover, mean progesterone and SHBG concentrations remained similar when compared with placebo, demonstrating that lumiracoxib did not interfere with the efficacy of Triphasil®-28.

## P - 199

Lumiracoxib Demonstrates High Absolute Bioavailability in Healthy Subjects

[1]Hartmann S., [2]Scott G., [1]Rordorf C., [3]Campestrini J., [1]Branson J., [4]Keller U.
[1]Novartis Pharma AG, Basel, Switzerland, [2]Novartis Pharmaceuticals, Horsham, UK, [3]Laboratoires Novartis S.A., Rueil-Malmaison, France, [4]Swiss Pharma Contract Ltd., Allschwil, Switzerland

This study assessed the absolute bioavailability of a lumiracoxib 200 mg tablet (Prexige®), a cyclooxygenase-2 selective inhibitor, following concomitant oral and intravenous (iv) administration. 12 healthy subjects (9 male, 3 female) received simultaneously $^{13}C$-lumiracoxib 100 mg iv (2.26 mg/mL potassium salt, infused over 30 minutes) and lumiracoxib 200 mg orally. Serial blood samples were withdrawn over 48 hours post dose to calculate non-compartmental pharmacokinetic parameters. Plasma $^{13}C$-lumiracoxib and lumiracoxib were analyzed simultaneously by HPLC-MS. Tolerability and monitoring of vital signs were assessed throughout. Subjects were of mean age 38.2 years and mean weight 77.7 kg. Estimates following iv and oral lumiracoxib were $C_{max}$ (14,625 vs 5,964 ng/mL), $T_{max}$ (0.5 vs 2.3 hours) and $AUC_{0-\bullet}$ (13,343 vs 20,036 ng∑h/mL), respectively. Distribution volume, clearance and absolute bioavailability were 9.0 L, 7.7 L/h and 74%, respectively. No discontinuations due to serious adverse events or relevant changes in vital signs occurred. In summary, this study showed that the clearance and volume of distribution of orally administered lumiracoxib is low and the absolute bioavailability is high (74%). Both oral and iv lumiracoxib were well tolerated.

## P - 200

Co-administration of Lumiracoxib and Warfarin does not Alter the Pharmacokinetic Profile of R- or S-Warfarin

[1]Bonner J., [1]Scott G., [2]Branson J., [3]Milosavljev S., [2]Rordorf C.
[1]Novartis Pharmaceuticals, Horsham, UK, [2]Novartis Pharma AG, Basel, Switzerland, [3]Novartis Pharmaceuticals Corporation, East Hanover, NJ, USA

Lumiracoxib (Prexige®), a novel cyclooxygenase-2 selective inhibitor, is metabolized by cytochrome P450 (CYP) 2C9. This study investigated the interaction between lumiracoxib and warfarin, a 'sensitive' CYP2C9 substrate. Subjects (n=24, 20 male, mean age: 33.5 years) genotyped as extensive CYP2C9 metabolizers received loading and maintenance doses of warfarin on Days 1–13. On Day 9, subjects were randomized to receive lumiracoxib 400 mg od or placebo for 5 days. On Day 8 and Day 13 blood samples were taken serially and urine collected for measurement of plasma R- and S-warfarin levels and urinary excretion of the warfarin metabolite S-7-hydroxy warfarin (HPLC). Prothrombin time (PT) was measured every 12 hours. Co-administration of lumiracoxib and warfarin did not significantly alter the pharmacokinetics of R- or S-warfarin, including AUC or $C_{max}$ for R- or S-warfarin or metabolite excretion. Lumiracoxib increased PT at Day 13 versus Day 8 (19.9 vs 17.5 seconds; placebo PT 17.8 vs 17.6 seconds, respectively). These results suggest that lumiracoxib has low potential for interaction with other CYP2C9 substrates. In accordance with standard clinical practice, the increase in PT suggests routine monitoring of coagulation should be performed during co-administration of lumiracoxib and warfarin.

## P - 201

Omeprazole and Maalox® Antacid do not Affect Lumiracoxib Pharmacokinetics in Healthy Subjects: an open-label, randomized crossover study

[1]Reynolds C.V., [2]Scott G., [1]Milosavljev S., [1]Langholff W., [3]Shenouda M., [4]Rordorf C.
[1]Novartis Pharmaceuticals Corp., East Hanover NJ, USA, [2]Novartis Pharmaceuticals, Horsham, UK, [3]MDS Pharma Services, Neptune, USA, [4]Novartis Pharma AG, Basel, Switzerland

This study evaluated the effect of co-administration of omeprazole (proton pump inhibitor) or Maalox® (aluminum hydroxide/magnesium hydroxide antacid) on the pharmacokinetic profile of lumiracoxib (Prexige®), a cyclooxygenase-2 selective inhibitor. Twelve fasted healthy volunteers (9 males) received 3 treatments each separated by a 7 day washout period: single oral-dose lumiracoxib 400 mg (Day 1); Co-administration of lumiracoxib 400 mg with omeprazole 20 mg od (preceded by 4 day's treatment with omeprazole, 20 mg od); and co-administration of lumiracoxib 400 mg with Maalox® (20 mL). Plasma was obtained pre dose and serially up to 48 hours post dose for lumiracoxib measurement (HPLC-MS). Subjects were of mean age 36 years and mean weight 76.8 kg. The ratio of the geometric means of $AUC_{0-\infty}$ and $C_{max}$ between lumiracoxib alone and both lumiracoxib plus omeprazole and lumiracoxib plus Maalox® were close to unity (0.95–1.11). The 90% CIs for $AUC_{0-\infty}$ and $C_{max}$ were within boundaries of 0.80–1.25, except for $C_{max}$ after Maalox® co-administration (0.95–1.31). The difference in $C_{max}$ was however not significant (p=0.261). In conclusion, in healthy subjects, co-administration of omeprazole or Maalox® with lumiracoxib does not affect lumiracoxib pharmacokinetics and dose adjustment of lumiracoxib is unnecessary.

## P - 202

Safety of Neuroleptics in Schizophrenic Patients in Correlation with the Total Oxidative Hepatic Capacity.

Ziganshina L.E., Kuchaeva A.V., Vedernikova O.O., Yakhin K. K., Gatin F.F.
Department of Clinical Pharmacology and Pharmacotherapy, Kazan State Medical Academy, Russia

The objective of the study was to evaluate the safety of neuroleptics' therapy at the psychiatric hospital on the basis of dosing analysis and total hepatic oxidative capacity.
Methods: 210 patients were followed for the period of 2000-2002 years. The total daily neuroleptics load was calculated with chlorpromazine equivalent and measured in mg of oral chlorpromazine. The total hepatic oxidative capacity was tested with the help of antipyrine test. The results were evaluated statistically with the Student's *t*-test.
Results: 33,3% of patients experienced side effects of neuroleptics with movement disorders being most problematic. Total daily neuroleptics' load in these patients was 563,2±246,35 mg of oral chlorpromazine which was not different from the same of the patients without side effects - 515,71±158,55.
The mean antipyrine half-life in patients with neuroleptics-induced side effects was longer than in patients without side effects: 17.49±0.15 vs 14.95±0.72, p<0,05. In all patients with antipyrine half-life 15 hours and more the mean daily neuroleptics' load was 263.25±45.69. In patients with antipyrine half-life less than 15 hours the mean daily neuroleptics' load was higher - 776.36±221.27 mg of oral chlorpromazine, P<0.05.
Conclusion: lower total hepatic oxidative capacity is one of the risk factors for the development of neuroleptics induced side effects; these patients require lower doses of neuroleptics for the therapeutic effect.

## ORAL

Light Evoked Pupillography - a Sensitive Clinical Biomarker for 5-HT1A Compounds

Boettcher M., Heinig R., Wensing G., Kuhlmann J.
Institute of Clinical Pharmacology, Bayer AG, 42096 Wuppertal, Germany

Light evoked pupillography (LEP) is a simple, non-invasive, valid method to quantify pharmacodynamic effects on the autonomic and central nervous system.
Method: The influence of the 5-HT1A-agonists (40-120mg Ipsapirone, 125µg-2.0mg Repinotan (CYP2D6 substrate)) on pupil reaction was investigated in 180 young, healthy male subjects by means of LEP (PupilscanTM). The initial pupil diameter (INIT) and reflex amplitude (RA) were related to plasma concentration and compared to body temperature and quantitative pharmaco-EEG (QPEEG).
Results: Both 5-HT1A-agonists showed a dose- and concentration-effect related reduction of the INIT and RA. This effect was more pronounced for Repinotan. In contradiction to the poor (counter-clock wise hysteresis), extensive and intermediate metabolizers show the same concentration-effect relationship. Therefore, LEP can be used to differenciate poor and extensive metabolizers. For Repinotan, significant effects were observed for the INIT at plasma levels > 4 µg/L, RA > 13µg/L, body temperature > 15µg/L and QPEEG >> 20 µg/L.
Conclusion: LEP is more sensitive but less specific than hypothermia and QPEEG. Therefore it should be discussed as a 'standard' to measure pharmcodynamic effects on 5-HT1a-compounds.

## P - 203

Pharmacokinetics (PK) of Melagatran, the Active Form of the Oral Direct Thrombin Inhibitor Ximelagatran, and the Relationship to Clinical Response in Extended Secondary Prevention of Venous Thromboembolism

[1]Cullberg M., [1]Clason S.M., [2]Eriksson H., [3]Karlsson M.O., [1]Lundström T., [1]Nyström P., [4]Schulman S., [1]Wåhlander K.
[1]AstraZeneca R&D Mölndal, Mölndal, Sweden; [2]Sahlgrenska University Hospital/Östra, Göteborg, Sweden; [3]Uppsala University, Uppsala, Sweden; [4]Karolinska Hospital, Stockholm, Sweden.

Purpose: To characterize the PK of melagatran, after oral dosing with ximelagatran (Exanta™, AstraZeneca), in extended secondary prevention of venous thromboembolism (VTE), and the relationship between exposure and clinical outcome.
Methods: PK data (3595 samples/596 patients) from THRIVE III, a randomized, placebo-controlled, double-blind study of patients with previous VTE receiving oral ximelagatran (24 mg bid) for 18 months after standard anticoagulation, were evaluated using a population model. Plasma samples were collected at 0.5, 3, 6, 9, 12, 15, and 18 months. The relationship between exposure and clinical outcome was evaluated using a proportional hazard model.
Results and Conclusions: PK of melagatran were consistent over 18 months. Population mean AUC was 1.8 h·µM (5th-95th percentile 1.1-3.6). Melagatran CLpo was correlated with CrCL. Smoking or comedications (13 classes tested) did not significantly influence melagatran PK. The hazard ratio [HR] for ximelagatran vs placebo was 0.16 (95% CI 0.09-0.30) for VTE and 1.19 (95% CI 0.93-1.53) for bleeding. There was no significant association between exposure and VTE risk (HR per unit AUC=0.55; 95% CI 0.21-1.46), or bleeding risk (HR=1.06; 95% CI 0.89-1.27). These results support the use of fixed-dose oral ximelagatran 24 mg bid for long-term secondary prevention of VTE, without drug monitoring.

## P - 204

Subdosing of Parenteral Antibiotics in General Practice (GP) in Serbia

[1]Samardzic R., [1]Divac N., [1]Bajcetic M., [2]Vujnovic M.
[1]Institute of Clinical Pharmacology, School of Medicine, Belgrade, [2]WHO Office Belgrade

Extremely high consumption of cotrimoxazole, ampicillin and gentamycine has been reported in Serbia over the last decade. The aim of this study was to investigate the pattern of prescribing and dosage of antibiotics in GP. In a retrospective, cross-sectional study, drug prescriptions issued to 1800 patients (58.3+-0.3 years of age; 60% females)during one visit to GP were analyzed. Total number of DDD of each antibiotic prescribed per one patient was calculated. Total of 415 antibiotic prescriptions (8.9% of all prescribed drugs) were given to 313 patients (17.3% of all patients), mostly diagnosed with acute upper respiratory and urinary tract infections. The most frequently prescribed antibiotics were penicillins (19.8%), cotrimoxazole (18.0%), aminoglycosides (14.2%), cephalosporins (13.7%), tetracyclines (11.3%), pipemidic acid (9.8%), cyprofloxacine (3.1%) etc. Average number of DDD per patient for oral antibiotics varied from 4.2 to 7.4. Parenteral antibiotics were prescribed to 98 patients (gentamicin 57, procain penicillin 25, lincomycine 13, amikacin 2, ceftriaxone 1). The number of DDD of parenteral antibiotics per patient was 2.9 (gentamicin), 4.6 (penicillin), 2.3 (lincomycin) and 1.0 (amikacin and ceftriaxone). These results indicate a restricted choice of antibiotics associated with serious subdosage of all parenteral antibiotics and of some oral fomulations.

## P - 205

Clinical and Pharmacoeconomical Outcomes of Posternotomy Mediastinitis due to Staphylococcus Aureus Methicillin-Resistant and Methicillin-Susceptible Infection

Kadusevicius E., Zaliaduonyte D., Zmuidaite V., Stankevicienė I., Benetis R.
Kaunas Medical Univesity Hospital, Department of Clinical Pharmacology, Cardiac Surgery Department, Eiveniu str.2, Kaunas 3000, Lithuania.

Objective: to evaluate clinical and pharmacoeconomical outcomes of poststernotomy mediastinitis (PSM) caused by methicillin-resistant and methicillin-susceptible Staphylococcus aureus (MRSA and MSSA, respectively).
Methods: we reviewed hospital records of 61 patients with S. aureus PSM who were treated from 1 January 1999 to 1 January 2002 at Kaunas University Hospital. Staphylococcus aureus was the infectious agent identified in the wound secretion or in the mediastinum, or both. PSM was caused by MRSA in 12 patients and by MSSA in 49. Both groups had similar perioperative characteristics.
Results: The median time from operation to the development of mediastinitis was 9 (9.24+/-1.13) days in MSSA pts. group vs.11 (11.83+/-2.14) days in MRSA group. In-hospital mortality rate in pts. with MRSA mediastinitis was significantly higher 0.33 % vs. to 0.04 % of pts. with MSSA, respectively (relative risk [RR], 8.17; 95% confidence interval [CI], (1,89 to 34,57); Number needed to treat [NNT] = -3,42; 95% [CI](-12,37 to -1,74). Duration in-hospital stay for pts. with MRSA mediastinitis - 63 (63.33+/-5.8) days vs. 43 (43.88+/-4.18) days for pts. with MSSA mediastinitis (p = 0,0169). Direct costs for antibiotic treatment for one patient in MRSA group was 880.85+/-158.86 €; 95%[CI] (534.72-1226.99) vs. 249.63 €; 95%[CI] (123.52-375.75), p<0.001. Incremental cost per one death avoided for antibiotic treatment (ICER) - 2176.62 €. 18 days treatment with vancomycin and fusidic acid was more successful that 9 days treatment with vancomycin alone in MRSA group. Relative risk reduction [RRR] = 0,65; 95% (-0,56-0,94) of PSM-related death and treatment failure.

## P - 206

Dermal Absorption of Permethrin Following Administration to the Haired Area of the Head

Lazar A., Tomalik-Scharte D., [1]Bastian B., 1Meins J., [1]Ihrig M., [2]Wachall B., Jetter A., Fuhr U.
Institute for Pharmacology, University of Köln; [1]Zentrallaboratorium Deutscher Apotheker, Eschborn; [2]Infectopharm Arzneimittel und Consilium GmbH, Heppenheim; Germany

Permethrin is an insecticide used in the treatment of lice and scabies infection. Although efficacy and safety are documented, pharmacokinetic data are sparse. The objective of the present study was to determine dermal absorption and elimination of permethrin from a hair rinse solution (Infectopedicul®) used to treat head lice. In 6 young healthy male volunteers with a hair length of 5 to 15 cm, 50 ml of the solution containing 215 mg of permethrin (cis/trans: 25/75) were administered to the haired area of the head. The hair was rinsed with clear water 45 min and washed with shampoo 48 hours thereafter. Urine was collected 0-8, 8-16, 16-24, 40-48, 88-96 and 160-168 hours postdose. The main metabolite of permethrin, 3-(2,2-dichlorvinyl)-2,2- dimethylcyclopropane carboxylic acid, and its conjugates were measured in urine using a specific and sensitive GC/ECD method. Pharmacokinetic parameters were estimated using WinNonlin, version 4.01. Maximal urinary excretion was reached during the 8-16 hours sampling interval. The terminal elimination half-life was 32.7 +/- 6.7 hours. Urinary recovery of the metabolite (extrapolated to infinity and for the intervals not covered by sampling) reached 0.35 +/- 0.12 molar % of the permethrin dose. The treatment was well tolerated. In conclusion, the extent of systemic exposure following this external administration is low and therefore does not cause a specific risk for systemic adverse effects.

## P - 207

Increased Concentrations of the Acyclovir Main Metabolite 9-Carboxymethoxymethylguanine (CMMG) in CSF in patients with Neuropsychiatric Side Effects

1Helldén A., 2Lycke J., 1Ståhle L.
1Division of Clinical Pharmacology, Department of Laboratory Medicine, Karolinska Institutet, Huddinge University Hospital, Stockholm, Sweden. 2Institute of Clinical Neuroscience, Department of Neurology, Göteborgs Universitet, Sahlgrenska University Hospital, Göteborg, Sweden

Introduction: Acyclovir-related neuropsychiatric side effects have frequently been reported in patients with acute or chronic renal failure. We have shown that the concentration in serum of the acyclovir (ACV) main metabolite CMMG was increased in patients with neuropsychiatric symptoms (1). The aim of this study was firstly, to investigate if CMMG could be found in the cerebrospinal fluid (CSF), and secondly if there was any difference in concentration between patients with neurological symptoms compared with patients lacking these symptoms.
Patients and methods: We collected CSF samples from 17 patients, 5 with and 12 without neuropsychiatric symptoms. Those with neuropsychiatric symptoms had acute or chronic renal failure. Patients with no symptoms had normal renal function. The samples were collected within 24 hours after previous dose. The CMMG concentrations were analysed with HPLC (2).
Results: The median concentration of CMMG in the CSF in patients with no symptoms was below the limit of detection (<0.2 μmol/L), compared with mean concentration of 2.46 μmol/L, (95% CI 0.21 to 4.71) in patients with neuropsychiatric symptoms.
Conclusion: The main finding in this study was that CMMG could be detected in the CSF. Secondly, we found that the concentration of CMMG in CSF was at least 7- to 70- fold higher in patients with neuropsychiatric symptoms compared with patients having no symptoms. These findings support our hypothesis that CMMG might be involved in the development of neuropsychiatric side effects in ACV-treated patients.

## P - 208

Flavonoids Modulate Endothelial Function and Have Protective Role on Cardiovascular System
Ilic K., Kuntic V.
Faculty of Pharmacy, Belgrade, Serbia and Montenegro

Flavonoids are group of more than 4 000 biologically active compounds with heterogeneous molecular structures. They are responsible for the colour and taste of many fruits and vegetables. Red wine, black tea, fruit juices, apples, onion, broccoli are particularly reach in flavonoids. Flavonoids demonstrate antioxidative, anti-inflammatory, antiallergenic, anticancer and cardioprotective effect. Flavonoids favourably affect endothelial function. The endothelium consists of cells that cover the inside of blood vessels. Normal endothelium regulates vasomotor tone, platelet activity, leucocyte adhesion and vascular smooth muscle proliferation via release of nitric oxide (NO) and prostaciclin. In endothelial dysfunction release of those factors is impaired. In atherosclerosis endothelial dysfunction is associated with increased oxidative stress and may be reversed by antioxidant treatment. The precise mechanism by which flavonoids improve endothelial function was not determined. Several mechanisms have been suggested. Inhibition of cyclooxygenase and scavenging of superoxide anions, which are strong inhibitors of prostacyclin production, seems to be essential. Experimental evidence shows that flavonoids improve endothelium-derived NO bioactivity. Recent research indicates that flavonoids modulate endothelial function and suppress release of proatherosclerotic factors, such as endothelin-1.

## P - 209

New and rapid LC-MS Method to Determine Piperacillin and Tazobactam in Sputum of Patients with Cystic Fibrosis
Trittler R., König A., Frank U., Kümmerer K.
Institute of Environmental Medicine and Hospital Epidemiology University Hospital Freiburg, Germany.

Piperacillin and Tazobactam are used in the therapy of patients with cystic fibrosis. It is important that adequate doses reach the location of the infection. Effective control can be achieved by monitoring the drug concentrations in sputum. The analysis of piperacillin and tazobactam in sputum with HPLC and UV-Detection is very difficult because of the high variability of different sputum samples. Not all substances which interfere UV-detection can be eliminated by solid phase extraction techniques. A new LC-MS method with integrated sample preparation was developed which allows the determination of piperacillin and tazobactam in sputum without interference with ms-detection. The method was used to determine piperacillin and tazobactam in sputum of 6 young adults which have been treated with 4,5g Tazobac administered as a 30-min intravenous infusion every 8h. It could be shown that in no case adequate doses at the place of infection was reached.

## P - 210

Impact of the Directive 2001/20/EC on Clinical Trial Regulation and Process in Hungary
Eggenhofer J., Borvendég J.
National Institute of Pharmacy Budapest, Hungary

Major objectives of the CT Directives are: harmonisation of EU regulations, ensure a legislative framework for GCP, shorten timelines, (single application format and concent for applicant to CA and EC, single EC opinion, harmonisation of AR-s reporting and impection procedures, establish an EU database. In Hungary: all of the CT-s has to be authorized by the CA (since the 70-s),documentations which should be submitted by applicant, and the content of the application form are "essentially similar" to those requested by the Directive, the "single ethical opinion" - given by an independent EC is part of the authoratization, released by the CA. The pharmacovigilance system, and inspection of CT-s are organised by the CA. The principles of the Directive 2001/20/EC have already been transposed into Hungarian legislation (24/2002/EüM). The present situation of authorization and ethical approvel of the CT-s in Hungary will be presented by the authors in detail.

## P - 211

Cystic Fibrosis: Pharmacoeconomic Analysis in Hospitalized Patients in the University Paediatric Hospital
Vitezic D., Rosovic-Bazijanac V., Rozmanic V., Ahel V.
University of Rijeka Medical School and University Hospital Centre Rijeka, Croatia.

The aim of the study was to obtain information concerning the most frequently prescribed drugs in defined daily doses (DDD) in patients with cystic fibrosis, and also to analyse financially the use of drugs (in Euro) in CF patients in the hospital setting. During the examined period seven patients with CF were hospitalized. The patients were aged between 2 and 19 years. The analysis showed that the most frequently prescribed drugs were antimicrobial drugs : meropenem (142 DDD; 8396.85 Euro), piperacillin and tazobactam (72.67 DDD; 4013.06 Euro), cefepime (34.00 DDD; 736.88 Euro), ceftazidime (33.75 DDD; 1263.96 Euro) and amikacin (14.00 DDD; 135.77 Euro). The next drug groups were J 02 with fluconazole (10.50 DDD; 152.93 Euro), R 03 and R 05 with salmeterol (12 spray lag.; 346.78 Euro) and dornase alfa (377.00 DDD; 10017.50 Euro). Because of malabsorption pancreatic enzyme replacement products were applied (22510000 IU; 705.18 Euro) and hypercaloric solution (377 L; 1371.76 Euro). The patients were also treated with the use of chest physiotherapy, exercise programs etc. For one year the cost of hospital treatment for our seven patients was 27140.67 Euro totally, and they were hospitalized for 53.86 days on the average (average length is 10.62 days). The used high-cost treatment with a considerable contribution of the specific drugs from J group and dornase alfa prolonged significantly the life of the patients with CF (life expectancy is more than 30 years of age) but the need for a separate budget is obviously needed for these specific and expensive medical conditions.

## P - 212

Regional Clusters in Antibiotic Consumption in Europe Monique

Elseviers M., Robert H., Stichele V., Ferech M., Goossens H.
ESAC management team, University of Antwerp, Belgium

Introduction Within the framework of the ESAC project (European Surveillance of Antibiotic Consumption, EU project granted by DG/SANCO), retrospective data of antibiotic use in ambulatory care (AC) and hospital care (HC) for the period 1997-2001 was collected on a quarterly base. Methods Consumption of antibiotics was expressed according to ATC/DDD classification (WHO, version 2002) and volume was presented in DDD/1000 inhabitants per day (DID). Antibiotic use data were provided by 26 countries; AC use data of 19 countries and HC use data of 22 countries were suitable for international comparison. European countries were geographically clustered in North (LT, LV, NL, NO, SE, DK, FI), South (ES, IT, PT, GR, MT, FR), Central (BE, LU), East (BG, HU, SK, SI, HR, PL) and West (UK). Antibiotic consumption between clusters was compared using ANOVA.
Results In 2001, total AC use (mean, range) differed significantly between regional clusters and was low in the North (14.5 DID (10.0-19.8)) and the West (14.6 DID), moderate in the East (20.6 DID (17.4-24.8)) and high in Central (25.3 DID (24.3-26.4)) and South (26.6 DID (18.8-32.9)). Large regional differences could be observed in the proportional use of different antibiotic classes. North was using low proportions of cephalosporins (CEP) and quinolones (Q) and higher proportions of tetracyclines (TET). In contrast, in South and Central, the proportional use of CEP, macrolides (M) and Q was exceptionally high. .
Conclusion In AC, the high variation in antibiotic use observed between different European countries was clearly related to geographical clustering. In HC, regional clustering of observed variation could not be documented.

## P - 213

A Tolerability and Pharmacokinetic Study of a New Formulation of Disodium Clodronate in Comparison with Two Marketed Formulations in Healthy Female Volunteers

[1]Mariotti F., [2]Corrado M.E., [1]Acerbi D.
[1]Chiesi Farmaceutici S.p.A., Pharmacokinetics Department, Parma, Italy
[2]Cross Research s.a., Phase I Unit, Arzo, Switzerland

Clodronate is a bisphosphonate that has demonstrated efficacy in patients with a variety of diseases of enhanced bone resorption. Intramuscular clodronate can cause pain at the injection site, it is therefore of particular usefulness to co-administer a local anaesthetic with clodronate to reduce pain at the injection site.The tolerability and pharmacokinetic of a new formulation of disodium clodronate 100 mg containing lidocaine 1% (test formulation) were investigated in comparison to a marketed formulation of disodium clodronate 100 mg containing benzyl alcohol 1% (reference A) and to a marketed formulation of disodium clodronate 100 mg without any compound added to reduce the perception of pain associated with intramuscular injection (reference B). Thirty healthy female volunteers were treated according to a single dose, double-blind, randomised three-way cross-over design. The local tolerability was investigated by assessing reddening and hardening at the injection site, and plasma creatinine phosphokinase (CPK) levels. Pain intensity was investigated on the visual analogue scale (VAS). Urinary clodronic acid concentrations were determined by using a validated specific GC/MS/NCI assay. CPK levels and occurrence of hardening at the injection site did not show statistically significant differences between formulations. No local redness was reported. The statistical analysis on pain assessment showed a significant reduction of pain intensity immediately and up to 2 hours after administration of the new formulation compared to the marketed ones. The statistical analysis on urinary excretion didn't show any difference among the formulations demonstrating comparable bioavailability. It was concluded that the investigated new formulation of disodium clodronate 100 mg containing lidocaine 1% was better tolerated than the marketed formulations.

## P - 214

Nonparametric Expectation Maximization (NPEM) population pharmacokinetic analysis of caffeine disposition from sparse data in adult

Terziivanov D., Bozhinova K., Dimitrova V., Atanasova I.
Clin Ther Clin Pharmacol, Univ Hosp «St. I. Rilsky», 15 D. Nestorov st., 1431 Sofia, Bulgaria

Objectives: To explore the ability of the NPEM method to deal with sparse data for elaborating of population pharmacokinetic model of caffeine in adult Caucasians to phenotyping CYP1A2 activity.
Design and Participants: Nonblind, single dose clinical investigation. Thirty four non-related adult Bulgarian Caucasians with normal and reduced renal function, 18 women and 16 men, between 18 and 62 years.
Methods: Each participant received 3mg.kg-1 p.o. caffeine. Two blood samples per individual were taken according to the protocol for measuring caffeine plasma concentrations. A total of 67 measured concentrations were used to obtain NPEM estimates of caffeine population pharmacokinetic parameters. Paraxanthine/caffeine (PX/CA) plasma ratios were calculated and correlated with clearance estimates.
Results: NPEM median estimates of caffeine absorption and elimination rate constants, KA=4.54h-1 and KEL=0.139h-1, as well as of fractional volume of distribution and plasma clearance, VS1=0.58 L.kg-1 and CLS1=0.057L.h-1.kg-1 agreed well with reported values from more «data rich» studies. Significant correlations were observed between PX/CA ratios at 3h, 8h and 10h and clearance (Spearman rank correlation coefficients, rs>0.74, p?0.04). There were no significant differences in clearance due to gender or renal function. Heavy smokers and drinkers showed 2-fold higher clearance values.
Conclusions: Collectively, the results show that the NPEM method is a suitable and relevant one for large-scale epidemiological studies for population phenotyping purposes by monitoring CYP1A2 activity based on sparse caffeine data.

## P - 215

Randomised Trial of Candesartan and Enalapril (RACE) in the Treatment of Hypertension

Cheung B.M.Y., Law C.Y, Fung P.C.W., Tsang K.W.T., Tan K.C.B., Kumana C.R., Lau C.P.
University Department of Medicine, Queen Mary Hospital, Hong Kong.

Introduction: We compared blocking the renin-angiotensin system with an angiotensin-converting enzyme inhibitor or an angiotensin II receptor blocker.
Method: 22 hypertensive patients (M:F, 16:6; age 47±10 yrs) were randomised to candesartan 8mg or enalapril 10mg daily for 3 months. The dose could be doubled for blood pressure control. Ambulatory blood pressure and echocardiography was performed at randomisation and 12 weeks. Flow-mediated dilatation (FMD) was measured at the brachial artery to assess endothelial function. Exhaled nitric oxide (NO) was measured by chemiluminescence. The coefficient of variation of left ventricular mass index (LVMI), FMD and NO measurement were 7%, 5% and 3% respectively.
Results: Candesartan and enalapril significantly lowered clinic and ambulatory systolic and diastolic pressure.

| | Baseline SBP | Baseline DBP | Baseline LVMI |
|---|---|---|---|
| candesartan | 158.2±5.7 | 100.3±3.9 | 139.8±12.5 |
| enalapril | 159.8±4.0 | 97.4±3.0 | 127.3±6.4 |
| | Final SBP | Final DBP | Final LVMI |
| candesartan | 134.5±4.3* | 85.3±3.2* | 134.9±11.1 |
| enalapril | 145.3±6.1* | 87.0±3.4* | 134.5±8.0 |

*p<0.05

The drugs did not differ in their effect on LVMI and exhaled NO. Changes in LVMI correlated with changes in ambulatory SBP (r=0.62, p=0.02) and DBP (r=0.61, p=0.02). FMD increased with enalapril but not candesartan (p=0.04). Neither treatment significantly altered plasma potassium, creatinine, renin and aldosterone. Fasting blood glucose decreased significantly from 5.6±0.4 to 5.1±0.3 mmol/L in the enalapril group (p=0.01) only.
Conclusions: Both drugs lower blood pressure efficaciously. Enalapril may have a favourable effect on blood glucose and endothelial function.

## P - 216

Effect of Renal and Hepatic Function on Oxaliplatin Pharmacokinetics: a Pilot-Analysis in Patients with Gastrointestinal Carcinoma

[1]Merkel U., [1]Zimmer M., [2]Wedding U., [3]Roskos M., [2]Höffken K., [1]Hoffmann A.
[1] Department of Clinical Pharmacology, [2] Clinic of Internal Medicine, [3] Department of Clinical Chemistry and Laboratory Diagnostics, Friedrich Schiller University Jena, Germany

In this pilot investigation, pharmacokinetics of oxaliplatin, measured as the levels of ultrafilterable platinum, the pharmacological active form, was evaluated on day 4 during chronomodulated infusion of oxaliplatin (25 mg/m²/d), 5-fluorouracil (750 mg/m²/d) and sodium folinate (150 mg/m²/d) over 4 days. The effect of renal and hepatic function on pharmacokinetics of ultrafilterable platinum was analysed in 12 patients with gastrointestinal tumours. Creatinine clearance of the patients (range 58.6 - 103.7 ml/min) as marker of renal function was calculated according to Cockcroft and Gault formula. Total clearance of ultrafilterable platinum was significantly related to creatinine clearance (r=0.807; p=0.003). $C_{max}$ did not correlate with renal function, but for $AUC_{0-24h}$ a trend was observed to a negative relationship. Hepatic function was characterised by aspartate aminotransferase (ASAT, range 0.13 - 1.61 µmol/l*s) and alanine aminotransferase (ALAT, range 0.09 - 1.11 µmol/l*s). Total clearance of ultrafilterable platinum was not dependent on hepatic function (ASAT p=0.480; ALAT p=1.0). Neither $C_{max}$ nor $AUC_{0-24h}$ correlated significantly with hepatic function. These results indicated that elimination of ultrafilterable platinum is significantly determined by renal function whereas hepatic function had no effect on the pharmacokinetics of ultrafilterable platinum.

This project is supported by German Cancer Aid (grant AZ-70-2445-Hö3).

## P - 218

Increase in Overall Use and Regional Differences in Prescription Pattern

[1]Christophersen A.B., [2]Andersen S.E., [1]Christensen H.R.
[1]Department of Clinical Pharmacology, [2]Centre for internal medicine; Geriatric Clinic, H:S Bispebjerg Hospital, Copenhagen, Denmark.

Background: There is increased use of cobalamin for preventing neuropsychiatric symptoms in the elderly. The criteria for commencing treatment are controversial and evidence for effect is inconclusive.
Methods: As part of a clinical audit regarding the use of cobalamin, we analysed data from the Danish Medicines Agency and data from Danish Statistics(1997-2001).
Results: National statistical data show a 1.3% increase in total population and 2.4/3.8% in people aged 60+/80+. Prescribing in DDD/1000 inhabitants/day shows extensive regional variation. Overall prescribing increased and 2 counties showed a doubling in DDD by 2001. The proportion of people aged 60+ and 80+ receiving cobalamin increased from 2.0-2.9/4.6-7.1% respectively (p<0.0001) by the year 2001. Direct drug costs of cobalamin increased from 12.2 to 15.6 million DKK during this period, with most of the cost related to use in the primary sector.
Discussion: Overall increased use of cobalamin and large regional differences in prescription pattern illustrate the problems related to implementation of poorly documented treatments. Although inexpensive and with few side effects, there are many related costs of e.g. homecare nursing. Otherwise healthy elderly are made dependent on the health care system. Furthermore, the possibility of designing studies to prove efficacy is obscured by current practice.

## P - 217

Drug Committee Work: To Recommend Or Not To Recommend Activated Protein C (Apc) In The Treatment Of Severe Sepsis

Victor J., Christophersen A.B., Christensen H.R.
Department of Clinical Pharmacology, H:S Bispebjerg Hospital, 2400 Copenhagen, Denmark.

A recurrent problem for drug committees is whether to recommend a new drug. Studies with methodological problems and/or limited indications for subpopulations are of great concern. During the trial of activated protein C several changes to the protocol were made and furthermore approval was only for a subset of patients. Several admendments took place half-way through the trial: the inclusion/exclusion criteria and endpoints were modified. Drug manufacturing procedures, placebo, and the number and location of investigational centers were changed. The treatment benefit was almost exclusively found in the second half of the study. Despite extensive analysis it was not shown that the changes made half-way through the study were responsible and the substantial better treatment benefit in the second half of the study could be caused by chance. Authorities have approved the drug for a subset of more severely ill patients due to the better treatment benefit in these. Alternatives would be to reject a drug depite efficacy in a subpopulation or to approve widely, including a population where efficacy/safety was in doubt. Despite the above problems, APC seems to have the claimed effect and can be recommended, taking the usual economic evaluations into consideration.

## P - 219

Cobalamin Prescribing in a Geriatric Outpatient Clinic; Old Drug, New Indication

[1]Andersen S.E., [2]Christophersen A.B., [2]Christensen H.R.
[1]Centre for internal medicine; Geriatric Clinic, [2]Department of Clinical Pharmacology, H:S Bispebjerg Hospital, Copenhagen, Denmark

Background: The use of cobalamin for preventing neuropsychiatric symptoms in the elderly is increasing. We anted to evaluate the clinical use of cobalamin in patients in a geriatric outpatient clinic. The clinic has a consensus-based guideline for diagnosing cobalamin deficiency.
Methods: We reviewed a random sample of case records from 99 (51%) of the 196 patients attending the clinic at the time.
Results: There were 78 female and 21 male patients. Mean age 81.7 (95% CI 80.2-83.2) years. Overall, 40 patients were receiving cobalamin. None of these for pernicious anemia. In 27 of 40 cases, treatment was initiated in this clinic. In 30 out of 40 patients treatment was administered by homecare nurses. Most prescriptions were in fair accordance with the clinic's guideline, but showed poor compliance with a second guideline in this hospital.
Discussion: Well-designed studies demonstrating efficacy of cobalamin on neuropsychiatric symptoms are lacking. The simultaneous existence of two different guidelines reflects this controversy. Overall, 40% of patients were in cobalamin treatment. Patients are prescribed life-long treatment, where there is no consensus regarding diagnosing and effect is undocumented. The results emphasize the urgent need for large clinical studies to clarify this issue.

P - 220

Correlation of Tramadol Pharmacokinetics in Relation to CYP2D6 Activity in Healthy Volunteers

[1]Perlík F., [2]Nobilis M., [1]Slanař O., [2]Květina J.
[1]Postgraduate Medical Institute and 1st Faculty of Medicine, Charles University, Prague, Czech Republic, [2]Inst. of Experimental Biopharmaceutics, PRO.MED.CS, Academy of Sciences Joint Inst., Hradec Králové, Czech Republic.

Tramadol is a widely prescribed analgesic, which is extensively O-demethylated through CYP2D6 to its main active metabolite (M1). Our aim was to assess the relationship between drug disposition and CYP2D6 phenotype. Blood samples of 10 extensive netabolizers (EM) and 2 poor metabolizers (PM) were collected for 32 hours after a rectal administration of 100 mg of tramadol for pharmacokinetics evaluation. The data were compared with dextromethorphan/dextrorphan metabolic ratio using Spearman correlation coefficient. The metabolic ratio significantly correlated to t1/2 and AUC ($r_s$ values 0.596 and 0.538, respectively), whereas correlation to $c_{max}$ was not significant. Nevertheless, there was a tendency to reach higher $c_{max}$ in PM (1.68 and 1.13 nmol/ml), while mean $c_{max}$ in EM was 0.98 nmol/ml (SD 0.38). It was previously shown that better tramadol efficacy but also higher incidence of ADR in EM than PM after a single dose is related to higher M1 concentrations. On the contrary, based on our preliminary data we can speculate, that after repeated doses ADR frequency could be higher in PM than EM due to accumulation of tramadol in organism. CYP2D6 phenotype can be a helpful criterion for tramadol dosing.
The study was supported by a IGA MZ ČR grant No. 7073-3.

ORAL

Documentation Grading - a Signalling and Quality Assurance Tool for International Adverse Reaction Data

Lindquist M., Kiuru A., Pettersson M., Meyboom R., Edwards R.
WHO Collaborating Centre for International Drug Monitoring, Uppsala Monitoring Centre, Uppsala, Sweden

In 1990, a publication listed criteria for the type of information needed for well-founded signals from the WHO ADR database. The case reports were categorized based on the amount of information in the reports. The analysis showed that agranulocytosis signals could have been identified before publication in the scientific literature in 7/15 instances. Based on these results, a new field 'documentation grading' was added to the WHO database to facilitate the signalling process. The documentation grading is also used for statistical purposes, and to identify problems related to missing data in the reports received. For instance, when investigating why there was a sudden change in the overall documentation grading scores from one country it was revealed that the 'indication' field was left empty. This was due to a change in the national database system, which had not been reflected in the data export files to the WHO database. The situation was quickly remedied. The newly implemented database system (Vigibase) at the UMC allows the capture of more detailed information on each case report. The criteria for the documentation grading have therefore been revised and will hopefully continue to be a useful tool for improving the quality of reports in Vigibase.

P - 221

Bioequivalence Study With Two Preparations Containing Selegiline

Skreblin M., Staresinic-Sernhorst I., Saric-Kuzina S.
BELUPO, Pharmaceuticals&Cosmetics, Koprivnica, CROATIA Regulatory Affairs Zagreb, I Savica 36

In a single-blind, single-dose (10 mg), randomised, two-period, cross-over study with 26 healthy male volunteers the bioavailability of two selegiline HCl products (Nozid® 5 mg tablets, Belupo, and reference product) was compared. Bioequivalence study was based on analytical evaluation of selegiline metabolites (desmethylselegiline /DMS/, methamphetamine/MA/ and amphetamine/A/) concentrations in plasma. The plasma concentrations of metabolites were determined by gas chromatography using a nitrogen-phosphorus detector (DMS, MA) and electron capture detector (A). Statistical analysis was made with 90% confidence intervals for next pharmacokinetic parameters: AUC, $C_{max}$, $T_{max}$ , for which bioequivalence acceptance limits in the range of 0.80 - 1,25 were required. Anova latin square confidence intervals on ln transformed data results were as follows: DMS : 0.822 - 1.193 for AUC (pg.hrs/ml), 0.892 - 1.177 for $C_{max}$ (pg/ml); MA : 0.806 - 1.135 for AUC (pg.hrs/ml), 0.954 - 1.141 for $C_{max}$ (pg/ml); A : 0.881 - 1.061 for AUC (pg.hrs/ml), 0.951 - 1.032 for $C_{max}$ (pg/ml). The results of this study are showing that pharmacokinetic parameters AUC, $C_{max}$, and $T_{max}$ for all 3 selegiline metabolites are completely fulfilling the requirements for bioequivalence. According to this results it can be concluded that Nozid® 5 mg tablets, *selegiline*,Belupo, is bioequivalent to the reference product.

P - 222

Succinate Treatment in Children with Lactic Acidosis

Globa O.V., Jourkova N.V., Kondakova O.B., Bacanov M.I., Maslova O.I., Balkanskaya S.V., Andreenko N.V., Basargina E.N.
Institute of Pediatrics Scientific Center of Children's Health RAMS, Lomonosovsky pr. 2/62,

Both inherited and acquired disturbances of mitochondrial energy generating system represent large group of heterogeneous disorders, which predominantly affect tissues with high energetic demands and often manifested in children. The majority of these diseases are accompanied by neuromuscular deficits. The clinical examination in 10 children with lactic acidosis (3,5-12 mmol/l) and metabolic acidosis revealed the neurological signs in 6 children and cardiological deterioration in 4 children. In prospective and DNA studies 5 children defined as MELAS. All children were treated by metabolic therapy in additional to symptomatic treatment. The metabolic therapy included riboflavin(100mg/day), coenzyme Q(30-90 mg/day), L-carnitine(200-1000mg/day). Supplementary the succinate 250-1000 mg/day orally depending of ages was used. The courses of succinate treatment were 1-3 months and longer depending on the gravity of diseases. Succinate was used with and without of other metabolic medications in some period of treatment. This therapy improved the neurological and somatic status. The gravity and frequency of headaches and seizures were decreased even to absence of syndromes in 80% of cases. In addition we treated children with lactic acidosis in episodes of metabolic acidosis following by the infections by high doses of succinate with positive effect. In conclusion: succinate aid in mitochondrial lactic acidosis detoxification.

P - 223

On the Classification of Sets of Experimental Points and Curves in Biopharmacy. Dissolution And Bioequivalence "Metrics".

Mircioiu C.
Dept. of Applied Mathematics and Biostatistics, University of Medicine & Pharmacy "Carol Davila", Bucharest, Romania

In biopharmacy in the last years were introduced a lot of "metrics", in order to compare or to measure the distances between sets of experimental points obtained for characterization of evolutions of different phenomena. The term "metrics" was chosen since is suggestive it concerns the objectives of these evaluations. Sometimes the proposed metrics are in accordance with the rigorous mathematical definition, corresponding to some particular, well known metrics derived from "norms" on vectors, which are useful to be identified since their properties are extensively studied. These correspond to functions of similarity and functions of dissimilarity, to semimetrics, quasimetrics, different "probabilistic metrics" etc., in a more general "theory of classification". Finally are proposed, starting from cubic norm and from Mahalanobis probabilistic metrics, some new pharmaceutical metrics for the evaluation of sets of dissolution or pharmacokinetic data.

P - 224

On Pharmacokinetic of Orally Administered Glyburide

[1]Mircioiu C., [1]Miron D.S., [2]Taranu B., [2] Mircioiu I.
[1]University of Medicine and Pharmacy "Carol Davila", Bucharest [2]Biopharmacy & Pharmacol Res, Bucharest

A single-dose, randomized, two-treatment, two-periods, two-sequence cross-over study under fasting conditions was performed for comparing equal doses of glyburide administered to 24 healthy volunteers. The good absorption of glyburide cannot be explained by mechanism of solubility and diffusion. It is probable that a great part of absorption is the result of embedding of glyburide molecules in micelles of cholic acid. This hypothesis is agreement with the fact that approximately half of glyburide is eliminated in bile. Time of maximum absorption of glyburide was found to be practically the same for both products, approximately 4 hours. Tested product achieve maximum concentration lower than reference product. A supplementary complication appeared from the saw-teeth aspect of curves in the zone of Cmax. Since the metabolism of glyburide means mainly hydroxylation and half of elimination is made by bile route, an enterohepatic circulation of conjugated metabolites is also probable. AUDs differences had a distribution very closely correlated with that of Cmax. Global examination gave the impression of two populations: a great one, of very similar results in both products, and a smaller one category of volunteers with large differences in AUD. Since variabilities were practically the same for both products, the separation in two classes seemed to rather a characteristic of glyburide than effect of formulation. But, if we take into consideration the dependence of absorption on the dimensions of particles of glyburide, (micronized or non-micronized) would be possible also to think to separation into two clusters following a non homogeneous distribution of particles size between different tablets.

P - 225

Comparative Bioavailability of Two Metoprolol Formulations in Healthy Volunteers

[1]Voicu V.A., [1]Mircioiu C., [1]Miron D.S., [2]Lovin I.
[1]University of Medicine and Pharmacy "Carol Davila", Bucharest,[2]Labormed Pharma, Bucharest

Metoprolol has a good solubility and also a good and rapid absorption, belonging theoretically to the class I in the biopharmaceutical classification of drugs, this assuring automatically bioequivalence. Practically, metoprolol is subject to considerable first-pass metabolism. Following a high variability of metabolism peak plasma concentrations vary widely and metoprolol is incriminated as a highly variable drug, though this variability is mainly intersubject variability. On other hand, metabolism is less dependent on formulation and appears the danger of imposing criteria of bioequivalence to the tested drug which are not achieved even if we compare reference drug with itself. Such a way interpretation of data has to be founded on a more refined analysis in order to separate clear the contribution of pharmaceutical formulation to variability. In a bioequivalence study concerning two metoprolol formulation on 26 healthy volunteer in a 24h interval, pharmacokinetics of metoprolol appeared to be highly variable interindividual (90% for AUC and 70 % for $C_{max}$). On the contrary, the apparent intra-individual variability (which is a sum of intrinsec intraindividual variability and formulation effect) was low, for AUC being 27%. In these conditions more reliable information on bioequivalence was the difference between experimental means than the composition of the large confidence interval with acceptance limits.

P - 226

Enterohepatic Circulation and Bioequivalence Evaluation

Voicu V.A., Mircioiu C.
University of Medicine & Pharmacy "Carol Davila", Bucharest, Romania

Enterohepatic circulation is analysed in connection with two phenomena of "flip-flop" balance in a reversible conjugation reaction and in embedding of drug molecules of billiary acids and possible dependence of these processes on the farmaceutical formulation. A first consequence of the enterohepatic circulation on the pharmacokinetics is the prolongation of the half-life of the drug in the living body. Another consequence is the appearance of more maxima in plasma levels. These effects lead to difficulties in evaluation of maximum concentration $c_{max}$ and half—time elimination $t_{1/2}$. First criterion of bioequvalence (BE) evaluation - $c_{max}$ is, in some cases really discredited. Another criterium - difference between areas under curve is also viciated due to propagation of uncertaintes in $t_{1\backslash 2}$ evaluation in uncertainties in extrapolated areas and implicitly to total areas. It remains as main method of BE evaluation the comparison of areas under experimental data. Joint with this evaluation it can be considered a comparison of zones of maxima using some models.

## P - 227

Purinergic Modulation of Voltage-Dependent Calcium Channels in Rat Dorsal Root Ganglion Neurons

[1]Borvendeg S.J., [1]Gerevich Z., [2]Gillen C., [1]Illes P.

[1]Rudolf-Boehm-Institute of Pharmacology and Toxicology, University of Leipzig, Härtelstraßse 16-18, D-04107 Leipzig and [2]Preclinical Research, Grünenthal GmbH, D-52088 Aachen, Germany

The inhibition of voltage-dependent calcium channels (VDCCs) mediated by $P2Y_1$ receptors and the co-localization of $P2X_3$ and $P2Y_1$ receptors in cultured small to medium-sized neurons were investigated in rat dorsal root ganglia (DRG). Whole-cell patch-clamp techniques and Fura-2 fluorescence measurements with additional isolectin $B_4$-labelling, were used. In patch-clamp recordings, the P2X/P2Y agonist ATP concentration-dependently inhibited the inward current through VDCCs. The $P2X_{1-3}/P2Y_1$ receptor antagonist pyridoxal-5-phosphate-6-azophenyl-2',4'-disulphonic acid (PPADS) and the $P2Y_1$ receptor antagonist 2'-deoxy-$N^6$-methyladenosine-3',5'-diphosphate (MRS 2179) markedly reduced the inhibitory effect of ATP. In $Ca^{2+}$-imaging experiments, the high external $K^+$-induced increase in $[Ca^{2+}]_i$ was inhibited both by ATP and ADP-b-S. In contrast, a,b-methylene ATP (a,b-meATP) potentiated the effect of high $K^+$ on $[Ca^{2+}]_i$. However, when given alone, ATP, ADP-b-S and a,b-meATP all increased $[Ca^{2+}]_i$. PPADS and MRS 2179 antagonized the effects of ATP and ADP-b-S, whereas TNP-ATP interfered with that of a,b-meATP. $P2Y_1$ receptor appears to act via G proteins and a membrane-delimited pathway. $P2X_3$ and $P2Y_1$ receptors appear to be co-localized on the same DRG cell population. $P2X_3$ and $P2Y_1$ receptor-activation may lead to increased transmitter release from the central neuronal processes and to counterbalancing inhibition of VDCCs, respectively, probably resulting in a finely tuned regulation of pain signal transmission.

## P - 228

The Influence of Drug Bulletins on Prescribing

Ksenija M.A., Igor F., Bozidar V.

Katalinic Romana Division of Clinical Pharmacology, Department of Medicine, University Hospital Centre Rebro, 12 Kispaticeva, Zagreb, Croatia

At the end of year 2002 Editorial board of the Hospital Drug Bulletin, the official bulletin of Hospital Drug Committee of the University Hospital Zagreb and Clinical Hospital Merkur decided to carry out a survey of its acceptance, use and influence on its readers. The Hospital drug bulletin is in the 27th year, appearing 10 times a year. Its target audience are hospital physicians esp. doctors of teaching hospitals. Plus that about 1300 doctors and pharmacists all over Croatia get it by subscription. The prepared questionnaire was sent to all doctors of these two hospitals. This survey, the fourth till now carried out by Hospital drug Committee, was performed with intention to learn the habits of doctors and their attitude to rational drug prescribing. All previously conducted surveys of Drug bulletin had a poor response (not more than 10% of readers responded). Some of the questions from questionnaire are listed bellow: 1.Are you a specialist (which specialisation?) or resident (which specialisation?) 2.Age? Sex? 3.How long do you practice medicine? 4.I read Drug bulletin: a) regularly; b) occasionally; c) don't read 5.Is the Drug bulletin critical enough and publish objective, comparative and independent information on drugs? 6.Does Drug bulletin increase your knowledge about rational pharmacotherapy? Does it influence your prescribing? 7.Does Drug bulletin help you in recognizing interactions and side effects of drugs? Do you report adverse drug reactions? 8.Do you trust the information published in Drug bulletin?

## P - 229

Randomised Controlled Trial of Low Salt Diet in the Treatment of Hypertension

Cheung B.M.Y., Law C.Y., Ho G.Y.Y., Ng P.P.Y., Kumana C.R., Lau C.P.

University Department of Medicine, University of Hong Kong, Queen Mary Hospital, Hong Kong.

Background: Non-pharmacological treatment is the preferred initial management of mild hypertension. We compared its efficacy with drug treatment.

Methods: 93 patients (M:F, 45:48; age 44 ± 11 yrs) with untreated mild essential hypertension were recruited. After a placebo run-in phase, 73 eligible patients were randomised to drug treatment (with hydrochlorothiazide 25 mg daily [n=19] or metoprolol 100 mg daily [n=14]) or low-salt diet for 6 months. Drugs were allowed after 12 weeks for blood pressure control.

Results: In the diet group, there was a significant decrease in sodium intake (56 ± 14 mmol/day) and body fat (1.7 ± 0.5%).

| | N | Diastolic BP | | Systolic BP | |
|---|---|---|---|---|---|
| | | baseline | final | baseline | final |
| diet | 38 | 95 ± 1 | 89 ± 1 | 142 ± 2 | 135 ± 3 |
| drug | 35 | 96 ± 1 | 83 ± 2* | 142 ± 2 | 122 ± 3* |

* $P < 0.05$

There were significant decreases in ambulatory systolic and diastolic pressure in the drug (16±2 mmHg and 10±2 mmHg) and diet group (10±2 mmHg and 6±1 mmHg). Change in sodium excretion correlated with diastolic pressure (r=0.44, p=0.02).

Conclusion: Non-pharmacological treatment reduces blood pressure slightly, but to a lesser extent than antihypertensive drugs. In patients with severe hypertension, it should be implemented in conjunction with medications.

## ORAL

Survey on Prescribing of Antimicrobial Agents (AA) in University Hospital in Two Consecutive Years

Francetic I., Bilusic M., Macolic-Sarinic V., Huic M., Mercep I., Erdeljic V., Makar-Ausperger K., Katalinic R., Likic R.

Division of Clinical Pharmacology, Department of Medicine, University Hospital Centre Rebro, Kispaticeva 12, Zagreb, Croatia

Over prescribing of antimicrobial agents (AA) is generally regarded as one of the major causes of growing resistance both in outpatient and hospital setting. In attempt to improve prescribing of AA in our hospital we did a survey of prescribing of AA in our hospital. In 2001 and 2002 during one day all the patients hospitalized were seen by clinical pharmacologists and checked for AA therapy. On Feb21st 2001 216 out of 714 patients (30.3%) and on Oct 23rd 2002 207 out of 891 (23.2%) were receiving AA. On both occasions gentamycin and cefuroxime were mostly prescribed AA representing nearly 25% of total AA prescribed. To determine whether AA were used appropriately a scoring system was used. Out of 243 courses of AA treatment 86 were restricted release antimicrobials in 2001 and 77/237 in 2002. . According to the robust scoring system in 2001 AA were properly used in 104 out of 138 pts for treatment (prophylactic use excluded) and in 2002 AA were properly used in 113 out of 149 pts. Questionable use of AA was very similar, 24% in both years. The results of the survey are the basis for the measures to be proposed by Hospital Drug Committee to improve AA prescribing in our Hospital. Taking into account that 25% of total drug bill goes to AA optimising of prescribing or diminishing even a part of unnecessary use of AA could save substantial amount of money not to speak about medical aspects of rational use of AA in the hospital.

## P - 230

Nasal Sumatriptan Effectively Relieves Migraine Attacks in Children

[1,2]Ahonen K., [1]Hämäläinen M.L., [3]Rantala H., [1,2]Hoppu K.
[1]Hospital for Children and Adolescents, and [2]Department of Clinical Pharmacology, University of Helsinki, Helsinki; [3]Department of Paediatrics, University of Oulu, Oulu, Finland

Objective: To Investigate The Efficacy Of Nasal Sumatriptan In Migraine Attacks Of Children And Adolescents.
Methods: A Double-Blind Placebo-Controlled Two-Way Crossover Trial With 8 To17 Years Old Children, With At Least Two Attacks (IHS 1988) Per Months And Duration Over Four Hours. The Study Treatment Was A Single Dose Of Sumatriptan Nasal Spray (Imigran®, GSK) Or A Matching Placebo At The Onset Of An Attack. Sumatriptan Dose Was 10-Mg (Body Weight 20 -39 Kg) Or 20-Mg (> 40 Kg). The Primary Efficacy Endpoint Was Headache Reduction By Two Grades On A Five-Grade Face Scale At Two Hours.
Results: Totally 129 Children Were Recruited. Of Them 83 Used Both Treatments And 11 Only The First. The Primary Efficacy Endpoint At Two Hours Was Reached Twice As Often After Sumatriptan (N=53; 64%) As After Placebo (N=32; 39%; P<0.01). However, At Two Hours, Only 30% (N=25) After Sumatriptan And 19% (N=16) After Placebo Became Pain-Free (P=Ns). Already At One Hour, Primary Endpoint Was Reached More Often After Sumatriptan (N=42; 51%) Than After Placebo (N=24; 29%; P=0.01). Subjectively, 57% (N=47) Preferred Sumatriptan And 34% (N=28) Preferred Placebo (P<0.05), While 8 Were Undecided. Rescue Medication Was Used By 35% (N=29) After Sumatriptan And 51% (N=42) After Placebo (P=Ns). No Serious Adverse Events Were Observed, 29% (N=26/90) Reported A Bad Taste After Sumatriptan And 3% (N=3/87) After Placebo (P<0.01).
Conclusions: Nasal Sumatriptan Is An Effective Treatment For Migraine Attacks In Children And Adolescents.

## P - 231

Orange Juice Greatly Reduces Plasma Concentrations of Celiprolol

Lilja J.J., Juntti-Patinen L., Neuvonen P.J.
Department of Clinical Pharmacology, University of Helsinki, FIN-00290 Helsinki, Finland

Background: Celiprolol is a beta-adrenoceptor blocking agent that is eliminated without a significant metabolism. We wanted to study the effects of orange juice on the pharmacokinetics of celiprolol.
Methods: Ten healthy volunteers drank in a randomized, two-phase cross over study either 200 ml normal-strength orange juice or water three times daily for two days. On the morning of day 3, the subjects ingested 200 ml orange juice or water. One hour later they received 100 mg celiprolol with 200 ml orange juice or water. In addition, the subjects drank 200 ml orange juice or water 4, 10, 23, and 27 hours after ingestion of celiprolol. Blood pressures and heart rate were measured before the administration of celiprolol and 2, 4, 6, and 10 hours later. Celiprolol plasma concentrations and its excretion into urine were measured up to 33 hours.
Results: Orange juice reduced the Cmax and AUC(0-33) of celiprolol by 89% (P < 0.01) and 83% (P < 0.01). In addition, the amount of celiprolol excreted into urine was reduced by 77% (P < 0.01) by orange juice. No significant differences were observed in the haemodynamic variables between the study phases.
Conclusion: Orange substantially reduced the Cmax, AUC and urinary excretion of celiprolol which indicates an impaired absorption of the drug. This food-drug interaction probably is of clinical importance.

## P - 232

Bioequivalence Study of Two Enalapril Formulations (20 mg) in Healthy Volunteers

Portolés A., García-Arenillas M., Terleira A., [1]Almeida S., Vargas E.
Phase I Study Unit, Clinical Pharmacology Service, Hospital Clínico San Carlos, Madrid, [1]Tecnimede SA, Prior Velho, Portugal

Objective: The objective of the present study was to compare the bioavailability of two commercial brands of enalapril tablets (enalapril from Tecnimede, vs Renitec® from MSD, 20mg), described as the rate and extent of absorption of the active moiety, in order to assess their bioequivalence.
Design: The study was conducted as an open, 2x2 crossover study, with two administration periods (20mg of enalapril, under fasting conditions) separated by a washout period of 7 days.
Setting: Phase 1 study unit. During each study period, a single oral dose of one of the formulations was administered, and 15 plasma samples were collected to determine enalapril and enalaprilat levels and calculate their kinetic parameters.
Subjects: 24 healthy volunteers of both sexes (12 males and 12 females), aged 22.83 ± 2.21 years, with an average weight of 65.1 ± 12.35Kg and height of 173 ± 10.18cm, were included in the study. Results: From the plasma levels of the drug and active metabolite the following kinetic parameters were calculated for each formulation: $C_{max}$, $AUC_t$, $AUC_{inf}$ and $t_{max}$. The 90% confidence intervals of the ln-transformed concentration derived parameters ($C_{max}$, $AUC_t$ and $AUC_{inf}$) were all within the 80-125% rule, both for enalapril and enalaprilat. No statistically significant model effect was found (formulation, sequence, period and subject within sequence). Time to maximum plasma concentration was also not statistically different and the 90% confidence interval calculated for $t_{max}$ by Wilcoxon's test, for the difference of the medians, was also within the predefined range.
Conclusions: both formulations can be considered bioequivalent both in extent and rate of absorption.

## P - 233

Incidence of Drug-Related Visits in a Hospital Emergency Room

Juntti-Patinen L., Kuitunen T., Pere P., Neuvonen P.J.
Department of Clinical Pharmacology, University of Helsinki and Porvoo Hospita, Finland.

Objectives: To determine the incidence of drug-related visits in a emergency department (ED) of a district hospital.
Methods: During the study period of six months there were altogether 7143 emergency department visits to the Porvoo hospital. The physician in duty or one of the authors (LJ-P) selected the suspeted drug-related visits for further scrutinization. The final decision whether the visit to the ED was drug-related or not was based on the patients files including laboratory and other test data. The probability of a drug´s relation to the visit was classified according to the WHO´s classification.
Results: The number of evaluable visits was 7113 (99.6 % of all the visits) and 168 of them (2.4 % of all visits) were classified as "certainly" or "probably" drug-related. There were 66 (0.9%) intentional overdose-related visits and 102 (1.4%) adverse drug event (ADE) -related visits. The most common ADEs were gastrointestinal symptoms caused by antibiotics or NSAIDs. The majority of overdose-related ED-visits were caused by psychotropics, mainly by anxiolytic drugs, but also antipsychotics and antidepressants were involved. Rate of hospitalisation was 40% in all drug-related visits.
Conclusions: Drug-related visits constitute a significant part of all visits in the ED. ADE-related visits lead considerably often to hospital admission. Majority of patients suffering from intentional overdose were discharged from the ED after few hour`s observation.

ORAL

## Do Medical Students Copy the Drug Treatment Choice of Their Teachers or Do They Think for Themselves ?

Richir M.C.
Department of Medical Pharmacology, VU Medical Centre, Amsterdam, Netherlands.

Aim To find out if students copy the drug treatment choice of their teachers, and if they differ from their teachers in the argumentation for that choice.

Methods 32 final year medical students and 103 medical teachers from all eight Dutch medical faculties first determined a (drug) treatment for a straightforward uncomplicated and a complicated written patient case. For each case, they indicated to what extent drug choice related factors played a role in the argumentation of their (drug) treatment. Finally, they filled out a questionnaire about teaching therapeutics.

Results For both cases, the students prescribed about the same number of specific drugs as general practitioners, but less compared to clinicians. There was no significant difference between the drug choice related factors and the level of the two patient cases. Clinicians used practically and drug oriented factors significantly more than students, while students relied more on education oriented factors. Both students and teachers agreed about the insufficient teaching regarding choosing drugs.

Conclusion The overall results indicate that students are less able to choose drugs themselves and tend to copy the drug choice behaviour of their teachers, most likely due to lack of experience and training in choosing drugs.

P - 234

## NSAIDs Sensitive to Radiant Tail Flick Test When Given Peripherally

[1]Dogrul A., [3]Gulmez S.E., [2]Ossipov M.H., [2]Porreca F., [3]Tulunay F.C.
[1]Department of Pharmacology, Gülhane Academy of Medicine, 06018-Etlik, Ankara, Turkey [2]Department of Pharmacology, Arizona Health Sciences Center, University of Arizona2, Tucson AZ 85724 USA [3]Department of Pharmacology and Clinical Pharmacology and Headache Research Center, Medical School of Ankara University, Ankara, Turkey

Several animal models have been used for preclinical evaluation of analgesic potency of the nonsteroidal anti-inflammatory drugs (NSAIDs). Historically, the tail-flick test has reliably predicted the antinociceptive activity of the opioids. In contrast, the NSAIDs, are not detected by this test when administered systemically. The anti-inflammatory and antinociceptive activities of NSAIDs are attributed to inhibition of the cyclo-oxygenase (COX) enzyme, thus blocking the synthesis of prostaglandins that promote inflammatory responses and enhanced sensitivity to pain at the site of tissue injury. Prostaglandin release at peripheral sites, such as the skin, sensitizes the nociceptors to noxious inputs, thus promoting pain.

Antinociceptive activity was determined by increased tail-flick latencies to noxious radiant heat applied to the tail of the mouse. NSAIDs were administered by subcutaneous (s.c.) injection, and radiant heat was applied at the site of injection. The s.c. injection of diclofenac, dipyrone, ketorolac and lysin acetyl salicylate over the dose range of 3-300 µg produced dose-dependent increases in tail-flick latency when the radiant heat source was focused directly over the injection site. The NSAIDs were not active when the heat source was directed 1 cm proximal or distal from the site of injection. The maximal antinociceptive responses produced by s.c. diclofenac, ketorolac and lysin acetyl salicylate were 98 %, 54 % and 82 %, respectively. The duration of antinociception was 120 min. The $ED_{50}$ values and 95 % confidence interval of diclofenac, ketorolac and lysin asetyl salisilate are found to be 10.71µg ( 7.88 to 14.57), 135.26 µg (48,75 to 374) and 228.9 µg (125,04 to 419,31), respectively. Importantly, the intraperitoneal injection of diclofenac, ketorolac or lysin acetyl salicylate given over the dose range of 100-300 mg/kg did not produce any detectable antinociception in the tail-flick test, consistent with previous studies.

Results: NSAIDs demonstrate a promonent localized antinociceptive effect at peripheral sites. Localized activity of NSAIDs is underscored by the observations that the s.c. NSAIDs did not block nociception when the heat stimulus was applied to the surrounding region, and relatively large i.p. doses of the NSAIDs were also without antinociceptive effect.

P - 235

## The Effect of Gemfibrozil on the Pharmacokinetics of Rosuvastatin

[1]Schneck D.W., [1]Birmingham B.K., [1]Wang Y., [1]Zalikowski J.A., [1]Mitchell P.D., [2]Lasseter K.C., [1]Raza A.
[1]AstraZeneca, Wilmington, Delaware, USA; [2]Clinical Pharmacology Associates, Miami, Florida, USA

Co-administration of statins and gemfibrozil is associated with increased risk for myopathy, which may be due in part to a pharmacokinetic interaction. This randomised, double-blind, 2-period crossover trial (4522IL/0095) assessed the effect of gemfibrozil on rosuvastatin pharmacokinetics. Twenty healthy volunteers were given gemfibrozil (600 mg b.d.) or placebo orally for 7 days. On the fourth morning of each period a single oral dose of rosuvastatin 80 mg was co-administered. Plasma concentrations of rosuvastatin, rosuvastatin-lactone, and N-desmethyl rosuvastatin were measured. Gemfibrozil increased rosuvastatin AUC(0-t) 1.88-fold (90% CI: 1.60–2.21), and Cmax 2.21-fold (90% CI: 1.81–2.69), compared with placebo. Pharmacokinetics of rosuvastatin-lactone were unchanged. N-desmethyl rosuvastatin AUC(0-t) and Cmax decreased by 48 and 39% respectively. The size of this interaction is similar to that reported for simvastatin acid (AUC(0-infinity) and Cmax increased 2.5- and 2.1-fold) and lovastatin acid (both AUC(0-24) and Cmax increased 2.8-fold), but substantially less than that for cerivastatin acid (AUC(0-infinity) and Cmax increased 5.6- and 3.1-fold) and lactone (AUC(0-infinity) and Cmax increased 4.4- and 1.8-fold). The reduced N-desmethyl rosuvastatin exposure could reflect gemfibrozil inhibition of CYP2C9. CYP2C9 metabolism is a minor rosuvastatin clearance pathway, inhibition of which could not account for the rosuvastatin interaction. The mechanism remains to be determined.

P - 236

## The Influence of Senna's Leaves Water Extract on Rat Liver Enzymes Activity

[1]Samajlik I., [1]Djakovıc-Svajcer K., [2]Popovic M.
[1]Dept of Pharm, Tox and Clin Pharm, Faculty of Medicine, Novi Sad, [2]Institute of Chemistry, Faculty of Natural Sciences and Mathematics, Universtity of Novi Sad, Serbia and Montenegro

Senna (Cassia senna L., C. acutifolia) is a well-known drug used in the treatment of constipation. Its purgative action is due to the presence of sennosides A and B. The aim of our assay was to examine the influence of senna water extract on rat liver enzymes activity and systems. We used rats, divided into 4 groups according to the duration of senna oral intake: C - control group, no senna intake; AC - group which received 1 mL of extract only once; CH3 - group which was receiving it during 3 days and CH7 group which was at the same regimen during 7 days, prior sacrificing. Senna's leaves water extract (maceration) consisted of about 2,9 mg sennosides B/mL. Results showed significantly great loss in body mass of animals after 1st and 3rd day, while it was less on 7th day. The activity of glutathione-peroxidase and lipid peroxidation were significantly increased, while the content of glutathione was decreased earlier, on 3rd day. The activity of liver peroxidase was increased after first application of senna and reached the maximum value on 7th day. These results may suggest on possible interactions and potentiation of oxidative action of other drugs/substances taken concomitantly during senna intake.

## P - 237

Consumption of Medicines in Southwestern Russian Medical or Social Disabled Person Population: The Most Reimbursed vs. Most Utilized Drugs

Tatarkin A., Kalinichenko V., Mamontov A., Kalinichenko D., Gorokhov S., Shevchenko N.
Regional Clinical Hospital # 1, Medical Information Center, Krasnodar Research Center of RAMN and Administration of Krasnodar Kray, Krasnodar, Russian Federation

About (mean+/-SD) 192 670 +/- 6543 (from total of 750000) residents of the city of Krasnodar are eligible to get their pharmaceuticals free of charge or with 50% reimbursement. We analysed 1817667 prescriptions to 344487 outpatients in 1999-2001 according to ATC/DDD methodology and reimbursed drug expenses. Average budget charges on each recipe (1999/ 2000/ 2001) have made - EUR 1,55.- / 2,09.- / 2,36.-. An annual average per capita expenditures were EUR 7,45.-/ 10,10.-/ 15,03.- respectively. The first ten most reimbursed pharmaceuticals in 2001 were as follows(INN/EUR): Enalapril (50491,61); Levodopa+Carbidopa (46267,56); Vinpocetine (41283,23); Captopril (36699,10); Desmopressin (23582,81); Valproic acid (19819,60); Fenoterol (19798,86); Carbamazepine (17506,62); Amiodarone (17376,31); Beclometasone (16378,38). And the first ten most utilized drugs were (2001, INN/DDDs): Amoxicillin+Clavulanic acid (3176160); Enalapril (990723); Drotaverine (349841); Digoxin (346407); Nifedipine (256592); Hydrochlorthiazide (246790); Cinnarizine (234839); Captopril (226311); Glyceryl trinitrate (221812); Verapamil (216261). In conclusion, the budget financing of Russian preferential medicinal provision is extremely poor, but has trend to grow. It was demonstrated significant consumption of medicines without evidence based actions.

## P - 238

The Infuence of Hormone Replacement Therapy on Bone Mineral Density and Risk Factors for Occurence of Osteoporosis

[1]Knezevic N., [1]Dragovic G., [2]Beljic T.
[1]Department of Clinical Pharmacology, Pharmacology and Toxicology; Medical School, University of Belgrade; [2]Department of Endocrinology, University Hospital Center, Zvezdarac Belgrade; Serbia and Montenegro (Yugoslavia)

Osteoporosis is an important cause of morbidity and mortality in the postmenopausal women. The aim of our study was to investigate the effect of hormone replacement therapy (HRT) on bone mineral density (BMD) and risk factors of osteoporosis in postmenopausal women. In this study we included 91 women who received HRT more than 12 months. BMD were measured at the lumbal spine (L2-L4) by dual-energy X-ray absorptiometry (DEXA). We investigated different risk factors for osteoporosis: smoking, family tendency, decreased body mass index (BMI), duration of postmenopausal period etc. The average number of risk factors in the group of 41 women who had normal BMD (T score more than - 1.0) was 2.05. The average number of risk factors in the group of 21 women who had osteopenia (T score between -1.0 and -2.5) was 2.76, and 3.17 in group of 29 women who had osteoporosis (T score less than -2.5). The results showed that smoking (RR=2.54) and duration of postmenopausal period (RR=1.91) were statistically significant risk factors. Family tendency and decreased BMI were important risk factors for osteoporosis, but were not statistically significant (p>0.05). The average value of T score before prospective follow-up was -2.98±1.06, and after 12 months of follow-up was -2.45±1.03 (t=10.86, p<0.01). Results of our study have showed that long-term HRT increases bone mineral density and has an important role in protection of osteoporosis.

## P - 239

Influence of CYP2C9, 2C19 and 2D6 Genetic Polymorphisms on Plasma Levels of Fluoxetine and Norfluoxetine Enantiomers

Scordo M.G., Spina E., Dahl M.L., Gatti G., Perucca E.
Department of Clinical and Experimental Medicine and Pharmacology, Section of Pharmacology, University of Messina (Italy), Division of Clinical Pharmacology, Karolinska Institutet, Huddinge University Hospital (Sweden), Department of Medical Sciences, Clinical Pharmacology, University Hospital, Uppsala (Sweden), Clinical Pharmacology Unit, Department of Internal Medicine and Therapeutics, University of Pavia (Italy)

The antidepressant fluoxetine is administered as racemic mixture of two enantiomers (S and R), equipotent in blocking serotonin reuptake. Conversely, the S-enantiomer of its active metabolite norfluoxetine is about 20 times more potent than the R-enantiomer. The metabolism of fluoxetine to norfluoxetine is claimed to be mediated by polymorphic CYP2C9, CYP2D6 and CYP2C19. Aim of the present study was to evaluate the impact of CYP2C9, CYP2C19 and CYP2D6 polymorphisms on the steady-state plasma levels of fluoxetine and norfluoxetine enantiomers in 78 depressed patients (26 males and 52 females, aged 18-76 years), receiving fluoxetine (10-60 mg/day). Genotyping for the main CYP2D6, CYP2C9 and CYP2C19 allelic variants was carried out by molecular biology techniques. Plasma levels of the four enantiomers were measured by HPLC. There was no statistically significant relationship between the CYP2D6 or CYP2C19 genotypes and the plasma levels of each enantiomer or their active moiety (sum of S- and R-fluoxetine and S-norfluoxetine), except for the finding of very low levels of S-norfluoxetine in the only CYP2D6 PM. A correlation ($p<0.05$) was found between CYP2D6 genotype and S-norfluoxetine/S-fluoxetine ratio. Statistically significant relationships ($p<0.05$) were found between CYP2C9 genotype and plasma concentration-to-dose (C/D) ratios of R-fluoxetine, and between CYP2C9 genotype and active moiety. Our results suggest that the polymorphic CYP2D6 and CYP2C9 may play a role in the broad interindividual variability in the fluoxetine kinetics at steady-state.

## P - 240

Rosuvastatin Pharmacokinetics in Heart-Transplant Recipients Administered Cyclosporin

[1]Simonson S.G., [2]Schneck D.W., [3]Martin P.D, [2]Mitchell P.D., [4]Jarcho J.A., [2]Raza A.
[1]AstraZeneca, Lund, Sweden; [2]AstraZeneca, Wilmington, Delaware, USA; [3]AstraZeneca, Alderley Park, Cheshire, UK; [4]Brigham and Women's Hospital, Boston, Massachusetts, USA

Cyclosporin increases the systemic exposure of statins. The effect of cyclosporin on rosuvastatin (Crestor®) pharmacokinetics was assessed in an open-label trial (4522IL/0021) involving 10 stable heart-transplant recipients (more than 6 months post-transplant) taking an anti-rejection regimen containing cyclosporin (Neoral® or Sandimmun®). Rosuvastatin AUC(0-24) and Cmax were determined on Days 1 and 10 of daily oral dosing with rosuvastatin 10 mg. Five of these subjects were then assessed while taking rosuvastatin 20 mg for 10 days. Rosuvastatin pharmacokinetic parameters were compared with controls (historical data from healthy volunteers).

Table 1 Rosuvastatin (RSV) steady-state pharmacokinetic parameters (gmean [CV%])

| | Rosuvastatin controls | Rosuvastatin+cyclosporin | | |
|---|---|---|---|---|
| | 10-mg n=21 | 10-mg n=10 | 20-mg n=5 | 10/20-mg ratio n=5 |
| AUC(0-24) ng.h/ml | 40.1 (39.4) | 284 (31.3) | 424 (21.7) | 1.38 (0.30) |
| $C_{max}$ ng/ml | 4.58 (46.9) | 48.7 (47.2) | 83.4 (37.3) | 1.49 (0.37) |

Compared to controls, AUC(0-24) and Cmax were increased 7.1- and 10.6-fold, respectively, in transplant recipients taking rosuvastatin 10 mg. In subjects taking rosuvastatin 20 mg, these pharmacokinetic parameters increased less than proportionally. The effect of cyclosporin on rosuvastatin exposure is not readily explained by metabolic inhibition since metabolism plays a minor role in rosuvastatin clearance. Inhibition of rosuvastatin hepatic transport processes by cyclosporin may contribute to the mechanism of the interaction.

## P - 241

### Calcitonin Gene-Related Peptide-Induced Vasodilation in the Human Forearm is Inhibited by $CGRP_{8-37}$

De Hoon J.N.J.M., Vanmolkot F.H.M.
Center for Clinical Pharmacology, University Hospital Gasthuisberg (K.U.Leuven), Leuven, Belgium

Introduction: In vitro and animal studies have shown that calcitonin gene-related peptide (CGRP)-induced vasodilation is inhibited by the CGRP fragment $CGRP_{8-37}$. The aim of this study was to investigate the effects of $CGRP_{8-37}$ on resting forearm blood flow (FBF) and on CGRP-induced vasodilation in vivo in humans.
Methods: Increasing doses of CGRP (1-3-10 $ng.min^{-1}.dL^{-1}$) were infused into the brachial artery of 12 healthy subjects. After washout, CGRP infusions were repeated during simultaneous infusion with placebo (NaCl 0.9%, n=6) or $CGRP_{8-37}$ (333 $ng.min^{-1}.dL^{-1}$, n=6). FBF and FBF-ratio (FBF infused / FBF non-infused arm) were assessed using bilateral venous occlusion plethysmography.
Results: CGRP increased FBF from 3.2±0.3 (baseline) to 4.8±0.3, 7.7±0.7 and 12.7±1.0 $mL.min^{-1}.dL^{-1}$, respectively (P<0.001, n=12). FBF-ratio during the first (1.9±0.2, 3.1±0.3 and 5.2±0.8) and second (2.1±0.1, 3.0±0.1 and 4.7±0.3) series of CGRP infusions did not differ. Baseline FBF did not change during $CGRP_{8-37}$ infusion (3.1±0.3 versus 3.1±0.3 $mL.min^{-1}.dL^{-1}$). $CGRP_{8-37}$ attenuated CGRP-induced increase in FBF-ratio (2.2±0.3, 3.3±0.2 and 5.7±0.4 versus 1.6±0.1, 2.0±0.3 and 3.5±0.6, P=0.012).
Conclusions: Intra-brachial CGRP infusion results in a dose-dependent and repeatable FBF response. The CGRP-receptor antagonist $CGRP_{8-37}$ does not affect resting FBF, but effectively inhibits CGRP-induced vasodilation in the human forearm.

## ORAL

### Quality Assured Sources in Knowledge Databases for Computerised Drug Prescribing

Eiermann B., Julander M., Gustafsson L.L.
Stockholm County Council, Division of Drug Management and Informatics, Sweden.

Background: Drug prescribing will change in the near future. Paper prescription will turn into electronically transferred messages. Information overflow for physicians is overwhelming and reliable information sources have to be available at their fingertips. Knowledge databases with quality assured sources supporting medical decision-making are important for the medical and economical outcome in drug therapy.
Method: About 15 different sources selected by general practitioners are used to construct a knowledge database with relevant content for choosing drug therapy. Information about available drugs on the market including dosage information and prices, local recommendation of drug committees, codes for the classification of diseases, drug interaction warnings, pregnancy and breast feeding alerts and treatment strategies are collected and used for database construction. Since most of the sources have different owners data quality and update frequency vary over a wide range. Sources have to be harmonised against each other and thereafter will result in a quality assured database. Irregularities in the sources are reported to the respective owner to improve future quality.
Result: The resulting database delivers relevant, updated and harmonised information needed for drug prescribing leading towards improved drug therapy.

## P - 242

### A Placebo-Controlled Study of the Inhibition of Pentagastrin-Induced Gastric Acid Secretion by Single Oral Doses of Pantoprazole

[1]Paul J., [1]McKeand W., [1]Abell M., [2]Baird S., [1]Mako B., [3]Smout A., [2]Patat A., [1]Wyeth-Ayerst Research, Clinical Pharmacology, Collegeville, PA; [2]Wyeth-Ayerst Research Clinical Pharmacology Paris, [3]Utrecht University Medical Center, Utrecht, Netherlands.

Pantoprazole is a proton pump inhibitor that suppresses gastric acid secretion and is currently used for the treatment of gastroesophageal reflux disease-associated erosive esophagitis. This study assessed the magnitude and time course of the inhibition of pentagastrin (PG) stimulated gastric acid secretion by a single oral 40mg dose of pantoprazole. This single-dose, double-blind, randomized, placebo-controlled study was conducted at 1 investigational site. Fifteen young healthy men were dosed with either 40-mg delayed release pantoprazole (n=10) or matching placebo (n=5) in a fasting state. PG was administered intravenously at a rate of 1.0 µg/kg/hr for 24 hours and was initiated simultaneously with pantoprazole administration. Gastric acid measurement, volume, and pharmacokinetic blood samples were collected at specific time intervals during the 24-hour period. Oral administration of 40mg pantoprazole reduced acid output to £ 10 mEq/hr within 8.2 hours with a mean duration at this target for an additional 6.8 hours, whereas placebo subjects maintained a high gastric acid output (mean 29 mEq/hr) over the same period. The mean cumulative acid output per 24 hours was 615 mEq for placebo and 319 mEq for pantoprazole. In conclusion, orally administered 40-mg pantoprazole successfully suppresses acid output as demonstrated in this hypersecretory disease model.

## ORAL

### Operational Problems of a Pilot Study in Usual Clinical Practice: Reasons for a Failure

Durán M., Morralla C. Vidal X. Laporte J.R.
Unitat d'Assaigs Clínics i Farmacoepidemiologia. Fundació Institut Català de Farmacologia. Departament de Farmacologia Clínica. Hospital Universitari Vall d'Hebron. Barcelona. Spain.

Introduction: We planned a follow up study in order to evaluate the antiemetic effectiveness of nabilone, a synthetic cannabinoid, in cancer chemotherapy induced nausea and vomiting. First, a pilot study was conducted to evaluate the use of an adapted version of the MANE (Morrow Assessment of Nausea and Emesis) questionnaire. The study was conducted in the hospital outpatient day clinic with data collection by nurses.
Objectives: (1) To identify reasons for lack of operation of the pilot study, and (2) to make recommendations for a properly conducting pilot study in this setting. . Methods: (1)The procedures followed during the study and (2) the interrelations between the various actors (promoter, principal investigator, coordinator, nurses and patients) were reviewed. 3) Expected vs actual enrolment and follow up was examined.
Results: Major problems identified in this review were (1) Failure of coordination between the nurse principal investigator and the other actors involved; (2) failures of communication between the nurses collecting patient data, the principal investigator and the coordinator, and (3) progressive loss of motivation in data collection by nurses. These operational problems translated into 50% (15/30) recruitment and follow up (8/15) expected rates.
Conclusions: Motivation of personnel responsible for data collection in studies performed in the usual clinical setting is basic in order to achieve study goals. Motivation can be impaired by problems in coordination and communication among the various actors of the study. More experiences of failures in study development should be evaluated and reported in order to avoid potentially unsuccessful research projects in usual clinical practice.

## P - 243

Novel Antioxidant L-2264 Prevents Insulin Resistance Development In Rats Ivanova O., Poltorak V., Gorbenko N., Lipson V., Leshchenko Z. Institute of Endocrine Pathology Problems, Kharkiv, Ukraine.

The aim of the study was to explore the effect of the new antioxidant L-2264 (heterocyclic amide of phenylpropionic acid) on the insulin resistance development in rats. Male Wistar rats (3-mo-old) were injected dexamethasone (D) (0.125 mg/kg s.c. 13 days). Control rats (C) were given vehicle alone. One group of D-treated animals received L-2264 (200 mg/kg) and another group was given placebo (CD). At the end of the study fasted rats were subjected to the GTT (3 g/kg i.p.). Oxidative status of experimental animals was assessed by determination of malonic dialdehide (MDA) contents in liver homogenate. At the tnd of the study there were no differences in basal blood glucose levels between all experimental groups. However, basal hyperinsulinemia was observed in CD rats (211.5± 9.2 pmol/l vs C: 67.2± 6.2 pmol/l, $p<0.05$). GTT revealed impairment of glucose tolerance in rats after D-administration (AUC/2h over GTT was 1245± 52 vs C: 960± 48 mmol·$l^{-1}$, $p<0.01$). L-2264-treatment prevented D-induced glucose intolerance development reducing AUC over GTT by 40 % ($p<0.05$) in comparison with CD rats. After L-2264 administration basal hyperinsulinemia and IR were significantly decreased (all $p<0.05$) in comparison with CD. L-2264-supplementation in diabetic animals reduced NEFA levels in plasma 2.5-fold ($p<0.05$) and reducing MDA contents 2-fold ($p<0.05$) compared to CD rats. We conclude: L-2264 prevents development of dexamethasone-induced insulin resistance.

## P - 244

Effect of Glipizide on Nephropathy Development in Streptozotocin-Diabetic Rats Poltorack V., Gorbenko N., Gladkih A. Institute of Endocrine Pathology Problems , Kharkiv, Ukraine

Glipizide (Gp) is the second-generation sulfonylurea compound that besides its hypoglycaemic effect could also improve lipid metabolism and vascular fibrinolitic activity in diabetic patients. The aim of the present study was to explore the influence of Gp on the nephropathy development in rats with long-term relative insulin insufficiency. The treatment with Gp (5 mg/kg/day per os) for 3 months) decreased basal hyperglycemia (6.0± 0.1 mmol/l vs 8.2± 0.2 mmol/l, $p<0.05$) and improve glucose tolerance ($p<0.01$) in comparison with non-treated diabetic animals. However, plasma insulin content was not differ from intact controls in all experimental groups. After Gp-supplementation it was revealed significant reduction of the total kidney weight (0.85± 0.15 g vs 0.97± 0.02 g, $p<0.02$) and microalbuminurea ($p<0.05$) compared to diabetic control. Histological examination of kidney revealed protective effect of Gp on microvascular complication development in diabetic rats. The thickness of capillary basement membrane ($p<0.02$) and mesangial expansion were decreased in comparison with non-treated diabetic controls. We conclude that Gp improves metabolic control and inhibits the development of nephropathy in rats with non-insulin dependent diabetes mellitus.

## P - 245

Antiatherogenic Effect of Novel Antioxidant Phensuccinal in Diabetic Rabbits Gorbenko N., Poltorak V., Gladkich A., Ivanova O.
Institute Of Endocrine Pathology Problems, Kharkiv, Ukraine

We have previously shown that the novel succinate derivative Phensuccinal (Ph), which is currently in clinical trials as antioxidant, attenuates the development of diabetic nephropathy. The aim of the study was to evaluate the impact of long-term treatment with Ph on the lipid profile in rabbits with dithizone-induced diabetes. Administration of Ph (50 mg/kg/day per os for 3 months) decreased basal hyperglycaemia by 40 % and increased basal plasma insulin ($p<0.02$) in comparison with diabetic controls (D). The treatment with Ph elevated HDL-cholesterol 1.5-fold ($p<0.01$) and diminished LDL-cholesterol by 37 % ($p<0.05$), compared to diabetic control group. Ph also provided reduction in free fatty acids, total cholesterol , triglycerides and lipid hydroperoxides levels (all $p<0.02$) in comparison with diabetic controls. Improvement of lipid profile in diabetic rabbits after Ph administration was accompanied by higher paraoxonase activity (59.0± 1.1 vs D: 37.6± 2.2; U/l, $p<0.01$). We suggest that Ph possesses antiatherogenic effect due to improvement of glycaemic control, lipid profile and enhancement of antioxidant defence in diabetic rabbits and may have implications in prevention of diabetic macrovascular complications.

## P - 246

Determination Of Ciprofloxacin In Gingival Crevicular Fluid And Plasma By High-Performance Liquid Chromatography

[1]Dincel A., [2]Yildirim A., 2Caglayan F., 1Bozkurt A.
[1]Department of Pharmacology, Faculty of Medicine, Hacettepe University, 06100, Ankara, Turkey. [2]Department of Periodontology, Faculty of Dentistry, Hacettepe University, 06100, Ankara, Turkey

A simple and selective high-performance liquid chromatographic (HPLC) method has been developed for determination of ciprofloxacin in gingival crevicular fluid (GCF) and plasma. Separation of ciprofloxacin was carried out with quinine sulfate as internal standard using Radial-pak, $C_{18}$ cartridge column (100 x 8 mm i.d., particle size 10 m with a mobile phase acetonitrile-sodium dihydrogen phosphate (pH 3.9; 0.1 M) (8:2, v/v) at a flow rate of 2 ml $min^{-1}$ at ambient temperature. The effluent was monitored on a fluorescence detector using an excitation and emission wavelength of 280 nm and 455 nm respectively. The retention times of ciprofloxacin and internal standard were 4.55 and 13.25 minutes respectively. The within-day and day-to-day reproducibilities were less than 9 % for ciprofloxacin at 0.1 and 0.5 g.$ml^{-1}$ ($n=6$) and the detection limit corresponding to signal-to-noise ratio of 2.5:1 was 30 ng $ml^{-1}$. This method was suitable and sensitive for determination of ciprofloxacin levels in human GCF and plasma.

## P - 247

Contribution of a Poison Information Centre (PIC) in the Evaluation of Adverse Drug Effects (ADEs) to the German National Pharmacovigilance System

[1]Mey C., [2]Hentschel H., [1]Hippius M., [3]Tiaden J.D., [3]Oerlinghausen B.M., [1]Balogh A.
[1]Department of Clinical Pharmacology, University of Jena, Dornburger Str. 159, 07743 Jena, Germany, [2]Poison Information Centre Erfurt, [3]Drug Commission of the German Medical Association

Objective: The aim of the study was to find out whether the national system of registration of ADEs by the Drug Commission of the German Medical Association (DCGMA) can be intensified and supplemented by the assessment of suspected adverse side effects of drugs practiced by the PIC Erfurt.
Method: All registered cases of assumed ADEs reported to the PIC in Erfurt were studied retrospectively and compared with ADEs reported to the DCGMA in the time period between 1995 and 1999.
Results: 317 inquiries received by the PIC concerned adverse effects (AEs) of drugs. After assessment 157 AEs were considered likely to be due to the administered drugs and therefore ADEs. 68 AEs seemed to be possibly connected with the drugs. The DCGMA registered 8.008 ADE reports. The comparison of ADEs showed differences in the ranking order of reported symptoms and frequencies of suspected drugs with the exception of reporting rates of metoclopramide. Interestingly, the PIC registered ADEs of newly released drugs and detected possible new drug risks.
Conclusions: PICs and Pharmacovigilance Centres should take advantage of their similarities in structure and scientific approach and therefore should co-operate for mutual profit.

## P - 248

Alfentanil-Induced Miosis in Patients

[1,3]Slanar O., [2]Urban M., [1]Roots I., [3]Perlík F.
[1]Institute of Clinical Pharmacology, Charité, Humboldt University, Berlin, Germany [2]Department of Anaesthesiology and Resuscitation, General Teaching Hospital, Prague, Czech Republic [3]Clinical Pharmacology Unit, 1st Faculty of Medicine, Charles University; General Teaching Hospital; and Institute for Postgraduate Medical Education, Prague, Czech Republic

Opioid drug alfentanil is an CYP3A4 substrate, whose clearance is used as an in vivo probe for this metabolic pathway. Alfentanil-induced miosis, correlating with the drug plasma levels, has been previously proposed as a possible noninvasive test for determining of hepatic CYP3A4 activity in healthy young volunteers. The aim of our study was to describe the influence of the patients´ age, color of their iris and smoking habits on the test results, as independent susceptibility factors affecting pupillar reactivity or CYP3A4 activity. Fifty-seven patients aged 24-79 years with CLL, non-Hodgkin, Hodgkin lymphoma, or multiple myeloma have been studied. The patients received analgosedative combination of intravenously addministred alfentanil 17 μg/kg and midazolam 42 μg/kg. Dark-adapted horizontal and vertical pupillar diameters in both eyes have been measured before the drugs administration (d0) and 90 minutes afterwards (d90). We observed a large interindividual variability of both d0 and d90. The d0 values decreased with increasing age of the patients, but there was no relationship between the difference of basal and 90 min. pupillar diameters (d0-90) and the age groups of the patients. Smoking reduced the miotic response of the eyes. The mean d 0-90 were 0,22±0,54 mm in smoking group (n=16), and 0,44±0,69 in nonsmokers (n=41) (p<0,05). The color of the iris did not affect pupillar reactivity, which was assesed by absolute values of d 0-90. Smoking habit can change alfentanil-induced miosis as a result of either possible increased clearance of the drug or reduced pupillar reactivity to miosis-inducing agents in smokers.

## P - 249

Prevalence of MRSA Infections in a Clinical Hospital Centre in Croatia

Bilusic M., Mercep I., Kalinic S., Francetic I., Macolic-Sarinic V., Huic M., Mimica S.
Section of clinical pharmacology, Departmenf Medicine, Department of Clinical microbiology, Clinical Hospital Centre Zagreb, Croatia

Since methicillin resistant staphylococcus aureus (MRSA) was first identifed in 1961,the number of patients with MRSA isolates have constantly been increasing. According to the Centers for Disease Control and Prevention's (CDC) the proportion of Staphylococcus aureus isolates resistant to methicillin in hospitals in USA increased from approximately 29% in the early 1990's to 47% in 1998. WE have also identified that MRSA infections in our hospital became an emerging problem. For this reason a 3 month survey have been conducted in Clinical Hospital Centre in Zagreb, Croatia during which we have monitored the incidence of infections caused by Staphylococcus aureus as well as the total share of those with isolated or colonized MRSA. During that period a total of 268 Staphylococcus aureus isolates were detected, while in 80 cases (29,8%) MRSA was isolated. From samples with Staphylococcus aureus, 44 were isolated in blood (16,5%), 160 (59,7%) in wound and 64 (23,8%) in respiratory discharge. An additional investigation of 27 samples with MRSA isolates, we found that the higest prevalence of MRSA infections occurred in Department of surgery (63%), followed by Department of urology (18.5%), Department of medicine (14.8%) and Neurosurgery (3.7%). Out of those 27 isolates 19 patients (70.4%) that showed signs of infection were treated with vancomycin, while other 8 (29.6%) were diagnosed as colonized by MRSA and did not require vancomycin therapy.

## P - 250

Teratogenic Effects of Diazepam Intake During Pregnancy to cleft palate & cleft lip

Takzaree N., Yarmohammadi K., Takzaree A.R., Semiyari H.
Dept. of Embryology, Tehran University of Medical Sciences, Faculty of Medicine, Tehran, Iran.

Diazepam is un sedetive that belongs to Benzodiazepines. It has been increasingly used recently. Itshould be noticed that Diazepam consumption during pregnancy may have teratogenic effects on embryo. Pregnantwomen use this drug in pregnancy pica, shortsleeping or necesserily in psychologic and neurologic disease. So inthis research we have studied Diazepam intake during pregnancy and its side effects leading to cleft lip, cleft palate- and anopsia. In our study the virgin rats of known age weight have been selected. After being pregnant they weredivided in three groups: Control group : 10 rats (injection of sterile water) First case group: 10 rats (sterile water andDiazepam 3 mg/kg/day Second case group : 10 rats (sterile water and Diazepam 8 mg/kg/day). These three groupstook the drugs daily, After embryonic period pregnant rats have been killed and their embryos have been divided alsoin the same three groups. After being studied macroscopically the embryos were observed microscopically. Thisshowed that some anomalies have been appeared in some cases. After analysing there were significant differencesbetween case and control groups (P value > 0.05). So it was proved that Diazepam is teratogen and is dangerous forpregnant women. Key Words:Diazepam, Teratogen, Cleft palate, Cleft lip

## P - 251

Study of Antiviral Activity of Cyclocitidinmonophosphate

Novikova I.V., Kevra M.K., Trukhacheva T.V., Boreko E.L.
Department of Clinical Pharmacology, Belarusian State Medical University, Minsk, Belarus

Objective: To study antriviral of modified cyclocitidinmonophosphate nucleoside (c-CMP) against herpes simplex virus, type 1.
Methods: Antiviral activity of c-CMP was tosted on fibroblastic cells culture as well as on the model of herpetic meningoencephalitis in white micc and in herpetic keratoconjuctivities in rabbits and guinea pigs.
Results: It was determined that c-CMP concentrations of 6-100 mg/ml inhibited multiplication of herpex simplex virus in fibroblastic cell culture. C-CMP doses of 10-100 mg/kg introduced intraabdominally produced therapeutic effect in herpetic meningoencephalitis in mice. 0.05-5.0% c-CMP aqueous solution and ophthalmic ointment had a marked therapeutic effect in experimental herpetic keratoconjuctivities in rabbits and guinea pigs. The tested preparation was also effective for viral strains resistant to acyclovir. The Health Ministry of Belarus approved clinical tests of c-CMP as a potential preparation for ophthalmoherpes. The first series of clinical tests revealed that 3% c-CMP ophthalmic ointment was tolerated by healty volunteers and had no marked side effects.
Conclusion: Cyclocitidinmonophosphate has a marked intiviral activity and is recommended for clinical study as a potential medical preparation in human ophthalmoherpes.

## P - 252

Synergism of NSAIDs with Pentoxiphylline in rheumatoid Arthritis Treatment

Kevra M.K., Dubovic B.V., Keura V.M.
Department of Clinical Pharmacology, Belarusian State Medical University, Minsk, Belarus

Objective: To assess the safety and effectiveness of tumor necrosis factor-alpha production inhibitor pentoxifylline in conbination with non-steroidal antiinflammatory drugs (NSAIDs) in patients with rheumatoid arthritis.
Methods: 120 patients, males and females, aged 20-72, were divided into three groups. The patients of each group were distributed in two equal amount subgroups (test and control). During 12 weeks the test subgroups subjects received NSAIDs monotheraphy: indomethacin 50 mg 3 times/day or naproxen 500 mg 2 times/day or diclofenac 50 mg 3 times/day. The test groups patients also received pentoxifylline (100 mg 3 times/day).
Results: It was shown that pentoxifylline supplement to NSAIDs treatment increased its effectiveness (pain, morning restraint duration, erythrocyte sedimentation rate, C-reactive protein and rheumatoid factor levels reduced faster) and diminished the potential risk of a NSAIDs-gastropathy development for 47,5 % ($p < 0,02$). No severe complications (bleeding, gastrointestinal tract ulceration) were observed in the patients receiving combined theraphy.
Conclusion: The combination of NSAIDs with pentoxifylline improves the effectiveness of rheumatoid arthritis theraphy and increases its safety.

## P - 253

Pentoxiphylline in Combination with Methylprednisolone in Treatment of Sepsis

Kevra M.K., Dubovic B.V., Leonovich S.I., Keura Zh.S.
Department of Clinical Pharmacology and Department of Surgery, Belarusian State Medical University, Minsk, Belarus

Objective: To assess the safety and effectiveness of tumor necrosis factor-alpha production inhibitors pentoxifylline and methylprednisolone in treatment of sepsis.
Methods: In addition to common treatment (antibiotics, plasma substitutes, pressor amines, inotropic agents) 38 patients with sepsis (men and women aged from 18 to 74) received intravenous infusions of pentoxifylline 5 mg/kg/d and methylprednisolone mg/kg/d. The criteria for assessment of this theraphy results were the survival rate, dynamics of clinical and laboratory data. Archive materials concerning results of sepsis common theraphy were used for comparison.
Results: Pentoxifylline and glucocorticosteroids supplement to common theraphy of sepsis essentially improved the results. 5 patients from the test group died (13,2%). The lethality in the control group (38 patients) was 36,8% (14 patients died). In patients receiving supplement theraphy temperature decreasing, improving of the cardiovascular, respiratory systems function and laboratory data registered earlier, within 24-72 hours.
Conclusion: The results of our study give the basis to recommend inclusion of pentoxifylline and methylprednisolone combination in complex theraphy of a sepsis.

## P - 254

Rationalization of Expenses for Lung Cancer Chemotherapy

Cervellino J.C., Araujo C.E., Fligman M.D., Pires E.A.
Chair of Pharmacology, School of Medicine, University of Buenos Aires (Argentina).

The development of new drugs for non-small cell lung cancer could be a big success in the treatment of this disease, improving objective response rate and quality of life. To cope with this formidable challenge, interest seems to be focused exclusively in the development of new molecules. But, what about the well known old agents combinations? Are they not useful anymore? generally speaking, modern cancer chemotherapy includes combination of new drugs exclusively. However, recent results are often quite similar to those achieved in the past at low cost and with mild toxicity. Comparison with the natural history of the disease could shed some light to the actual value of trials' result. According to P. Bunn (ESQ Monograph, 1991), median survival for non-small cell lung cancer was 27 weeks, which is quite similer to data obtained in the last 20 years (Table). On the other hand, because of the higher cost of new drugs and their severe toxicity, the cost-benefit relationship does not seem to be better. In several reports, median survival time (MST) was similar to the national history of the disease. If the therapeutic benefit over old treatments is null, is the benefit obtained from an economic analysis? Again, the answer is negative (Table)

| Chemotherapy | Obj. Response % | MST ( months) | 6 cycles dollar cost |
|---|---|---|---|
| Gemcitabine+DDP | 30 | 9.8 | 30.006 |
| Paclitaxel+Carbopt | 32 | 9.9 | 40.200 |
| Ifosfamide+Epi | 51 | 12.0 | 16.938 |
| Cyclophosphamide | 38 | 9.0 | 540 |

Probably a smarter approach could be to combine both old and new agents, in order to achieve better results when analyzed from the patient's point of view.

## P - 255

The Efficacy of Adsorbent's Mixture in Protection of Animals Poisoned with Bromadiolone

[1]Cupic V., [2]Dobric S., [2]Milovanovic Z., [2]Bokonjic D.
[1]Faculty of Veterinary Medicine, [2]National Poison Control Center, Military Medical Academy, Belgrade, Yugoslavia

The aim of this study was to evaluate the efficacy of adsorbent's mixture (5 g of activated charcoal, 2.5 g of tannin, 2.5 g of caoline, 2.5 g of magnesium oxyde and distilled water to 100 g), as an unspecific antidote, in protection against acute poisoning with bromadiolone, one of the widely used anticoagulant rodenticides. The experiments were performed on adult Wistar rats, both sexes starving for several hours before administration of bromadiolone (1.3 LD-50, p.o.). The protected animals were given adsorbent's mixture in doses of 1 ml/kg p.o. or 3 ml&kg p.o., immediately after bromadiolone; as well as in a dose of 3 ml/kg p.o. immediately, and 1h, 2h and 3h after bromadiolone. (totally four doses of 3 ml/kg). The efficacy of activated charcoal was estimated by means of mean lethal time (LT-50) of protected animals in comparison with that of the control one. The results demonstrated that adsorbent's mixture, regadless of given dose, failed to protect animals poisoned with bromadiolone. Moreover, the LT-50 values of the protected groups were even lower than that of the control one. Our results suggest that adsorbent's mixture could not offer any protection in animals acutely poisoned with anticoagulant rodenticides.

## P - 256

Comparison of Serious Adverse Drug Reactions (ADRs) Associated with Non-Selective and Selective COX2-Inhibitors

Haase G., Kohlen K., Riethling A.-K., Drewelow B.
Institut of Clinical Pharmacology., University of Rostock, Germany

Objective: Comparison of ADRs leading to hospital admission caused by non-selective NSAIDs and selective COX2-inhibitors.
Methods: Comprehensive ADR-monitoring using established trigger symptoms of all non-elective hospital admissions to the Departments of Internal Medicine, University Hospital Rostock and Hospital South Rostock (» 300.000 residents) Causality assessment was performed according of Begaud. Analysis of all NSAID-induced ADRs excl. ASS. Via the annual prescription frequency in Germany incidences were assesed.
Results: From 2000 to 2002 199 NSAID-associated ADRs were observed, 159 caused by non-selective NSAIDs, (n=89 diclofenac) and 40 by COX2-Inhibitors (n=33 rofecoxib). The majority of this patients (62%/66%) was > 65 years and predominantly female (63%/61%).

| Affectet organs/symptoms | NSAID-ADR (%) | COX2-I-ADR (%) |
|---|---|---|
| GI affections | 76,7 | 60,0 |
| Liver/biliary tract | 4,4 | 0 |
| Renal function | 3,8 | 7,5 |
| Immune system | 3,8 | 2,5 |
| Blood dyscrasias | 2,5 | 10,0 |
| Thromboembolism | 0 | 7,5 |
| Other | 8,8 | 12,5 |

Discussion: Compared to the annual prescription frequency in Germany (Mio. DDD) the incidence of COX2-Inhibitor associated ADRs were not lower than those of non-selective NSAIDs. Supported by BfArM Germany, Z12.01-68502-201

## P - 257

Serious Adverse Drug Reactions (ADR) Associated with Herbal Drugs

Haase G., Riethling A.-K., Drewelow B.
Inst. of Clin. Pharmacol., University of Rostock, Germany

Objective: Analysis of ADRs leading to hospital admission associated with herbal drugs.
Methods: Comprehensive ADR-monitoring using established trigger symptoms of all non-elective hospital admissions to the Departments of Internal Medicine, University Hospital and Hospital South Rostock (» 300.000 residents). Causality assessment was performed according of Begaud. All ADRs associated with the use of herbal drugs recorded between 2000 and 2002 were analysed.
Results: Out of 1332 ADRs only 31 (2,3%) were associated with herbal drugs. Gingko biloba was used in 9 cases, of which 6 patients suffered from bleed-ings. However, in 5 of them Gingko was co-administered with drugs associ-ated with a risk for bleeding events. 6 ADR cases were detected with Hyperi-cum spec. (gastritis haemorrhagica, livertoxicity, thrombosis), 2 cases with Aesculus hippocastaneum (livertoxicity, gastritis), 1 case with Kava Kava (liver failure with transplantation) and 1 case with Harpagophytum spec. (myalgia).
Discussion: With regard to prescription frequency in Germany (e.g. Gingko: 117 Mio. DDD in 2001) and assuming a high self-medication rate, the analysis shows a low incidence of ADRs associated with herbal drugs.
Supported by BfArM Germany, Z12.01-68502-201

## P - 258

Pharmacokinetics of Gapapentin in Neonates and During Lactation

[1]Öhman I., [1]Vitols S., [2]Tomson T.
Department of Medicine, Division of [1]Clinical Pharmacology and [2]Clinical Neuroscience, Karolinska Hospital, Stockholm, Sweden

Purpose: To investigate the pharmacokinetics of gabapentin (GBP) in the neonatal period and during lactation.
Methods: GBP concentration is plasma and breast milk were analysed with high-performamce liquid chromatography (HPLC) in two women with epilepsy treated with gabapentin, and in their offspring. Samples were obtained at delivery, the first days after birth and at breastfeeding at two weeks or three months postpartum.
Results: Maternal GBP plasma concentrations in the first patient were 30 mmol/L at delivery. GBP plasma levels in the newborn declined rather rapidly. At 24 h the concentration was 45% lower than the GBP level at 6 h postpartum. At sampling 2 weeks after deliveryi maternal GBP plasma concentrations were 10 mmol/L before dose intake and 20 mmol/L in sample collected 2 hours after dose intake. Milk concentrations were 6 mol/L in sample collected 2 hours after dose intake. Milk concentrations were 6 mmol/L and 9 mmol/L respectively. The milk/plasma concentration ratios were 0.6 and 0.45 respectively. In the second patient, GBP level in the umbilical cord was 61 mmol/L and the concentration in the neonate was 5 mmol/L 48 h postpartum. Three months after parturition the milk/plasma concentration ratio was 1.1. The infant's plasma concentrations were below the quantification limit.
Conclusions: Our limited observations suggest extensive excretion of GBP into breastmilk and that newborns seem to have a reasonable capacity to eliminate GBP. No adverse effects were observed in the infants.

## P - 259

CYP3A5*3 Polymorphism as Risk Factor for Prostate Cancer

[1]Karypidis H., [2]Söderström T., [1]Lundgren S., [1]Rane A.
[1]Dept of Clinical Pharmacology, Huddinge University Hospital, Stockholm, Sweden [2]Dept of Clinical Pharmacology, Uppsala University Hospital, Uppsala Sweden

Background: Androgens has a permissive role in the development of prostate cancer. In contrast to CYP3A4 (which has a low expression), CYP3A5 is markedly expressed in human prostate and metabolises testosterone to 6b-hydroxytestosterone. The CYP3A5*3 allele generates an aberrantly spliced mRNA with a premature stop codon and might therefore modulate the risk of prostate cancer.
Methods: We performed a case-control study in Swedish men. We included 176 cases and 161 age matched controls. Genotyping was performed using TacManÒ real time PCR.
Results: 159/176 cases and 141/161 controls were homozygous for the CYP3A5*3 allele, OR 1.33 (95%CI 0.67-2.63). Two cases but no controls lacked the *3 allele. The cases were in Hardy-Weinberg disequilibrium ($p<0.05$).
Conclusion:Putative CYP3A5 activity due to *3 heterozygosity is a rare event in our material, limiting the clinical use of this marker in Sweden. Given the high frequency of controls homozygous for *3 (87.5 %), we could only detect an OR of 3.5 or higher with 80% power.

## P - 260

Computer Simulations of the Regional Manufestation of Asthma

[1]Apiou G.S., [2]Lemaire M., [3]Katz I., [4]Conway J., [5]Floming J., [6]Martonen T.
[1]Claude Delorme Research Center, France, [2]Air Liquide Sante International,France, [3]Department of Mechanical Engineering, Lafayette Collage, U.S.A, [4]Department of Medicine, Southampton University, U.K, [5]Departments of Medical Physics and Bioengineering, Southampton General Hospital, U.K, [6]Department of Medicine, University of North Carolina, U.S.A

Asthma presents serious medical problems of global proportions. Clinical data suggest that the disease occurs preferentially at regions designated by large ($0\leq I\leq 5$), central ($6\leq 6\leq 11$) and small ($12\leq 6\leq 16$) airways, where I defines branching generations within lungs. Our straightforward hypothesis, therefore, was that the efficacies of pharmacologic grugs proposed for the treatment and prophylaxis of asthma would be enhanced via their largeted delivery to appropriate sites. Hence, we have developed a mathematical model describing the behaviour and fate of inhaled acrosols. Original algorithms have been derived to detail the physical manifestation of asthma as distinct components of smooth muscle constriction and inflammation. Different intensities of asthma were simulated by reducing airway diameters by prescribed amounts. A range of ventilatory parameters (e.g. tidal volumes) was employed to account for intersubject variabilities in aerosol theraphy protocols. We have conducted a systematic analysis of the relative effects of morphology, ventialtion, and particle size on aerosol deposition. Regarding therapeutic implications, it is clear that discase-induced changes in airway morphologies have pronounced effects on the administration of inhaled drugs. Likewisw, ventilation affects both the total aerosol mass deposited and its relatice spatial distribution among airways. By formulating these effects, the computer code allows drugs (e.g., bronchodilators for constriction, steroids for inflammation) to be selectively deposited. We suggested, therefore, that the code be used in a complementery matter with clinical studies and be integrated into aerosol theraphy regimens.

## P - 261

Psychologic Profile of Patients wiih History of Drug Hypersensitivity

[1]Sarinic V.M., [2]Herceg M., [1]Bilusic M., [1]Francetic I., [1]Huic M., [1]Mercep I.
[1]Division of Clinical Pharmacology, Department of Medicine, Clinical Hospital Centre Zagreb, Zagreb, Croatia [2]Psychiatric Hospital Vrapce, Zagreb, Croatia

From October 2002 till February 2003 48 patients (82% women and 18% men, mean age 46 years) with a history of drug hypersensitivity were hospitalised in the Division of Clinical Pharmacology to be biologically tested for drug hypersensitivity. All patients have concluded MMPI test consisting of 201 questions. The patients were divided into two groups (A): one with convincing history of drug sensitivity and the other with doubtful history of it (B). In group A 50% of patients had a pathological finding of MMPI test compared to patients in group B (35%). In group A pathologic values were found ranging from hypochondria (43%), hysteria (21%), hypomania (14%) to depression (7%). These findings belong to the group of minor psychic disorders that can appear secondary as reaction to existing objective problem. In the 35% of group B patients with positive MMPI test we found that their pathology findings were more severe compared to the group A. Besides hypochondria (57%), hysteria (57%), depression (28%) the scales of psychastenia (28%), paranoia (15%) and schizophrenia (15%) were abnormal. It can be concluded that 50% of patients with convincing history of drug hypersensitivity also suffer from mood disorders and anxiety as a secondary reaction to previous allergic experience, while from the 35% patients with positive MMPI test, 15%-28% suffer from severe disorder in which the symptoms of hypersensitivity are actually the symptoms of the primary psychiatric disease.

## P - 262

New Applications of Nebulizers in the Treatment of Asthma

[1]Martonen T., [2]Apiou G.S., [3]Lemaire M., [4]Katz I., [5]Conway J., [6]Floming J.,
[1]Department of Medicine, University of North Carolina, U.S.A, [2]Claude Delorme Research Center, France, [3]Air Liquide Sante International,France, [4]Department of Mechanical Engineering, Lafayette Collage, U.S.A, [5]Department of Medicine, Southampton University, U.K, [6]Departments of Medical Physics and Bioengineering, Southampton General Hospital, U.K,

Asthma presents serious medical problems of global proportions. Clinical data suggest that the disease occurs preferentially at regions designated by large ($0\leq I\leq 5$), central ($6\leq 6\leq 11$) and small ($12\leq 6\leq 16$) airways, where I defines branching generations within lungs. Our straightforward hypothesis, therefore, was that the efficacies of pharmacologic grugs proposed for the treatment and prophylaxis of asthma would be enhanced via their largeted delivery to appropriate sites. Hence, we have developed a mathematical model describing the behaviour and fate of inhaled acrosols. To show the real clinical applications of modeling we have simulated the performance of an available nebulizer (MobyNeb from Markos-Mefar). We sampled the Markos-Mefar nebulizer and we used its output as an input for our mathematical model. We have conducted a systematic analysis of the relative effects of morphology, ventilation and particle size on the deposition patterns of inhaled aerosols produced by the Markos-Mefar device. For evaluating performance capabilities of the device, our simulations were limited to considerations of doses normalized to airway surface areas. The polydisperse aerosol produced by the Markos-Mefar device actually has a quite narrow particle size distribution. That is, for all practical intents and purposes, it approaches being a monodisperse aerosol. The results of our simulations demonstrate that, when expressed as a function of patient breathing parameters, the device can effectivelt target drugs to the congested airways. The device has the operating characteristics neccessary to be successfully employed in the delivery of drugs used in the treatment of asthma in adults.

## P - 263

Inhibitory Effect of 5-Fluorouracil in CYP2C9 Activity

[1]Güneş A., [2]Coşkun U., [3]Börüban C., [2]Günel N., [3]Sencan O., [4]Bozkurt A., [5]Rane A., [6]Hassan M., [1]Zengil H., [4,5]Yasar U.
[1]Dept of Pharmacology, Gazi University, Medical Faculty, Ankara, Turkey, [2]Dept of Oncology, Gazi University, Medical Faculty, Ankara, Turkey, [3]Dept of Oncology, SSK Ankara Hospital [4]Dept of Pharmacology, Hacettepe University, Medical Faculty, Ankara, Turkey [5]Dept of Clinical Pharmacology, Karolinska Institutet, Huddinge University Hospital, Stockholm, Sweden [6] Division of Haematology, Karolinska Institutet, Huddinge University Hospital, Stockholm, Sweden

Introduction: 5-Fluorouracil (5-FU) is a commonly used anticancer agent for the treatment of gastrointestinal, breast, head and neck tumors. Drug interactions have been reported between 5-FU and two clinically important cytochrome P450 2C9 (CYP2C9) substrates, S-warfarin and phenytoin. The mechanism of this interaction has not been identified yet. Recently, urinary losartan/E-3174 (carboxy metabolite of losartan) ratio has been suggested as a marker for CYP2C9 metabolic activity. The aim of this study was to determine the influence of 5-FU on CYP2C9 activity.
Subjects & Methods: Sixteen colorectal cancer patients received 5-FU (425 mg/m$^2$) plus folinic acid (20 mg/m$^2$) for 3 to 5 days with three weeks interval. A single oral dose of 25 mg losartan was given to the patients two days before and during the 5-FU protocol. Losartan and E-3174 in 8-hour urine were assayed by HPLC. Losartan/E-3174 ratios before and during the treatment protocol were compared for each subject.
Results: 5-FU increased the urinary losartan/E-3174 ratio in 75% of the patients, up to 15-fold (2.7-fold ± 0.9; mean ± SEM, p=0.02).
Conclusion: 5-FU seemed to inhibit CYP2C9 activity in these patients as assessed with losartan as a probe drug. The inhibition of CYP2C9 activity might be the possible explanation for the 5-FU drug interactions with CYP2C9 substrates.

## P - 264

Role of Cytochrome P450 2C9 in the Metabolism of Ketobemidone

Annas A., Yasar U., Svensson J.O., AL-Shurbaji A.
Division of Clinical Pharmacology, Department of Laboratory Medicine, Karolinska Institutet at Huddinge University Hospital, Stockholm, Sweden.

Ketobemidone is a potent opioid analgesic frequently used in Scandinavia. Despite long time of use, its metabolism has not been characterized in detail. In the present study, we have investigated the role of major cytochrome P450 enzymes in the formation of the main metabolite norketobemidone from ketobemidone. This was studied in human liver microsomes prepared from 20 livers as well as in yeast expressed recombinant CYP2C9 variants. When compared to 11 different CYP enzyme activities, the formation of norketobemidone from ketobemidone (1 mM) correlated best with CYP2C9 activity, measured as losartan oxidation ($r_s$=0.83, n=20, P<0.001). The formation of norketobemidone from 1 mM ketobemidone in human liver microsomes was clearly affected by CYP2C9 genotype. The formation was three times higher in the wild type (CYP2C9*1*1) (0.7 pmol/mg protein/min) compared to CYP2C9*1*2, CYP2C9*1*3 and CYP2C9*3*3 (approximately 0.2 pmol/mg protein/min) (P<0.01). In a recombinant enzyme system, the intrinsic clearance (Vmax/Km) was 0.47 in CYP2C9*1, 0.11 in CYP2C9*2 and 0.08 in CYP2C9*3. Our data suggests that CYP2C9 is the major enzyme in the formation of norketobemidone from ketobemidone at clinically relevant concentrations and that genetic polymorphism of CYP2C9 may have a significant impact on the elimination of ketobemidone.

## P - 265

Caffeine as a Probe for the Assessment of CYP1A2, CYP2A6, NAT2 and Xanthine Oxidase Activities in Turkish Subjects

[1]Dincel A., [1]Yasar U., [1]Babaoglu M.O., [1]Bozkurt A., [2]Basci N., [1]Kayaalp S.O.
[1]Department of Pharmacology, Faculty of Medicine, [2]Department of Analytical Chemistry, Faculty of Pharmacy, Hacettepe University, Ankara, Turkey

Caffeine is commonly used as a probe to assess the metabolic activities of CYP1A2, CYP2A6, N-acetyltransferase and xanthine oxidase. The metabolic activities of these enzymes were determined in the urine samples collected at fifth hour after caffeine intake. Caffeine, 1,7-dimethylxanthine (17X), 1,7-dimethyluric acid (17U), 1,3-dimethyluric acid (13U), 3-methylxanthine (3X), 1-methylxanthine (1X), 1-methyluric acid (1U), theobromine (37X), and 5-acethylamino-6-formylamino-3-methyluracil (AFMU) were analysed by using HPLC. Urine samples were extracted with chloroform/isopropanol (85:15, v/v) and separated on a reversed phase $C_{18}$ column with acetic acid/tetrahydrofuran/acetonitrile/water (1:2.5:44:925, v/v). Peaks were monitored with UV detection at 280 nm. The CYP1A2, CYP2A6, NAT2 and XO activities were calculated from the ratios (AFMU+1X+1U)/17U, 17U/(17U+17X+1U+1X+AFMU), AFMU/1X and 1U/1X+1U, respectively, in 18 healthy volunteers (15 males and 3 females). The enzyme activities of CYP1A2, CYP2A6, NAT2 and XO were 2.52±1.18, 0.23±0.06, 0.32±0.16, and 0.59±0.10 (mean±SD), respectively. The activities of NAT2 (0.41±0.11 versus 0.17±0.06; p<0.05) and XO (0.66±0.14 versus 0.56±0.07; p<0.05) were significantly induced in smoker subjects (n=5) compared to the non-smokers (n=13). These results are comparable to those reported previously.
This study was supported by TUBITAK (SBAG-COST B15-2356).

## P - 266

Effect of Ketoconazole on the Pharmacokinetics of Erlotinib (TarcevaTM) in Healthy Adult Male Subjects

Abbas R., Fettner S., Riek M., Davis S., Hamilton M., Frohna P., Rakhit A.
Hoffmann-La Roche Inc, Nutley, NJ, OSI Pharmaceuticals, Inc, Boulder, CO, Genentech, Inc, New Jersey, U.S.A

Erlotinib (TarcevaTM) is an epidermal growth factor receptor (HER1/EGFR) tyrosine kinase inhibitor being developed for the treatment of various solid tumors. Erlotinib is metabolized mainly by CYP3A4. Therefore, the potential for drug-drug interactions exists when erlotinib is co-administered with drugs that are CYP3A4 inhibitors. The objective of this study was to assess the effect of ketoconazole, a potent inhibitor of CYP3A4, on the pharmacokinetics of erlotinib. Twenty four subjects were randomly assigned (1:1) to two treatment groups (1, 2), both receiving single oral doses of erlotinib (100 mg) in two treatment periods separated by a two-week washout. In Group 1, the subjects also received ketoconazole 200 mg orally twice daily for 5 days, starting one day prior to the second dose of erlotinib. Following co-administration of ketoconazole, exposure (AUC0-inf) to erlotinib increased by 86% (p-value=0.0001) compared to that without ketoconazole. Peak plasma concentration (Cmax) also increased by about 100% (p-value=0.0031). Plasma half-life, however, did not change to an appreciable extent (9.2 vs 8.9 hr) in spite of 35% decrease in oral clearance (CL/F) in presence of ketoconazole. These results indicate that a dose adjustment may be necessary when erlotinib is co-administered with potent CYP3A4 inhibitors such as ketoconazole.

## P - 267

Academic Fluoroquinolone Prescribing, Resistance and Impact of Guidelines

[1,2]Mol P.G.M., [1,2]Panday P.V.N., [3]Degener J.E., [4]Van Der Werf T.S., [1]Haaijer-Ruskamp F.M., [4]Gans R.O.B.
[1]Department of Clinical Pharmacology, University Groningen, the Netherlands [2]Pharmacy Department, University Hospital Groningen, the Netherlands [3]Department of Clinical Microbiology, University Hospital Groningen, the Netherlands [4]Department of Internal Medicine, University Hospital Groningen, the Netherlands

Introduction: Excessive ciprofloxacin use has recently been linked with the emergence of drug-resistant organisms like vancomycin-resistant enterococci. In our university teaching hospital, we observed over the past twelve years an increase in ciprofloxacin prescriptions that was mirrored by an emergence of drug-resistant enterobacteriacaeae.
Objective: We studied whether guideline-recommended antimicrobials could be used as effectively as ciprofloxacin for empirical treatment of infectious diseases.
Methods: Prescribing data were collected for 795 patients (1,822 antimicrobial prescriptions) admitted to the internal medicine department of our hospital from February 2001 - February 2002 with an infectious disease. An independent observer assessed adherence of every prescription.
Results: In a one year period only 50 of 199 (25%) ciprofloxacin prescriptions (144 patients) were in accordance with the guideline. Guideline-recommended antimicrobials were equally effective (78%) as ciprofloxacin(66%) as empirical therapy judged by in-vitro sensitivity testing of finally cultured pathogens. Moreover, we found that with culture results available doctors still started less effective therapy with ciprofloxacin in six patients.
Conclusion: Cultured pathogens are well covered by guideline recommended antimicrobial agents, therefore no reason exists to deviate from guideline-recommendations. Antimicrobial therapy should be targeted at known resistance patterns of likely or cultured pathogens, which is the very justification of antimicrobial guidelines.

## P - 268

When are Antimicrobial Treatment Guidelines Not Followed?

[1,2]Mol P.G.M., [1]Denig P., [1,2]Panday P.V.N., [4]Gans R.O.B., [3]Degener J.E., [2]Laseur M., [1]Haaijer-Ruskamp F.M.
[1]Department of Clinical Pharmacology, University Groningen, the Netherlands [2]Pharmacy Department, University Hospital Groningen, the Netherlands [3]Department of Clinical Microbiology, University Hospital Groningen, the Netherlands [4]Department of Internal Medicine, University Hospital Groningen, the Netherlands

Objective: Adherence to antimicrobial treatment guidelines is often only moderate. This study explored the impact of clinically relevant patient-characteristics on adherent prescribing.
Methods: Prescribing data were prospectively collected for 527 patients with sepsis, urinary tract infections (UTI), or respiratory tract infections (RTI) admitted to the internal medicine department of our hospital from February 2001- February 2002. An independent observer assessed adherence of every prescription. The guideline recommends for empirical treatment of sepsis and RTI mainly broad-spectrum antibiotics. When in-vitro culture results become available the guideline suggests narrowing-down initial broad-spectrum therapy. For UTI mostly narrow-spectrum antibiotics are recommended.
Results: Adherence varied from 37% for UTI, 53% for sepsis to 75% for RTI. The most prescribed drug was the broad-spectrum antibiotic ciprofloxacin for UTI (39%) and sepsis (24%), and co-amoxiclav for RTI (46%). This drug-choice was not adherent for UTI and sepsis, but adherent for RTI. Patient-characteristics like disease-severity and co-morbidity could not explain differences between adherent and non-adherent cases. Availability of culture results led to less adherence for RTI (OR: 0.5 [0.34–0.77]) and more adherence in UTI (OR: 3.24 [1.59–6.63]).
Conclusion: Doctors seem to prefer broad-spectrum antibiotics in many cases, irrespective of type of infection and patient-characteristics. This leads to low adherence in areas where narrow-spectrum antibiotics are recommended.

## P - 269

The Patient Administration System Registry Contained Several Severe Adverse Drug Reactions Never Reported to the Regulatory Authorities. Shame or Opportunity?

[1,2]Grundmark B., [2]Göransson V., [2]Söderström T.
[1]Medical Products Agency, Sweden .[2]Department of Clinical Pharmacology, Uppsala University Hospital, Uppsala, Sweden

Background The main diagnoses of all patients hospitalized at the Uppsala University Hospital are registered in a patient administration system (PAS) with its corresponding ICD-10-code. Physicians are by law compelled to report ADRs leading to hospitalization, to regulatory authorities. We compared the ADR diagnoses registered in the PAS with those reported.
Methods PAS was searched for patients hospitalized with ADR diagnosis during 2002. The Swedish pharmacovigilance database (SWEDIS)was searched for reports from the same hospital and time period.
Results The routine PAS records of Uppsala University Hospital identified several severe ADRs that had not subsequently been reported to SWEDIS. Examples of severe ADRs not reported were 2 cases of anaphylactic chock, 3 myopathies, 8 ovarian hyperstimulation, 4 drug induced osteoporosis fractures and 21 cases of digoxin intoxication.
Conclusion Using PAS, patients hospitalized due to severe ADRs can be identified. This system, albeit presently imperfect, can with modifications be developed into a new concept of ADR reporting complementing the spontaneous reporting.

## P - 270

Impaired Gastric Motility in the Gastroesophageal Reflux Rat Model: An in Vitro Study

Yıldız F., Tugay M., Utkan T., Gacar N.
Kocaeli University Medical School, Department of Pharmacology Kocaeli, Turkey

The present study investigated the effects of acid and mixed reflux on the responsiveness of gastric smooth muscle in the rat model using organ chambers. Three groups of rats were studied encompassing a gastric acid reflux, mixed reflux and sham operation. Serotonin- and carbachol-induced contractile responses of gastric fundus smooth muscle reactivity was significantly decreased with decreased Emax and pD2 values in the acid and mixed reflux groups compared with the sham operated group. The contractile response to KCl was also decreased especially in the acid reflux group compared with the sham operated group. Relaxant responses to nicotine significantly increased with increased Emax and pD2 values in the acid and mixed reflux groups compared with the sham operated group. However, sodium nitroprusside- and papaverine-induced-relaxant responses were similar in the all groups and there was no change in agonist potency. The present study indicated decreased contractile response and increased nicotine-induced relaxant response of the gastric smooth muscle in the presence of acid and mixed reflux. These findings suggested that impaired gastric smooth muscle contractility and overproduction of the nitric oxide is, at least in part, responsible for the gastric motor dysfunction seen in gastroesophageal reflux.
Index words: Gastroesophageal reflux, gastric motility, in vitro, rat.

## P - 271

Chronic Unilateral Cavernous Nerve Denervation-Related Changes in Neurogenic- and Endothelium-Dependent Relaxant Responses of Rabbit Corporal Smooth Muscle

Sarıoğlu Y., Utkan T., Yıldırım S., Yıldız F.
Kocaeli University Medical School, Department of Pharmacology Kocaeli, Turkey

We investigated the effect of unilateral cavernous nerve denervation on the reactivity of corporal smooth muscle in the male albino white rabbit. 18 rabbits were randomly divided into two groups. In the sham-operated control group (n=9), a pelvic exploration was conducted without division of the cavernous nerve. In the denervation group (n=9), a five mm segment of cavernous nerve excised unilaterally. The reactivity of corpus cavernosum tissue from the denervated animals and the control animals was studied in organ chambers at 4 weeks. In the denervation group, endothelium-dependent relaxation of cavernosal tissue to carbachol was significantly increased compared with the control group. In addition, the sensitivity (i.e. pD2) of denervated strips to carbachol was also increased compared to controls. Electrical field stimulation-induced neurogenic relaxation was significantly reduced in the denervated group. Relaxation to NO donor sodium nitroprruside and papaverine was similar in cavernosal tissue from two groups. There was no change in agonist potency. However, denervation had no effect on KCl-induced contractile responses. When tissue contraction was produced with phenylephrine for the study of relaxation to various stimuli, the tension induced was similar in the denervated and the control group. This data indicate that unilaterally chronic cavernous nerve denervation causes significant functional changes to the penile erectile tissue of rabbits and may contribute to the development of impotence.
Index words: penis, smooth muscle, denervation, rabbits impotence.

## P - 272

Ambiguous Diagnoses in the ICD-10 Classification System Make it an Unsatisfactory Tool in the Development of Quality Indicators of Drug Use

[1]Göransson V., [1,2]Grundmark B., [1]Söderström T.
[1]Department of Clinical Pharmacology, Uppsala University Hospital & [2]Medical Products Agency, Uppsala, Sweden

Background: Reporting of adverse drug reactions (ADRs) is mandatory in Sweden. It is well known that there is a great underreporting of ADRs. Therefore, we performed a systematic review of the diagnoses in the ICD-10 classification system to investigate if this, in combination with patient administration systems, could be a useful tool in creating a complementary ADR reporting system.
Methods: All diagnoses in the ICD-10 classification system were manually searched for any drug relation.
Results: A total of 266 drug related diagnoses were identified. Several of the diagnoses where ambiguous. It was impossible to distinguish drugs prescribed for medical purposes from drugs of abuse or other toxic substances. Only 142 of the diagnoses were unambiguous.
Conclusion: The ICD-10 classification system cannot always distinguish whether a diagnosis is iatrogenic or not. Therefore it is not, in its current form, a satisfactory tool in the development of quality indicators of drug use.

## P - 273

Renal Impairment and Dose Adjustment

[1]Lafay C., [1]Raylet D., [2]Barrière M., [1]Favrelière S., [1]Perault M.C.
[1]Pharmacologie clinique [2]Biochimie et Toxicologie - CHU Poitiers, France.

Patients with renal impairment have a high risk of developing adverse effects, since they are usually treated with many drugs whose elimination may be impaired. The purpose of this study was to assess the frequency of medication misuse in hospitalized patients developing renal impairment. From July to October 2002, a prospective study was conducted in 20 departments of Poitiers hospital. 207 patients with a minimum serum creatinine level of 150 µmol/L were included. The mean age and weight were respectively 75 years and 74 kg. The renal impairment was severe (clearance $< 30$ mL/min) in 54%. The results of the first 100 patients are described. 734 prescriptions were analysed corresponding to 194 different drugs. 85.3% of those 734 prescriptions include drugs with renal metabolism or excretion, 12.4% with potential nephrotoxicity and 59.3% with guidelines for dose adjustment in the Vidal® dictionnary. Taking those guidelines, 31.7% of those 435 prescriptions were inappropriate: 14.7% being inappropriate dosage and 17.0% being contra-indicated. Among the 56 patients with severe renal impairment, 39.5% of the prescriptions were inappropriate. The frequency of misuse is high and probably underestimated. This preliminary analysis shows that physicians have to pay more attention to patients'renal function and the medication prescribed.

## P - 274

Effect of Losartan on the Cardiovascular Response to Cold Pressor Test in Healthy Volunteers

Israel A., Zavala L.E.
School of Pharmacy, Laboratorio de Neuropéptidos, Universidad Central de Venezuela, Caracas and School of Medicine, Universidad Nacional Experimental, Francisco de Miranda, Coro, Venezuela.

Renin secretion and consequently circulating levels of angiotensin II (ANG) play an important role in the regulation of blood pressure and are increased in a number of stress paradigms. It is suggested that ANG is involved in the regulation of sympathetic nervous system and could have a facilitatory role in stress-induced cardiovascular responses. ANG exerts virtually all its cardiovascular effects via the stimulation of AT1 receptor subtype. In this study we investigated the interplay between the RAS and sympathetic nervous system stimulation, in a model of acute stress known to increase arterial pressure and heart rate, the cold pressor test (CPT), applied to healthy volunteers. In addition, we assessed the role of the AT1 receptor in the cardiovascular response to the cold pressor test subjects treated with two AT1 receptor selective antagonists: losartan (LOS) and valsartan (VAL). Thirty four normotensive subjects (24 women and 10 man), aged 21 to 59, were studied. The cold pressor test was performed 90 minutes after administration of LOS (50 mg PO), VAL (80 mg PO) or control (placebo 1 tab PO). The hemodynamic parameters were determined 30 minutes before and after CPT. In the basal state, LOS and VAL produced a significant decrease in mean arterial pressure whereas heart rate was not modified. In control groups the increase in blood pressure during CPT was 11.2 + 2 mmHg. Treatment with LOS or VAL significantly reduced the pressor response to CPT, while no changes were observe in heart rate response. Our results suggest that the AT1 receptor play a facilitator role in the sympathetic response to stress.

## ORAL

**Use of the "Pharmapac" Tool in a Regular Course in Clinical Pharmacology for Medical Students**

Törnqvist E., Böttiger Y., Lars L. Gustafsson. Division of Drug Management and Informatics, Stockholm County Council, Huddinge Department of Clinical Pharmacology, Karolinska Institute, Huddinge University Hospital, Stockholm, Sweden.

Background: The PharmaPac tool for presenting computer based, interactive patient cases was developed in 2000-2001 in collaboration with the Stanford School of Medicine. The basic structure of the tool allows for the creation of any form of web based, interactive flow of questions and answers, including various media, and with the opportunity of internet linkage. We have now introduced the Pharmapac tool into the regular course of clinical pharmacology for medical students at the Karolinska Institutet, with focus on the difficult task of drug choice and drug evaluation.

Aim: The aim of introducing the Pharmapac tool is to set the practice of drug choice and drug evaluation into a realistic learning environment, to gain the dual purpose of improving knowledge of pharmacotherapeutic principles and improving the ability of the students to search and evaluate medical information. This will lead to a learning situation, which will mirror their future work, when pharmacotherapeutic knowledge will have to be continuosly updated. A further gain is to develop teacher skills within the field of drug evaluation and informatics, as clinical pharmacologists in training are involved as seminar leaders.

Method: Both qualitative and quantitative evaluations have been performed by students and teachers.

Conclusion: Basic properties of the case in use, as well as student and teacher evaluation of this course will be presented.

## P - 275

**Lack of a Pharmacokinetic (PK) Interaction Between Sirolimus (SRL) And Cyclosporine (CsA) When SRL is Administered 2 Hours Before CsA**

[1]Parks V., [1]Patat A., [2]Zimmerman J.J., [3]Richards J.
[1]Wyeth Research, Paris, France; [2]Collegeville, PA, United States; [3]PPD Development, Leicester, United Kingdom

SRL (Rapamuneâ) is an effective immunosuppressant currently marketed worldwide for kidney transplant patients. The interaction between SRL 5 mg oral solution and CsA (Neoralâ) 300 mg capsules when administered simultaneously and 2 hrs apart was assessed in a randomized, open-label, 5-period crossover study in 33 healthy subjects (age 18-45 years, weight 58-89 kg) who received a single oral dose of SRL alone (A), CsA alone (B), SRL and CsA together (C), SRL 2 hrs after CsA (D), and SRL 2 hrs before CsA (E). Whole blood SRL was assayed by HPLC mass spectroscopy, and whole blood CsA by immunoassay. Geometric least-squares (GLS) mean ratios and 90% confidence intervals (CIs) were computed for group comparisons. Reference treatments for equivalence tests were either A (SRL alone) or B (CsA alone). A GLS mean ratio between 80 and 125% showed equivalence.

GLS MEAN RATIOS (90% CI) FOR WHOLE BLOOD SRL PK PARAMETERS

| | C vs A | D vs A | E vs A |
|---|---|---|---|
| $C_{max}$ | 217 (196-241) | 226 (204-251) | 98 (88-109) |
| AUC | 283 (257-311) | 241 (219-265) | 99 (90-109) |
| $t_{max}$ | 147 (131-162) | 147 (131-162) | 95 (79-111) |
| $t_{1/2}$ | 87 (82-91) | 87 (83-92) | 97 (92-103) |
| CL/F | 35 (32-39) | 42 (38-46) | 101 (92-111) |

SRL Cmax and AUC increased 2- to 3-fold when coadministered or administered 2 hrs after CsA but did not vary when SRL was given 2 hrs before CsA. SRL terminal half-life (t1/2) was equivalent among all treatment comparisons. The PK of CsA were not affected by coadministration of SRL regardless of the timing of administration. In conclusion, there was a PK interaction when SRL was administered simultaneously with or 2 hrs after CsA. However, no significant PK interaction was observed when sirolimus was administered 2 hours before CsA.

## P - 276

**Absolute/Relative Bioavailability of Bazedoxifene Acetate in Healthy Postmenopausal Women**

[1]Bellaire S.B., McKeand W., Patat A., [2]Ermer J., [3]Le Coz F.
[1]Wyeth Research, Clinical Pharmacology Paris, [2]Wyeth Research, Clinical Pharmacokinetics Collegeville, PA, [3]Biotrial, Rennes, France

Bazedoxifene (BZA) is a potentially best in class selective estrogen receptor modulator that is being developed for the treatment and prevention of postmenopausal osteoporosis. In preclinical models BZA has shown positive skeletal effect, no increase in vasomotor activity, and a superior uterine profile. The objective of this open-label, randomized, 3-way crossover study conducted in 18 healthy post-menopausal women was to assess the absolute bioavailability of two oral formulations of BZA, a 10 mg tablet and two 5 mg capsules, and a 3 mg IV formulation, as well as to assess the relative bioavailability of the two oral formulations. Doses were administered under fasting conditions. Blood samples were collected up to 168 hours after dose administration. Each period was separated by a 2-week washout interval. Non-compartmental PK methods were used to analyze BZA plasma concentrations and a 90% confidence interval (CI) were calculated for the geometric least squares mean ratio of the AUCT values. The absolute bioavailability of BZA was 6.2% for both oral formulations. The geometric least squares mean ratio and 90% CI of AUCT of the oral formulations was 99 (88-111). The concentration-time profiles for the two oral formulations were virtually superimposable. These results indicate that the oral bioavailability of BZA is approximately 6.2% and that both tablet and capsule formulations are bioequivalent with respect to AUC.

## P - 277

**Esophagitis Impairs Esophageal Smooth Muscle Reactivity in the Rat Model: An in Vitro Study**

Yıldız F., Tugay M., Utkan T.
Kocaeli University Medical School, Department of Pharmacology Kocaeli, Turkey

Reflux esophagitis is a condition in which the esophageal epithelium is damaged by gastroesophageal reflux (GER) of predominantly acid and pepsin. Impaired esophageal body motility like diminished peristalsis during GER is a common finding with a prevalence of 25% in patients with mild disease and up to 50% in patients with severe disease. Also increased exposure of the duodenal content may be associated with severe reflux esophagitis, and sometimes both acid and bile reflux occurs synchronously. However It is not clear; what type of reflux material impairs esophageal motor function much more than the other. In this study, we investigated esophageal smooth muscle reactivity in vitro after creating acid and mixed-reflux-induced-esophagitis in the animal model. Three groups of rats were studied encompassing a gastric reflux, duodenogastric reflux and sham laparatomy. Contractile responses of esophageal smooth muscle to carbachol and KCl were decreased in the gastric reflux and duodenogastric reflux groups. Relaxant response to Isoproterenol was also decreased in the gastric reflux and duodenogastric reflux groups with significantly decreased pD2 values compared with the sham control group. Relaxant responses to serotonin and papaverin were similar in the three groups. Our study revealed impaired esophageal smooth muscle reactivity following esophageal injury induced by acid or mixed reflux. We can assume that similar mechanisms may accuse for esophageal motor dysfunction seen in acid or mixed reflux induced esophagitis. This could explain to some extent the abnormal esophageal motor function seen in human GER disease.

Index words: Gastroesophageal reflux, duodenogastric reflux, in vitro, rat

## P - 278

Esophageal Smooth Muscle (Tunica Muscularis Mucosae) Reactivity in Diabetic Rats

Yıldız F., Utkan T., Ulak G., Gacar N., Goçmez S.
Kocaeli University Medical School, Department of Pharmacology Kocaeli, Turkey

In most diabetic patients, the motor functioning of the esophagus is impaired. But the contractile and relaxant mechanisms of esophagus in diabetes have not been investigated in-vitro. Therefore, in this study; the responses of the esophageal smooth muscle (tunica muscularis mucosae) strips isolated from diabetic rats to agonists were examined in-vitro. Diabetes was induced in male Wistar rats (250-300 g) by a single injection of STZ (65 mg/kg, ip). In a separate series of experiments, esophageal muscles isolated from untreated rats were mounted under 0.5 g tension for isometric recording, and incubated for 6 h in Krebs solution containing elevated glucose (44.1mM) (elevated glucose group). KCl and carbachol induced contractions were significantly decreased in the diabetic group compared with the elevated glucose and control group. Isoproterenole, serotonine and papaverine produced concentration dependent relaxation in submaximally precontracted (10-6 M Carbachol) esophageal strips obtained from diabetic, elevated glucose and control group. The relaxations elicited by serotonin or papaverine were similar in three groups. There were no significant changes in the Emax and pD2 values. Isoproterenole induced relaxation was significantly decreased in the diabetic group compared with control group. However, relaxation of esophageal strips to isoproterenole in the elevated glucose group was significantly decreased compared with the diabetic and control group. The concentration-response curve for isoproterenole was shifted to the right with significantly lower Emax and pD2 values. In conclusion, our findings suggest that diabetes may impair contractile and relaxant responses of esophageal smooth muscle, leading to esophageal disorders seen in diabetes mellitus.

Index words: Diabetes mellitus, rat, esophagus, in-vitro

## P - 280

Chronic Ethanol Consumption Impairs Cholinoreceptor-Mediated Contractions and Nanc-Mediated Relaxations of Isolated Rat Lower Esophageal Sphincter and Tunica Muscularis Mucosae

Yıldız F., Utkan T., Tugay M.
Kocaeli University Medical School, Department of Pharmacology Kocaeli, Turkey

It is known that acute ethanol causes esophageal dysmotility in humans and animals but the mechanism is not known. The present study was to designed to determine the effect of chronic alcohol consumption on reactivity of tunica muscularis mucosae and lower esophageal sphincter smooth muscle. Male rats received ethanol (7.2 % v/v) in a modified liquid diets for 4 weeks. Two control groups were assessed, eight rats in one group were fed sucrose and received a liquid diet and eight rats in the second group received standard rat chow and water for 4 weeks. The reactivity of tunica muscularis mucosae and LES smooth muscle strips from ethanol-fed and control animals was evaluated in organ chambers. Contractile responses of LES smooth muscle to serotonin or 80mM KCl and relaxant responses to papaverine or isoproterenole were similar in the control groups and the ethanol-fed group. The relaxation response elicited by nicotine or sodium nitro prusside (SNP) or contractile response elicited by carbachol was unaffected in the both control groups while it was significantly inhibited with decreased maximum responses and pD2 values, in the ethanol-fed group. The relaxation response elicited by serotonin or the contractile response elicited by carbachol or 80mM KCl was unaffected in both control groups while it was significantly inhibited in the ethanol-fed group. Our findings suggest that chronic alcohol consumption impairs relaxant and contractile responses of both tunica muscularis mucosae and LES smooth muscle strips and it may be responsible for gastroesophageal reflux commonly seen after alcohol binges.

## P - 279

Effects of Various Agonists on Lower Esophageal Sphincter Strips Isolated from Diabetic Rats

Yıldız F., Utkan T., Ulak G., Gacar N.
Kocaeli University Medical School, Department of Pharmacology Kocaeli, Turkey

Diabetes mellitus has been reported to cause reduced lower esophageal sphincter pressure, the mechanism of which is unknown. Therefore, we investigated the effect of diabetes on the responsiveness of the rat LES smooth muscle. Diabetes was induced by a single injection of streptozotocin (65 mg/kg, ip) (diabetic group). In addition, the effect of in vitro exposure to elevated glucose has been investigated on responsiveness in muscles from untreated rats (elevated glucose group). KCl, carbachol and, serotonine induced contractile responses were significantly decreased in the diabetic group compared with the elevated glucose and control group ($p<0.05$). The concentration-response curves for agonists were shifted to the right with significantly lower Emax and pD2 values ($p<0.05$). Nicotine, Sodyum nitro prusside (SNP), isoproterenole and papaverine produced concentration-dependent relaxation in submaximally precontracted (10-6M Carbachol) LES strips obtained from diabetic, elevated glucose, and control group. NO-mediated relaxation to nicotine and to SNP, an NO donor, was significantly decreased in the diabetic group compared to elevated glucose and control group ($p<0.05$). The concentration response curve for nicotine or SNP was shifted to the right with significantly lower Emax and pD2 values ($p<0.05$). Isoproterenole and papaverine-induced relaxant responses were similar in all groups and there was no significant changes in the Emax and pD2 values. In conclusion, it has been suggested that diabetes may affect alimentary tract motility through impaired contractility of LES smooth muscle by alterations in the NO/cGMP pathway or by alterations in voltage-dependent Ca++2 channels and/or receptor or post receptor mechanisms.

Index words: Diabetes mellitus, rat, lower esophageal sphincter, in-vitro

## P - 281

Ecstasy (MDMA) is a Mechanism-Based Inhibitor of CYP2D6

Heydari A., Rowland Yeo K., Rostami-Hodjegan A., Lennard M.S., Tucker G.T.
Molecular Pharmacology and Pharmacogenetics, Royal Hallamshire Hospital, University of Sheffield, Glossop Road S10 2JF, UK

Methylenedioxymethamphetamine (MDMA), more commonly known as Ecstasy, is metabolized predominantly by cytochrome P450 2D6 (CYP2D6) [Tucker et al. 1994]. More recently, Wu et al. [1997] reported that MDMA is a potent competitive inhibitor of CYP2D6 in human liver microsomes. In addition, it was observed that the inhibitory effect was enhanced by preincubation with microsomes, suggesting that MDMA may produce a metabolite complex with CYP2D6. Thus, the aim of this study was to characterise the mechanism of inhibition of CYP2D6 by MDMA.Yeast microsomes expressing CYP2D6 were preincubated with MDMA in the presence of an NADPH generating system. Incubates were then assayed for remaining CYP2D6 activity using dextromethorphan as the substrate (20 μM). Inactivation parameters were determined by varying the preincubation time (0,1,2,3,4,5 minutes) as well as the concentration of MDMA (0,1,2,5,10 μM). Time and concentration dependent inhibition was demonstrated. Estimates of the MDMA concentration required for half-maximal inactivation (KI) and the maximal rate constant of inactivation (kinact) were 3.23 μM ± 0.89 (SE) and 0.29 min-1 ± 0.03 (SE), respectively (GraFit, version 5.0). The results of this study confirm that MDMA is a mechanism-based inhibitor of CYP2D6.

Tucker et al (1994) Biochem Pharmacol 47:1151-6 Wu et al. (1997) Biochem Pharmacol 53:1605-12

## P - 282

The Effects of Age and Gender on Fluvoxamine Caffeine Interaction in Rats

Eminoglu O., Kalkan S., Guven H., Benker T., Gelal A., Gidener S.
Dokuz Eylul University Faculty of Medicine, Department of Pharmacology, Izmir, Turkey.

The objective of this study was to asses effects of the age and gender on fluvoxamine (CYP1A2 inhibitor ) and caffeine (CYP1A2 substrate )interaction in rats. A total of 280 male and female rats (35 rats of each gender per age group) in two age groups of (young and elderly )used. Each of these were divided into two groups as control and fluvoxamine. Fluvoxamine (20 mg/kg) dosed orally for 7 days and control groups received tap water. At the 7th day all groups were given caffeine 25 mg/kg orally. Blood samples were drawn at 0, 1, 2, 3, 6, 10 and 24th hours from five rats per groups. Serum caffeine levels was determined with GC/MS. The blood level of caffeine shown to be significantly higher at 1 and 6 hours in elderly female fluvoxamine group compared to other female groups. Among male rats, serum caffeine concentrations were reduced significantly in elderly fluvoxamine group, compared to their controls. In female elderly fluvoxamine group 2, 3, 6, and 10 hours caffeine concentrations were significantly higher than elderly male. In conclusion, serum caffeine levels increases after fluvoxamine administration in females but not in males.

This study was supported by Dokuz Eylul University Research Foundation with the grant number 0909.01.00.03

## P - 283

The Effects of Gender and Menopause on Serum Lidocaine Levels in Smokers

[1]Oztekin S., [2]Kalkan S., [1]Mavioglu O., [2]Elmas T., [1]Elar Z., [2]Guven H.
Dokuz Eylul University School of Medicine [1]Department of Anesthesiology and Reanimation [2]Department of Pharmacology. Turkey.

The activity of the human cytochrome P450 (CYP) is affected by gender (CYP1A2, CYP3A4) and menopausal status (CYP3A4). Lidocaine is commonly used during anesthesia to protect patients against sympathomimetic reactions and metabolized by CYP3A4 and CYP1A2. Smoking is known to be an inducer of CYP1A2. The aim of the study was to determine the effect of gender and menopause on serum lidocaine levels in smokers under general anesthesia. Eighteen subject were enrolled into the study. Men, premenopausal women, and postmenopausal women (respectively 44.3 ± 4.5, 32.0 ± 2.5, and 50.0 ± 2.3 years ) received i.v. lidocaine (1mg/kg) before induction of anesthesia. Serum lidocaine concentrations were measured using the EMIT at 1, 5, 10, 20, 40 and 60 minutes. Statistical analysis were performed using Mann-Whitney U test. There were no significant differences in lidocaine concentrations, AUC (0-60) *g/ ml /min and t 1/2 ( min ) among the groups. These results suggest that gender and menopause have no effect on serum lidocaine levels in smokers ( $p>0.05$).

## P - 284

Dextromethorphan Test and Enzyme Inhibition - Comparative Results with Urine and Serum Analysis

[1]Kuhn U.D., [1]Kirsch M., [1]Merkel U., [2]Eberhardt A.M., [3]Beier T., [3]Maurer I., [4]Härtter S., [4]Hiemke C., [3]Volz H.P., [1]Balogh A.
[1]Institute of Clinical Pharmacology, [2]Institute of Psychology, [3]Department of Psychiatry, University Jena, Germany; [4]Department of Psychiatry, University Mainz, Germany.

Eleven healthy male volunteers (none CYP 2D6 poor metabolizer) ingested 30 mg paroxetine once daily for 11 days. CYP2D6 phenotyping (30 mg dextromethorphan [DM] orally) was performed on day 11 (treatment period [TP]) and repeated after 3 weeks washout time (control period [CP]). Both times, divorced was sampled for 8 hours and serum taken at 2 hours after DM administration (with/without paroxetine). DM and metabolites (dextrorphan [DXT], 3-methoxymorphinan [MM] and 3-hydroxymorphinan [HM]) were measured by HPLC and metabolic ratios (MR) calculated (DM/DXT, MM/HM for CYP2D6, DM/MM and DXT/HM for CYP3A4 activity). Significant correlation between serum levels and urine excretion or between derived serum/urine MR was only seen during TP (with DXT and HM and with all MR except DM/MM). Both in urine and serum, paroxetine treatment led to an increase of DM and MM (and derived MR DM/DXT, MM/HM, but also DM/MM) and a decrease of DXT and HM, indicating CYP2D6 inhibition. MR increases in urine were more expressed than in serum (more prominent changes especially of DM and MM in urine). Paroxetine trough levels (day 10/11) correlated with both serum and urine DM/DXT MR from TP (but not from CP). Enzyme inhibition was recognized both with urine and serum analysis.

## P - 285

Adrenomedullin Suppresses Migration Inhibitory Factor Production and Cytokine Response of Rat Macrophages to Lipopolysaccharide

Cheung B.M.Y., Wong L.Y.F., [1]Li Y.Y., [1]Tang F., [2]Lan H.Y.
[1]Department of Medicine & Department of Physiology, [2]The University of Hong Kong; Baylor College of Medicine, Texas, USA.

Adrenomedullin (AM) is a vasorelaxant peptide that is also involved in inflammatory response. Macrophage migration inhibitory factor (MIF) is a critical mediator of inflammatory diseases that is released from pituitary and macrophages in response to inflammatory stimuli. We investigated the interactions between AM and MIF production and the cytokine response of AM on rat macrophages. Rat macrophages (NR8383) were activated by LPS in the absence and presence of AM at 1 to 1000ng/mL. The cytokine response of MIF, TNF-alpha, IL-1beta, and IL-6 was measured by ELISA at 1, 3, 6 and 24 hours. The effect of AM on MIF production from resting macrophages was determined from cell cultures containing RPMI medium and AM alone. AM (at 1 to 1000 ng/mL) increased release of MIF from resting macrophages dose-dependently by 36.3% to 75.7 % in the first hour while further production in subsequent 24 hours was not significantly affected by the presence of AM. For LPS-stimulated macrophages, AM increased MIF secretion in the first hour by 13.5% to 35.4 %, but reduced further production of MIF by 22.6+6.8% at 24 hours. The suppressive effect was observed even at 1ng/mL of AM. TNF-alpha production from LPS-stimulated cells was reduced by 15.6% to 66% with addition of AM at 1000 ng/mL but no significant effect was observed for AM at low concentrations (1 to 100 ng/mL). Our results suggest that AM modulates cytokine response from LPS-stimulated macrophages and may have a regulatory role in inflammation.

## P - 286

The Interaction of the Diltiazem with Oral and Intravenous Cyclosporıne in Rats

Kalkan S., Gumustekin M. , Aygoren O., Tuncok Y., Gelal A., Guven H.,
Dokuz Eylul University Faculty of Medicine, Department of Pharmacology, Izmir, Turkey.

The aim of the present study was to determine the effect of diltiazem on pharmacokinetics of cyclosporine (CsA) administered by orally and intravenously in rats. The diltiazem group received 60 or 90 mg/kg diltiazem by orally for 3 days, where as the control group received normal saline. Each experimental group divided into 2 equal groups. The first group received a single oral dose of CsA (10mg/kg), while the second group was injected as a bolus (6mg/kg). Pharmacokinetic parameters of CsA were measured (Table 1, 2). Statistical analysis was performed by nonparametric analysis of variance.

Table1. Oral group

| Parameter | CsA (alone)(n=4) | CsA+Diltiazem (60)(n=5) | CsA+Diltiazem (90)(n=5) |
|---|---|---|---|
| $AUC_{0-24}$(μg.h.mL) | 16.5 ± 1.8 | 18.7 ± 2.6 | 22.9 ± 1.7 |
| $AUC_{0-\infty}$(μg.h.mL) | 17.5 ± 2.3 | 29.8 ± 5.7 | 37.8 ± 3.6* |
| $t_{1/2}$ (h) | 5.7 ± 0.9 | 16.6 ± 3.4 | 18.2 ± 0.8* |
| $CL_{i.v}$(L/h/kg) | 0.105 ± 0.0 | 0.053 ± 0.0 | 0.039 ±0.0* |

Table 2. Intravenous group

| Parameter | CsA (alone)(n=5) | CsA+Diltiazem (60)(n=5) | CsA+Diltiazem (90)(n=5) |
|---|---|---|---|
| $AUC_{0-24}$(μg.h.mL) | 5.5 ± 0.4 | 2.5 ± 0.5* | 1.9 ± 0.3* |
| $AUC_{0-\infty}$(μg.h.mL) | 6.6 ± 0.3 | 2.8 ± 0.5* | 2.5 ± 0.3* |
| $t_{1/2}$ (h) | 9.3 ± 1.2 | 10.9 ± 2.3 | 11.4 ±2.8 |
| $C_{max}$(mg/mL) | 0.4 ± 0.1 | 0.2 ± 0.1 | 0.1 ± 0.0* |
| $t_{max}$(h) | 4.8 ± 0.8 | 3.6 ± 0.4 | 5.6 ± 0.9 |
| $F_{p.o}$ (%) | 22.6 | 9.6 | 8.5 |

*$p<0.05$ vs CsA(alone)

Diltiazem decreased the bioavailability of oral CsA, while it increased the bioavailability of intravenous CsA. This interaction must be considered in administering oral and intravenous CsA concomitantly with diltiazem.
This study was supported by Dokuz Eylul University Research Foundation with the grant number 0909.20.02.15.

## P - 287

Relation of Caffeinated Beverage Consumption With Serum Liver Enzymes, Serum Lipids and Caffeine Levels: A Preliminary Study.

[1]Güven H., [1]Gumustekin M., [1]Balkan D., [1]Benker T., [1]Eminoglu E., [1]Arslan S., [2]Musal B., [3]Tunca M.
[1]Dokuz Eylül University, Medical Faculty, Department of Pharmacology. Balçova-Izmir-Turkey [2]Dokuz Eylül University, Medical Faculty, Department of Medical Education. Balçova-Izmir-Turkey [3]Dokuz Eylül University, Medical Faculty, Department of Internal Medicine. Balçova-Izmir-Turkey

To examine the effect of caffeinated beverage consumption on serum liver enzyme levels and serum lipids in relation to smoking in volunteers. Patients applied to internal medicine outpatient clinic, from October 2001 to march 2002, without liver disease or any other chronic diseases were evaluated. Coffee drinking was ascertained by a self-administered questionnaire. Serum liver enzymes (ALT, AST, GGT), serum lipids (TG, total cholesterol) and caffeine levels were measured by Hitachi 912 and GC-MS (Hewlett Packard, 5973 MSD- 6890 GC). A total of 169 patient's data were collected, mean age was 51.1 ± 1.14 (Range: 17-88), men were 35.3 % and 64.7 % women. Housewife was the most prominent occupation among the volunteers (44.9 %). All patients were controlled for Hepatitis A, B and C and all of them were healthy. Alcohol consumption was 5.4 %, coffee 48.5 %, tea 91.6 %. The types of consumed coffee were; 25.7 % Turkish coffee, 15.6 % granulated coffee, 7.2 % mixed. Most of the consumed tea was; 87.3 % black tea. Caffeine, GGT, total cholesterol and TG levels were statistically significantly higher in caffeinated beverage consumers than non-consumers. Among caffeinated beverage consumers, caffeine and TG levels were statistically significantly higher in smokers than non-smokers.

## P - 288

The Comparison of Pharmacotherapy of Epilepsy in the Czech Republic and in Sweden

Koristkova B., Grundmann M., [1]Bergman U., [1]Sjöqvist F.
Dept. of Clinical Pharmacology University Hospital and Medico Social Faculty University of Ostrava, Ostrava, Czech Republic, [1]Division of Clinical Pharmacology, Huddinge University Hospital, Stockholm, Sweden

The treatment of epilepsy in the University Hospitals in Ostrava and Huddinge was compared. Request forms for therapeutic drug monitoring were used as data source. 2789 blood samples from 1108 in-patients (60% children, mean age 15±15 years, mean body weight 38±25 kg) were analysed during 1995-1999 in Ostrava. 10543 samples from 3232 out- as well as in-patientes (11% children, mean age 43±23, body weight unknown) were analysed in Huddinge.
The treatment of epilepsy was very similar. Monotherapy was the most common pattern (Ostrava-Huddinge: 50%-59% samples) followed by combination of two drugs (33%-29%). 60% of patterns involved carbamazepine, valproic acid and phenytoin in monotherapy, and combination of valproic acid or phenytoin with carbamazepine in both hospitals. Phenytoin was more frequent in adult patients, while children were treated more often with valproic acid. Higher ratio of adult patients in Huddinge caused the only difference – higher frequency in usage of phenytoin in Huddinge.

## P - 289

Antibiotic Prescribing in Pediatric Hospitalized Patients

Radosevic N., Bajcic P., Palcevski G., Ahel V., Francetic I., Vlahovic-Palcevski V.
University Hospital Center Rijeka, Croatia

Monitoring of antibiotic drug prescribing is of growing concern due to resistance, adverse reactions and cost. Thus, strict antibiotic policies are warranted. Prior to their implementation, detailed knowledge of antibiotic prescribing patterns is required. In this prospective, pilot study the utilization of antibiotics at the Pediatric Clinic, University Hospital Center Rijeka, Croatia has been analyzed. During a period from 8 January-15 February, 2003, patient charts were reviewed with regard to antibiotic prescription. Antibiotics were prescribed to 88 patients. In 72% of the patients antibiotics were given empirically, and only 20% had proven bacterial infection. More than one antibiotic was prescribed to 15%, and it was changed in 42% of the patients. In total, 150 antibiotic courses were prescribed. Restricted antimicrobials were given in 67% of the courses. Third generation cephalosporins were most commonly prescribed (48% of courses). Ceftriaxone was the single most prescribed drug (29%). Since it is not recommended to use a combination of drugs or a restricted antimicrobial as a first choice in empiric treatment, further diagnose-linked analysis is necessary. It also needs to be assessed whether the reason for such an extensive number of switches in antibiotic agents was a reflection of treatment failure.

## P - 290

Identification of Cytochrome P4503A4 and 2C9 as the Major Catalysts of Phenprocoumon Hydroxylation

Ufer M., Tybring G., Svensson J.O., Rane A.
Huddinge University Hospital, Karolinska Institute, Stockholm, Sweden.

This in vitro study aimed to identify hepatic cytochrome P450 (CYP) enzymes catalyzing the hydroxylation of the oral anticoagulant phenprocoumon (PPC) to pharmacologically inactive metabolites. In line with previous in vivo data, kinetic studies in human liver microsomes revealed (S)-7-hydroxyphenprocoumon as the quantitatively most important metabolite. Biphasic Eadie-Hofstee plots were indicative of more than one responsible enzyme catalyzing PPC hydroxylation. A correlation analysis of PPC hydroxylation rate with the catalytic activity of microsomes from 19 individual human liver specimens towards various CYP probe substrates was performed and used as a screening tool for relevant CYP enzymes. Significant correlations with CYP3A4 and CYP2C9 activity were obtained. Moreover, 4-, 6-, and 7-hydroxylation rates of the separate enantiomers were highly correlated arguing for a non-stereoselective metabolism. Specific inhibitors of CYP3A4 (triacetyloleandomycin) and CYP2C9 (sulfaphenazole) strongly inhibited PPC hydroxylation with CYP3A4-mediated inhibition being more potent. Experiments with cDNA-expressed human recombinant enzymes revealed (S)-PPC as a high-affinity substrate of CYP2C9 with $K_m$ values <1 µM, but CYP3A4 catalyzed with low affinity ($K_m$ >100 µM).
Thus, CYP3A4 and CYP2C9 were identified as major catalysts of phenprocoumon hydroxylation and drug interactions are predicted with substrates of these enzymes that may give rise to serious bleeding complications.

## P - 291

Essential Drug Lists a Way Towards a Rational Use of Medicines. A Venezuelan Model.

Landaeta L., Valdivieso L.H., Briceño E.
Ministry of Health and Social Developing, Caracas, Venezuela

The rational use of medicinal drugs is critical to the most important primary and preventive health care measures but this has not been possible in our country recently because of many adverse circumstances. We have created a Therapeutic Committee (TC) which has selected a list of drugs, after the study of those used to treat particular conditions, and a comparison of the value they give in relation to their cost by the National Public Health System. Among those particular conditions, 16 groups of morbidity were chosen and they account for the majority of the consultations which attend our health care centers. The availability of essential drugs, selected according to the level of ambulatory care, has been estimated in about 1500 therapeutics products, which means 26-31 % of the total Pharmaceutical Venezuelan Market, which has around 5700 presentations. According to the Intercontinental Marketing Services (IMS Health Venezuela) the average price of all the pharmaceutical products is 5,30 $ , with the selection of list of essential drugs, at ambulatory level, we have dropped the price to 3,64 $ The essential drug list will permit us to implement a pharmacovigilance program to follow up the security of those medicines and we consider that the essential drug concept, with its focus on equity and meeting real health needs, becomes even more convincing. National drug policies and essential drugs programs are now the best means we have available of pursuing and eventually attaining the dual objectives of rational management of drug resources with a better security profile of the drug and therefore a better health for all.

## P - 292

The Effects of Age and Gender on Fluvoxamine Caffeine Interaction in Rats

Emınoglu O., Kalkan S., Guven H., Benker T., Gelal A., Gıdener S.
Dokuz Eylul University Faculty of Medicine, Department of Pharmacology, Izmir, Turkey.

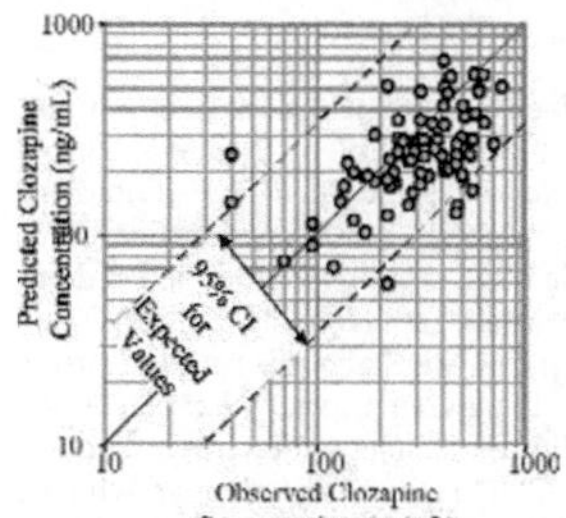


The objective of this study was to asses effects of the age and gender on fluvoxamine (CYP1A2 inhibitor ) and caffeine (CYP1A2 substrate )interaction in rats. A total of 280 male and female rats (35 rats of each gender per age group) in two age groups of (young and elderly )used. Each of these were divided into two groups as control and fluvoxamine. Fluvoxamine (20 mg/kg) dosed orally for 7 days and control groups received tap water. At the 7th day all groups were given caffeine 25 mg/kg orally. Blood samples were drawn at 0, 1, 2, 3, 6, 10 and 24th hours from five rats per groups. Serum caffeine levels was determined with GC/MS. The blood level of caffeine shown to be significantly higher at 1 and 6 hours in elderly female fluvoxamine group compared to other female groups. Among male rats, serum caffeine concentrations were reduced significantly in elderly fluvoxamine group, compared to their controls. In female elderly fluvoxamine group 2, 3, 6, and 10 hours caffeine concentrations were significantly higher than elderly male. In conclusion, serum caffeine levels increases after fluvoxamine administration in females but not in males.

This study was supported by Dokuz Eylul University Research Foundation with the grant number 0909.01.00.03

ORAL

## Validation of a Predictive Model for Individualizing Clozapine Dose

[1]Rostami-Hodjegan A., [2]Ros J.E., [2]Van Der Weide J., [3]Flanagan R.J., [1]Lennard M., [1]Tucker G.T.

[1]Molecular Pharmacology & Pharmacogenetics, University of Sheffield, UK, [2]Clinical Chemistry St Jansdal Hospital, Harderwijk, the Netherlands, [3]Medical Toxicology, Guy's & St Thomas' Trust, London

Background: The therapeutic response to clozapine is associated with a predose ('trough') plasma clozapine concentration of 350 ng/mL or more and concentrations above 1000 ng/mL are associated with a markedly increased risk of CNS toxicity. However inter-individual variability in plasma concentrations is large and thus dose selection is difficult.
Method: Using the results of an analysis in a database of over 4000 samples, we developed a model for predicting clozapine concentrations based on individual patient characteristics[1]. We have now validated this model using an independent data set for which dose, age, sex, body weight and smoking habit were known for 80 patients[2]. Since plasma clozapine/norclozapine ratios were not available mean values of 1.0 and 1.6 obtained from previous studies were entered into the model for smokers and non-smokers, respectively.
Results: The predicted and observed values of trough clozapine concentrations were correlated significantly ($r = 0.57, p < 0.001$) and only 7.5% of predictions fell outside the 95% CI for expected concentrations (see Figure).
Conclusion: The results demonstrate that the model can facilitate rapid individualization of clozapine dosage

ORAL

## Comparison of Quality of Life with Nebivolol and Losartan

Van Bortel L., Mäkel W., Fici F.
Dept of Pharmacology, Ghent University, Ghent, Belgium

The present study investigates quality of life (QoL) with the angiotensin receptor blocker losartan (L) compared to QoL with the third generation NO-release facilitating beta-blocker nebivolol (N) in patients with essential hypertension. 298 patients with mild-to-moderate hypertension were randomised to L 50 mg once daily (n=151; male/female: 94/57; age: 56±8 yrs) or N 5 mg once daily (n=147; male/female: 92/55; age: 56±9 yrs). If after 6 weeks diastolic blood pressure was not normalised, hydrochlorothiazide (HCTZ) 12.5 mg once daily (o.d.) was added. QoL was measured as health index using a validated questionnaire. The higher the score, the better the QoL. Statistical analysis was performed using analysis of variance.
Results: Health index scores (95% confidence intervals) were 0.868 (0.850-0.886) at baseline, 0.881 (0.863-0.899) after 6 weeks of treatment, and 0.877 (0.857-0.896) after 12 weeks with N. With L these were 0.873 (0.855-0.891), 0.875 (0.857-0.893), and 0.878 (0.857-0.897), respectively. Health index did not differ between L and N neither at 6 nor at 12 weeks of treatment.
Conclusions: Quality of life expressed as health index does not differ between N (5 mg o.d.) and L (50 mg o.d.). This remains after adding HCTZ 12.5 mg o.d. in patients with elevated diastolic blood pressure after 6 weeks of monotherapy.

P - 293

## Tropical Climatic Conditions Affect Bioavailability of Diclofenac Formulations

Van Bortel L., Risha P.G., Van den Abeele W.M., Vergote G., Vervaet C., Remon J.P.
Ghent University, Belgium; Muhimbili University College of Health Sciences, Dar es Salaam, Tanzania

The present study investigates the influence of tropical climatic conditions (40°C, 75% humidity) on the oral bioavailability of 2 enteric coated diclofenac 50mg tablets (Voltaren® [Novartis] and Diclo 50® [Camden]) available in Tanzania. Twelve healthy subjects (8 males/4 females, 19-38 years) were given in a 4-period double blind cross-over study in randomized order: Voltaren and Diclo stored under standard (Vs, Ds, resp.) and under tropical conditions (Vt, Dt, resp.). Statistical analysis was done using a two-way ANOVA and Scheffe test. Drug content was 99.2±0.3 % and 97.8±0.3 % in Vs and Ds, resp. and did not change under tropical conditions. Cmax was lower ($p<0.05$) with Dt (1043±197 ng/ml) than with Ds (1597±327 ng/ml) and Tmax was lower ($p<0.05$) with Ds (0.9±0.3 hr) than with Vs (2.0±1.0 hr). Other kinetic parameters did not differ between the test drugs.
Conclusions: Tropical climatic conditions did not change drug content but reduced Cmax of the Camden formulation and not of the Novartis formulation. Drugs for the tropical market should be tested for stability under tropical conditions.

P - 294

## Utilization of Fluoroquinolones and the Development of Bacterial Resistance

[1]Urbanek K., [2]Kolar M.
[1]Department of Pharmacology, [2]Department of Microbiology, Faculty of Medicine, Palacky University, Czech Republic

The aim of this study was to evaluate the dependence of the development of bacterial resistance on fluoroquinolones utilization in Olomouc region in comparison with Teaching Hospital Olomouc. During the period of 1997-2001, utilization of fluoroquinolones in the region was obtained from the data of regional General Health Insurance Company and expressed in a defined daily doses per 1000 patients per day. Hospital consumption data were obtained from the database of the Department of Pharmacology and expressed as a defined daily doses per 100 bed-days. Bacterial strains were isolated from clinical material of community and hospitalized patients, susceptibility to antibiotics was assessed by disk diffusion method and standard microdilution method. In the community, utilization of fluoroquinolones increased from 0.14 DDD/1000/d in 1997 to 0.89 in 2001. Occurrence of E. coli strains resistant to ofloxacin increased from 1% to 8%, resistance of P. mirabilis increased from 21% to 34%. According to linear regression analysis, increase in the resistance depends significantly ($p<0.01$) on fluoroquinolones utilization. Hospital fluoroquinolones consumption increased from 2.50 to 3.54 DDD/100, while the resistances increased from 2% to 4% in E.coli and from 5% to 16% in P.mirabilis. The study documents the dependence of increasing bacterial resistance on the utilization of fluoroquinolones. Supported by grant MSM 151100002.

## P - 295

The Role of Endothelin in Rat Gastric Mucosal Injury by Nonsteroidal Anti-inflammatory Drugs

[1]Murat N., [1]Gidener S., [2]Koyuncuoğlu M.
[1]Dokuz Eylul University School of Medicine Department of Pharmacology, [2]Dokuz Eylul University School of Medicine Department of Pathology, Turkey.

The aim of this study is to make clear the role of endothelin in NSAIDs-induced gastric mucosal injury, the effect of selective COX-2 enzyme inhibitors on gastric mucosa and the role of endothelin at this effect. In group I Indomethacin NS398 andvehicle were administrated. In group II, bosentan, PGE1 and vehicle were given 30 minutes before the administration of endothelin-1. In group III, bosentan were given 2 hours before the administration of indomethacin and NS-398. In group IV, nitric oxide synthase inhibitor were given 30 minute before the administration of NS-398. In our study we investigated that indomethacin-induced mucosal injury was significantly different from NS398 and control group. Endothelin-1 caused gastric damage which couldn't prevent by intragastric administration of bosentan completely but prevented by a cytoprotective PGE1 analogue. Pretreatment with bosentan didn't diminish indomethacin-induced gastric damage. On the contrary pretreatment with bosentan caused gastric damage in NS-398 group. Also, pretreatment with L-NAME caused gastric damage in NS-398 group as bosentan did. These results suggested that selective COX2 inhibitors doesn't cause gastric damage contrary to conventional NSAIDs. Endothelin-induced ulcer isn't completely receptor dependent. Our findings also point to indomethacin doesn't cause ulcer via ET receptors but inhibition of ET receptors caused COX2 inhibitor-induced ulcer. Protective effects of COX2 inhibitors may be via ET receptor related NO releasing.

## P - 296

Detection of Sulbactam Ampicilin Susceptibilty with Microdilution Method in Proteus, Citrobacter and same Gram Negative Bacteria

Uraz G., Öncül Ö.
Gazi University, Faculty of Science and Arts, Department of Biology, Teknikokullar, Ankara, Turkey

Antimicrobial susceptibility tests are being used to get the best effectual results in antimicrobial drug treatmets. The broth dilution method (MIC) has been regarded as a good alternative test for detection of antimicrobial agent susceptibilities.The minimal inhibitory concentration method that has given quantitative results is being selected specially for this study. In this research, antimicrobial activity of sulbactam ampicilin (SAM) was investigated on Proteus, Citrobacter, Morganella and some gram negative isolates. Thus, the drug solution was doubly diluted to give final concentrations from 256-0,125 μg/ml. Qualtiy control was performed by testing the a number of strains according to the recommendations of NCCLS Documents. The isolate collection included 91-gram negative isolates. In conclusion, 47 (%51,66) isolates were found sensitive (<8/4 μg/ml) to SAM, 13 (%14,28) isolates were found intermediately sensitive (16/8 μg/ml) to SAM and 31 (%34,06) isolates were found resistant (>32/16) to SAM.
In our study, some of the isolates which found sensitive to SAM and their MIC ranges are summarized in the table.

| Organism (no. tested) | MIC Range(μg/ml) | Sensitive |
|---|---|---|
| *Citrobacter freundii* (11) | 0,5-128 | 3 |
| *Eikonella corrodens* (2) | 0,5-1 | 2 |
| *Enterobacter cancerogenus* (1) | 1 | 1 |
| *Enterobacter cloaceae* (3) | 1-4 | 1 |
| *Morganella morgani* (8) | 0,5-4 | 3 |
| *Pseudomonas flourescens* (7) | 1-8 | 4 |
| *Pseudomonas maltophilia* (1) | 1 | 1 |
| *Proteus mirabilis* (13) | 0,5-32 | 8 |
| *Proteus penneri* (6) | 0,5-128 | 4 |
| *Proteus vulgaris* (6) | 1-16 | 5 |
| *Salmonella choloroseus* (2) | 0,5-16 | 1 |

The resuls of our study show that SAM was highly active (0,5-1μg/ml) aganist *E. corrodens*.

## ORAL

Multidisciplinary Medication Review among Nursing Home Residents - What are the Most Significant Drug-Related Problems? The Bergen District Nursing Home (BEDNURS) Study

[1]Ruths S., [2]Straand J., Nygaard H. A.
[1]Section for Geriatric Medicine, Department of Public Health and Primary Health Care, University of Bergen, Norway; [2]Section for General Practice/Family Medicine, Department of General Practice and Community Medicine, University of Oslo, Norway

Aim: Based on a multidisciplinary drug utilization review among nursing home residents, this study aimed to identify the most frequent clinically relevant medication problems, and to analyse them according to involved drugs and types of problems. Materials and Methods: Cross-sectional study auditing drug use among 1354 residents in 23 nursing homes in Bergen, Norway. Data were collected in 1997. A physician/pharmacist panel performed a comprehensive medication review with regard to indications for drug use, and active medical conditions. The drug-related problems were subsequently classified according to involved drugs and types of problems (i.e. indication, effectiveness, and safety issues). Results: 2445 potential medication problems of 1036 (76%) residents were identified. Psychoactive drugs accounted for 38% of all problems; anti-psychotics were the class most often questioned. Multiple psychoactive drug use was considered particularly problematic. Potential medication problems were most frequently classified as risk for adverse drug reactions (26%), inappropriate drug choice for indication (20%), and under-utilisation of beneficial treatment (13%). Conclusions: Three of four nursing home residents had clinically relevant medication problems. Psychoactive drugs accounted for most problems. Most frequent concerns were related to adverse drug reactions, drug choice, and probable under-treatment.

Keywords: nursing homes, multidisciplinary medication review, drug-related problems.

## P - 297

Pharmacokinetics and Pharmacodynamics of Subcutaneous Interferon Alpha-2b

Kinzig-Schippers M., [1]Jetter A., [1]Tomalik-Scharte D., [1]Szymanski J., [1]Fuhr, Illauer M., Skott A., Sörgel F.
IBMP - Institute for Biomedical and Pharmaceutical Research, Nürnberg-Heroldsberg, [1]Institute for Pharmacology, University of Köln; Germany

Interferon (IFN) alpha-2b is mainly used in the treatment of chronic hepatitis C infection, usually combined with ribavirin. However, long-term therapy related to many important adverse effects results in cure rates of only approximately 50 %. The present evaluation was carried out to address a possible use of pharmacokinetics to predict individual response as assessed by surrogate pharmacodynamic parameters. Eighteen healthy young volunteers (8 females, 10 males) received a single 38.5 μg (10 MIU) IFN alpha-2b dose by subcutaneous injection. IFN alpha-2b, beta2-microglobulin and neopterin were analyzed by precise enzyme immunoassay. Pharmacokinetic and pharmacodynamic parameters were determined by noncompartmental methods, and their relationship was examined by correlation analyses. Results (mean & SD): IFN alpha-2b: Cmax 159.5 +/- 53.5 pg/mL, AUC 2129 +/- 818.0 pg*h/mL, t1/2 6.7 +/- 3.7 h; beta2-microglobulin: Cmax 8.2 +/- 4.8 mg/L, AUC,0-216h 903.6 +/- 255.8 mg*h/L, t1/2 537 +/- 201 h, neopterin: Cmax 10.6 +/- 2.3 ng/mL, AUC,0-216h 1045 +/- 133.2 ng*h/mL, t1/2 174 +/- 50.3 h. There was no meaningful correlation between individual pharmacokinetic parameters of interferon and any of the pharmacodynamic metrics, suggesting that differences in individual signal transduction are more important than differences in individual IFN alpha-2b pharmacokinetics in subjects receiving identical doses. In conclusion, this evaluation provides no evidence for a role of INF alpha-2b pharmacokinetics to personalize INF doses.

## P - 298

### Role of Amoxicillin Prophylactic Therapy in Third Molar Surgery

[1]Sillet M., [1]Orellana A., [2]Mathison Y.
[1]School of Odontology and J.M. Vargas [2]School of Medicine, Universidad Central de Venezuela, Caracas, Venezuela

The use of antimicrobial prophylaxis in third molar surgery is widespread, but controversial. While there is some evidences that these drugs can reduce the incidence of postoperative complications, other findings suggest that they do not. We therefore designed a study to test the efficacy of two dosing regimen of antimicrobial prophylaxis whit amoxicillin during the removal of impacted third molar. The study was prospective, randomized, placebo-controlled. Patients gave consent for the study, which was approved by the local Ethics Committee. A total of 45 patients, aged 18-35 having impacted third molar, was randomized allocation into three groups: placebo (n=15), amoxicillin 2g orally, 1 hour preoperatively (n=15), or amoxicillin 500 mg orally eight hourly for 7 days postoperatively (n=15). Patients were assessment on the second, third and seventh postoperative days for pain, interincisal mouth opening (mm), swelling and whether there was purulent discharge from the wound or a dry socket. Three patients in the placebo group shown infection process and required antibiotic rescue (azitromicin), while no patients in the other group had infection; this difference was statistically significant (ANOVA) . Our results suggest that amoxicillin prophylaxis reduce morbidity after removal of third molar.

## P - 299

### Predicting Drug Clearance Allowing For The Influence Of P-Glycoprotein Activity Using SIMCYP™

Howgate E.M., Proctor N.J., Rostami-Hodjegan A., Tucker G.T.
University of Sheffield Section of Molecular Pharmacology & Pharmacogenetics, Royal Hallamshire Hospital, Sheffield, UK

The SIMCYP™ programme was used to predict total human unbound plasma clearances (CLu) for nine drugs for which suitable *in vitro* and *in vivo* data were available in the literature. Values of Vmax and Km for different metabolic pathways were obtained from reports using single expressed cytochrome P450 systems. Genetic, physiological, demographic and ethnic variability, relevant to the *in vivo* studies, was then incorporated to produce population distributions of predicted CLu values. These were then compared with weighted *in vivo* CLu values to determine their accuracy. $CLu_{po}$ and/or $CLu_{iv}$ were determined for alprazolam, imipramine, midazolam, R-verapamil, S-verapamil, caffeine, dextromethorphan, diltiazem and erythromycin. The ratio of median predictions ($CLu_{pred}/CLu_{obs}$) ranged from 0.20 - 1.10 for $CLu_{iv}$ and from 0.57 - 4.93 for $CLu_{po}$. The corresponding values for the ratios of 95% confidence intervals were 0.58 - 8.22 and 1.15 - 151.09, respectively. As several of these compounds are known to be substrates of P-glycoprotein, the relationship between prediction accuracy and *in vitro* transport was also examined. This indicated a significant ($p < 0.05$) negative correlation ($r = 0.81$) between bias (as expressed by the natural logarithm of the ratio described above) and affinity to P-glycoprotein (as assessed by relative flux).

## P - 300

### Comparative Study of Initial and Acquired Drug Resistance in Pulmonary Tuberculosis in National Research Institute of Tuberculosis and Pulmonary Disease

Arami S., Mansoori D., Mirabolhasani Z., Farnia P.
National Research Institute of Tuberculosis and Pulmonary Disease (NRITLD) Shahid Beheshti Medical university, Tehran, Iran

Background and Objective : Resistant to anti-tuberculosis agents is an important obstacle in the treatment and control of tuberculosis in the world. The present study was undertaken to assess the pattern of resistance at a referral center in Tehran, Iran.
Methods : Between Sep. 1996 and March 2000 for 273 smear and culture positive pulmonary tuberculosis patients (both old = 86/273 and new = 187/273) pretreatment susceptibility tests of isolated bacilli to INH, RIF, EMB and STM were performed by standard proportional method and the results were classified in three groups: I) Newly diagnosed without any history of treatment II) Patients with history of treatment with one course III) Patients with history of treatment for two or more courses supposed to be MDR cases. The results were collected for each drug individually and different combinations of two, three and four medications.
Results : Resistance was significantly increased in group III in comparison to group II and I, also significantly increase in group II when compared to group I. We observed a high rate of primary resistance to INH and STM in group I and II and a high rate of MDR (INH and RIF resistance) in groups II and III.
Conclusion : The duration of bacilli exposure to anti-tuberculosis agents in the past is a major factor in developing resistance. Due to high rate of primary resistance especially to STM in our area, we recommend a more conservative approach with six drugs for treatment of patients whose initial four-drug regimens have been failed (group II).
Key words : Tuberculosis, drug resistance, initial, acquired

## P - 301

### Influence of Long-term Anticonvulsant Drug Therapy on Bone Mass Status in Childrens: A Quantitative Ultrasound Study

Pedrera J.D., [1]López-Lafuente A., [1]López-Rodríguez M.J., Borrella S., Rodríguez T., Canal M.L.
Departamento de Enfermería Universidad de Extremadura, [1]Servicio de Pediatría Hospital San Pedro de Alcántara, Cáceres, Spain

Objetive: The objetive of the study was to evaluate bone mass status in children on long-term anticonvulsant therapy.
Patients and methods: We measured and compared the basal serum levels of 25(OH)D3, parathyroid hormone and phalangeal bone ultrasound (Ad-SOS) in 40 children (8.39± 3.35 years old), 28 patients in treatment with valproic acid (VA) and 12 in treatment with carbamazepine (CBZ), with a control group of similar age and sex.
Results: In the group patients, height, 25(OH)D3 and Ad-SOS values were significantly lower ($p=0.0485$, $p<0.0001$ and $p<0.0001$ respectivamente). The low Ad-SOS values for the patients were independent of the treatment, and values for 25(OH)D3 and total alkaline phosphatase (AlPh) were significantly lower in patients treaties with VA ($p=0.0146$ and $p=0.0009$. For stepwise regression taken AD-SOS as dependent variable, only the height values are significant in patients treated with VA (beta = 198.83, $p=0.0019$), and in patients treated with CBZ, are significant height values, AlPh and tartrate-resistant acid phosphatase (beta=14.88, 0.196 and 0.971, $p=0.0005$).
Conclusions : Theses findings justify the need to assure adequate vitamin D intake, especially in children in treatment with VA, in order to prevent osteomalacia and low growth.

## P - 302

Ultrasound Bone Mass in Patient Treated with Long-Term Oral Anti-Coagulants

Pedrera JD, Canal ML, Bote JL, Morales ML, Retortillo C, Lavado JM
Departamento de Enfermería, Universidad de Extremadura, Cáceres, Spain

Objective : The objective of this work is to determine the effects that produces the chronic treatment with oral anti-coagulants (ACO-K) on bone mass, valued by means of quantitative bone ultrasound.
Method : 99 patients in chronic treatment with ACO-K (56,96 ± 34,30 months of treatment) have been studied (71,48±4,6 years of half age) and have been compared to control group of similar age and sex. We measured and compared osteocalcine, tartrate-resistant acid phosphatase, coagulation study, international normalized reason (INR) and time of activated partial tromboplastine. The bone mass has been valued by means bone speed transmission of the ultrasound of phalanges (Ad-SoS) and the attenuation of the bone ultrasound in calcaneus (BUA).
Results : The analysis of stepwise regression among the Ad-SoS in relation to biochemical variables, antropometric factors and BUA was significant and positive with the INR, BUA, urea and total alkaline phosphatase (ß=74,151; 1,468; 0,635 and 0,103 respectively; F=12440,897; p=0,0067).
Conclusions : According to the results, the bone mass in patient in chronic treatment with ACO-K is not affected if the INR is among the values 1,42 and 4,30. it is necessary to carry out wider longitudinal studies with object of knowing the effect of the ACO-K more correctly on the bone mass

## P - 303

Ultrasound Bone Mass in Schizophrenic Patients on Long-Term Neuroleptic Therapy

Rey P., Lavado J.M., Morales M.L., Rodríguez T., Borrella S., Pedrera J.D.
Departamento de Enfermería, Universidad de Extremadura, Cáceres, Spain

Objetive: The objetive of the study was to evaluate bone mass status in patients on long-term neuroleptic therapy. Patients and methods: A total of 66 schizophrenics patients (46 males, mean age 61.4±12.8 years; 20 females mean age 59.1±15.1 years) who were taking neuroleptic drugs and 66 healthy subjects control of similar age and sex were included in the study. Bone status was assessed by phalangeal bone ultrasound (Ad-SOS) and the attenuation of the bone ultrasound in calcaneus (BUA)
Results: Significant differences don't exist among patient and controls in the Ad-SOS and BUA. For stepwise regression, in patient's group the Ad-SOS in taken as dependent variable and the rest independent variable, in females' group are significant age and weight (beta = -4.78 and -3.15 respectively, p=0.0002) and in males; group are significant BUA and body mass index (beta = 1.33 and -3.45 respectively, p=0.0130). In the control group only is significant the age in females and males (beta = -3.23 and -3.20 respectively, p <0.0001 in both)
Conclusions: In schizophrenics; patients on long-term neuroleptic therapy, the weight should be controlled with object of avoiding the possible negative effects on the bone mass

## P - 304

The Influence of Sibutramine on the Therapy of Obese Patients Representing Different Behaviour Patterns

Bogdanski P., Szulinska M., Pupek-Musialik D.
Department of Internal Diseases and Metabolic Disorders, University of Medical Sciences, Poznan, Poland

Objectives: In Poland almost 70% of adult population is overweight or obese. Obesity is a complex phenomenon, because it is conditioned by many genetic, metabolic, psychological and social factors. The aim of this study is influence of sibutramine on the therapy of obese patients representing different behaviour patterns.
Methods: Studied group included 60 patients aged 28-52 years (F/M 32/28) with obesity (body mass index (BMI)- 38,4+/-4,8kg/m2). In all of them comparable complex 3-month non-pharmacological treatment of obesity was introduced. 40 of them were given also Sibutramine (10mg/day). BMI, WHR (waist hip ratio) and fat content in organism were measured before and after treatment. All patients were asked to fill up a questionnaire concerning specific behaviour patterns. On a basis of the questionnaire they were divide into to groups: group A- strong desire to change; further education and medical help necessary and group B- full readiness and motivation to continue dieting.
Results : 1. In the studied group significant weight loss was observed (P<0.05). 2. A greater loss of body weight was observed among patients taking Sibutramine in comparison to others (P<0.05). 2. Significantly greater weight loss was observed in patients representing B type of behaviour (P<0.05). 3. Men, more often than women, were classified as B types.
Conclusions: 1. Sibutramine improves effectiveness of non-pharmacological treatment of obesity. 2. Obesity treatment results (both non-pharmacological and pharmacological) depend on behaviour patterns. 3. Behaviour patterns are highly associated with sex.

## P - 305

Evaluation of Blood Pressure Values in 3-Month Obesity Treatment with Use of Sibutramine

[1]Bogdanski P., [1]Pupek-Musialik D., [1]Bryl W., [1]Luczak M., [2]Jabecka A.
[1]Department of Internal Diseases and Metabolic Disorders, [2]Clinical Pharmacology, University of Medical Sciences, Poznan, Poland

Objectives : One of potential Sibutramine adverse effect is blood pressure increase. The aim of the study was evaluation of Sibutramine influence on blood pressure values depending on range of weight loss.
Methods : 50 patients with mild to moderate essential hypertension (35,5+/-11,2lyears, BMI 39,2+/-8,9kg/m2) were studied. After 3-month individualised hypertensive treatment blood pressure was normalised. After that patients were divided into two groups, 25 patients each (comparable according to age, sex, BMI, systolic -SBP and diastolic -DBP blood pressure). In the first group 3-month non-pharmacological treatment and the pharmacological one (Sibutramine 10mg/day) was started. The second group was treated with comparable non-pharmacological methods without Sibutramine.
Results : 1. After one month obesity treatment in the first group comparing to the second one: higher weight loss (p<0.05) and increase of SBP (p<0.07) were observed. 2. After 3- month obesity treatment in the first group comparing to the second one: higher weight loss (p<0.01) and no differences in SBP and DBP were observed.
Conclusions : 1. Blood pressure increase (not significant) during the first month of Sibutramine therapy was observed. 2. Potential hypertensive Sibutramine effects observed during the first month of the therapy was balanced with blood pressure decrease in the next months associated probably with farther weight loss.

## P - 306

Evaluation of Influence of Angiotensin Converting Enzyme Inhibitor Treatment on Blood Pressure and Serum Endothelin-1 Concentration in Young Hypetensives During 6-Month Therapy.

Bryl W., Miczke A., Bogdanski P., Luczak M., Cymerys M., Pupek-Musialik D.
Department of Internal Disease and Metabolic Disorders, University of Medical Sciences, Poznan, Poland

Growing evidence suggest that, endothelin-1 (ET-1) because of its vasoconstrictor action can play a role in pathogenesis of hypertension. The aim of study was to assess the influence of ACEI therapy on ET-1 plasma concentration in young patients with essential mild-to-moderate hypertension.
Methods : 15 young men, the average age 17.1+/- 1.2 years. In all hypertension-stadium 1 or 2 according to VI Report of JNC was diagnosed. They were treated with ACEI-trandolapril (2 mg once-a-day) for 6 months. Before and after 3rd- and 6th-month therapy the SBP and DBP (systolic and diastolic blood pressure) and ET-1 serum concentration were measured. ET-1 was measured by radioimmunoassay using Amersham RPA 545 England kit.
Results : In analyzed group both SBP and DBP decreased significantly after 3-month ($P<0.05$) and 6-month therapy ($P<0.001$). Tendency to decrease ($P=0.08$) after 3-month and significant reduction ($P<0.05$) after 6-month trandolapril therapy in ET-1 concentration was detected. 6-month trandolapril therapy did not influence serum lipid profile significantly. Serum uric acid decreased but not significantly.
Conclusions : 1. 6-month hypertensive treatment with ACE-inhibitor (trandolapril) caused significant SBP and DBP reduction. 2. 6-month trandolapril therapy was effective in serum ET-1 concentration reduction.

## P - 307

Prescribing and Health Care Utilisation – Is it Possible to Analyse the Effects of Interventions Using Aggregate Data?

[1]Wettermark B., [2]Krakau I., [1]Bergman U.
[1]Karolinska Institute, Department of Medical Laboratory Sciences & Technology, Division of Clinical Pharmacology, Huddinge University Hospital, and [2]Research Center of General Medicine, Department of Internal Medicine, Karolinska Hospital, Stockholm, Sweden.

The main caregivers in Stockholm County, Sweden, are 185 Primary Health Care centres (PHCs) with over 900 general practitioners (GPs). In 2000 and 2001 an intervention with the aim to increase quality of care by reducing the number of listed patients/doctor to 1/1500 was carried out at 10 PHCs. We evaluated effects on drug prescribing and health care provided. The study was performed on routinely collected data from pharmacy- and county council databases. Time periods for analyse were Oct-Dec 1999, 2000 and 2001. Drug data was analysed by age using the ATC/DDD-methodology. In 2001, between 248 and 420 inhabitants/1000 in the catchment areas had visited the local PHC. The local PHCs accounted for between 14 and 36% of all doctor-consultations and between 20% and 41% of all prescriptions to the inhabitants in the surrounding area. There was no clear improvement of the prescribing doctors´ compliance with recommended guidelines from the County Council, neither with the utilisation of health care in the catchment areas.
Conclusion: It was feasible to analyse aggregated prescription- and health care data on a population level. However, the effects on quality of care by allocating increasing primary care resources have to be analysed in a broader context.

## P - 308

Paracetamol Poisoning and N-Acetylcysteine Treatment in Patients without Liver Damage. Which one Modifies the Prothrombin Time?

[1]Lopez-Torres E., [1]Seoane J., [1]Verge C., [2]Martinez A.,[3]Andrade R.J., [1]Sánchez de la Cuesta F., [1]Lucena M.I.
[1]Servicio de Farmacología Clínica, [2]Servicio de Documentación Clínica y [3]Unidad de Hepatología, Hospital Clínico Universitario, Facultad de Medicina, Málaga. Spain.

Background: N-acetylcysteine (NAC) has been implicated in a decrease in prothrombin time (PT) in patients with paracetamol poisoning without evidence of liver damage. Aim: (1) to identify if there is a time-dependent effect of paracetamol on PT and, (2) To explore the effect of intravenous NAC on the time course of prothrombin activity in patients with paracetamol overdosage and a normal liver profile. Material & Methods: a retrospective case series study was undertaken to examine all admissions with a diagnosis of paracetamol poisoning in a tertiary care center between 1989 to 2002. A structured protocol was implemented that included demographic data, dose of paracetamol taken, drug levels, time of onset and ending of NAC treatment and all PT values and alanine transaminases concentrations post ingestion.
Results: Of 60 admissions with paracetamol poisoning during this period, 29 (48%) met the inclusion criteria. Median quantity of paracetamol ingested was 162,9 mg/kg (range 50-357). Seven patients drank alcohol. Mean baseline PT was 91% (range 62-107) on a median time of six hours postingestion. The mean differential decrease of the PT after initiation of NAC treatment (n=20) was 19,4 (range 5-53). The timecourse of the PT was a sharp fall at the start of NAC followed by a slow recovery. Conclusions: Most of the observed effect on PT seems to be due to the great overload of NAC infused at the beginning since this effect was not apparent in patients who did not receive NAC.

## P - 309

Reproducibility of Prostaglandin $D_2$ Induced Nasal Obstruction Using Active Anterior Rhinomanometry in Healthy Subjects

[1]Van Hecken A., [1]de Hoon J.N., [1]Depré M., [2]Ragab A., [3]De Lepeleire I., [3]Laethem T., [4]Deutsch P., [4]Mazina K., [4]Thach C., [4]Hartford A., [2]Clement P.
[1]Center for Clinical Pharmacology, [2]U.Z.Gasthuisberg (K.U.Leuven), Leuven, Belgium and Otorhinolaryngology department, [3]Free University of Brussels, Belgium; Merck Research Laboratories, Brussels, [4]Belgium and Rahway NJ, USA

Introduction: As prostaglandin (PG) $D_2$ is known to reproduce the nasal blockade experienced by seasonal rhinitis, intranasal challenge with $PGD_2$ can be an interesting tool for evaluating DP receptor antagonists. This study assesses the intersession reproducibility of PD75, which is the provocative dose of intranasal $PGD_2$ resulting in a 75% increase in total nasal airflow resistance ($NAR_T$).
Methods: In an open-label, 2-period, non-randomized study, 17 healthy subjects received saline followed by 2, 4, 8, 16, 32 and 64 µg of $PGD_2$/nostril, administered at 15-minute intervals. $NAR_T$ was measured at 4, 8 and 12 minutes after each challenge, until $NAR_T$ increased 75% above baseline or until the maximum $PGD_2$ dose was reached. Linear regression was applied to each individual's $NAR_T$ to estimate their PD75. Reproducibility was assessed by within-subject standard deviation (SD) and by the Pearson (r) and intraclass (ICC) correlation coefficients.
Results: Overall mean (± SD) PD75 was 15.8 ± 22.5 µg/nostril in period 1 and 10.6 ± 8.5 µg/nostril in period 2. Within-subject SD was 12.0 µg/nostril [95%CI (8.8, 18.9)]. Good correlation was obtained between the 2 sessions (r=0.82 and ICC=0.75).
Conclusion: PD75 can be assessed in a reproducible and reliable way in healthy subjects. The obtained information allows for power calculations for future studies evaluating DP receptor antagonists.

## P 310

Effect of Aprepitant on the Pharmacokinetics and Pharmacodynamics of Warfarin

[1]Depré M., [1]Van Hecken A., [1]Oeyen M., [2]De Lepeleire I., [2]Laethem T., [3]Rothenberg P., [4]Petty K., [5]Majumdar A., [3]Crumley T., [4]Panebianco D., [5]Bergman A., [1]de Hoon J.N.
[1]Center for Clinical Pharmacology, U.Z.Gasthuisberg (K.U.Leuven), [2]Leuven, Belgium and Merck Research Laboratories, Brussels, Belgium; [3]Rahway, NJ, [4]Blue Bell, PA, and [5]West Point, PA, USA

Design: Aprepitant is a $NK_1$-receptor antagonist developed as an antiemetic for chemotherapy-induced nausea and vomiting. A double-blind, placebo-controlled, randomized, 2-period, parallel-group study was designed to investigate the effect of aprepitant on steady-state warfarin pharmacokinetics and pharmacodynamics. In period 1, warfarin was individually titrated to a stable prothrombin time (expressed as International Normalized Ratio, INR) from 1.3-1.8. Subsequently, the daily warfarin dose remained fixed for 10-12 days. In period 2, the warfarin dose was continued for 8 days, and on days 1-3 administered concomitantly with aprepitant (125 mg on day 1, 80 mg on days 2 and 3) or placebo. At baseline (day -1 of period 2) and on day 3, warfarin pharmacokinetics were investigated. INR was monitored daily. In period 2, warfarin trough concentrations were determined daily.
Results: Steady-state pharmacokinetics of warfarin enantiomers after aprepitant versus baseline did not change. However, compared to placebo, trough R(+)warfarin concentrations slightly increased on day 3 (18 %, $p<0.01$) while S(-)warfarin concentrations decreased on days 5 to 8 (maximum decrease 34% on day 8, $p<0.01$). INR displayed a downward trend after aprepitant (maximum decrease on day 8, 11% versus placebo, $p=0.011$).
Conclusion: These data are consistent with a slight induction of CYP2C9 metabolism of S(-) warfarin by aprepitant. Subsequently, the INR should be closely monitored after a 3-day regimen of aprepitant.

## ORAL

Smart Choice List : A New Concept to Reach the Prescribers with Evidens-based Recommendations

Sjoberg S., Bahr C., Bergman U., Granberg-Stange M., Jagre I., Persson P., Tryselius R., Thornwall G., Gustafsson L.L.
Stockholm Regional Drug & Therapeutic Committee and Division of Drug Management and Informatics, Stockholm County Council, Stockholm, Sweden.

Background : The concept of essential drug recommendations is established since years. Still selection and use of drugs are influenced by marketing activities by drug companies towards prescribers and public. This is one factor explaining a steady increse in drug costs 10 to 15 % annually in Sweden in recent years.
Smart Choice List concept : The Essential Drug List was relaunched and marketed as Smart Choice List in Stockholm in 2000. The aim has been that doctors and public becomes aware that there is no point in using new, expensive drugs that are no better than old drugs. A special edition for patients has proven to be a strong channel, as well as strengthening the role of the drug experts of the committee in media.
Acheivements : Interviews with general practitioners verify a high level of acknowledgement of the Smart Choice List campaign and strong support of campaigns towards the public. Interviews with the public shows increasing levels of appreciation of Smart Choice List campaign and awareness of increasing drug costs in society. As many as 90% want their own Smart Choice List and 7 out of 10 would like the doctor to prescribe from the list. Leading medical journalists acknowledge both the Smart Choice List and the website of the Regional Drug & Therapeutic Committee of Stockholm www.janusinfo.org.
By introduction of the concept of Smart Choice List and adopting a media strategy, the Regional Drug and Therapeutic Committee has strengthened the image of the essential drug concept. Adherence to recommendations has improved.

## P - 311

Therapeutic Drug Monitoring in North Eastern Greece: Focus on Digoxin and Cyclosporin

Manolopoulos E.G.
Democritus University of Thrace, Medical School, Lab Of Pharmacology, Elexandroupolis, Greece

The University Pharmacology laboratory in Alexandroupolis was first in introducing systematic measurement of therapeutic agents in the North-East region of Greece (Thrace) in 1992 and it remains the only laboratory in this area offering a complete range of tests. Furthermore, it is one of the very few clinical pharmacology laboratories in the country that is familiar with the concept of therapeutic drug monitoring and implements many of each principles to daily practice. It is equipped with 2 Abbott automatic analyzers (TDX and AxSYM) and routinely performs a broad range of assays, including antibiotics, anticonvulsants, methotrexate, digoxin, cyclosporin A, acetaminophen, salicylate and theophylline, as well as a complete screen for drugs of abuse. Besides the clinical work, the laboratory has introduced a special course for the training of medical students and other lab personnel to the principles and practise of TDM. Finally, the laboratory is involved in clinical research projects as well as epidemiological studies regarding the use of certain drugs in the area of Thrace. The results from two pharmacoepidemiological studies will be presented dealing with a) the prescription practices for digoxin in a local rural population, b) study of the transplant recipients in the area receiving cyclosporin.

## P - 312

Circadian Change in Ondansetron (Zophren®) and in Oxaliplatin Toxicities in Mice

[1]Khedhaier A., [2]Ben Attia M., [2]Sani M., [2]Gadacha W., [1]Chouchane L., [1]Boughattas N.A., [3]Bouzouita K.
[1]Faculté de Médecine, 5019 Monastir, Tunisia; [2]Faculté des Sciences de Bizerte, 7021 Zarzouna, Tunisia; [3]Faculté de Médecine, 1006 Tunis, Tunisia.

Ondansetron (OND) is a serotonin antagonist, used as adjuvant to prevent nausea and vomiting caused by several anticancer agents, such as Oxaliplatin (l-OHP). The aim of this study is to determine the circadian rhythm in lethal toxicity of OND or l-OHP in mice. A lethal dose of OND (3.5 mg/kg; i.p.) or l-OHP (17 mg/kg; i.v.) was injected at 4 circadian times (1, 7, 13 or 19 Hours After Light Onset- HALO). Male swiss mice (20 mice/time-point/drug) aged 10-12 wks and synchronized by light-dark cycle (L/D:12/12 hr) have been used. Statistical analysis of survival was performed by Cosinor and Chi-square test. The 24-hr mean survival rates (S.R) of OND and l-OHP were respectively 80% and 65%. A significant circadian change in SR was validated for OND or l-OHP ($p < 0.05$). The highest SR was 80% when I-OHP was injected at 19 HALO, time which corresponded to the lowest value for OND (50%). The optimal tolerance occurred when OND was injected during the light-rest span. OND exhibited an inversed circadian rhythm as compared to l-OHP. These results should further allow a clinical optimization of cancer chemotherapy based on circadian rhythms. Supported by the SERST (MD 06) and the MES (Tunisia).

## P - 313

Antibiotic Resistance in Catheter-Associated Urinary Infections at the Clinical Center of Banja Luka - Bosnia and Herzegovina

[1]Verhaz A., [2]Skrbic R., [2]Stojisavljevic-Satara S., [2]Babic-Djuric D., Stojakovic N., [2]Nezic L.
[1]Clinic for Infection diseases, Clinical center of Banja Luka, Banja Luka, Bosnia and Herzegovina, [2]Department of Pharmacology and Clinical pharmacology, Faculty of Medicinel, University of Banja luka, Banja Luka, Bosnia and Herzegovina

Catheter-associated urinary infections are the most common nosocomial infections of the urinary tract, and one of the most common nosocomial infections in general. The major problems of these infections are increased resistance to the antibiotics and enormous direct and indirect costs of the treatment. A retrospective study on major causes of infections and antibiotic resistance was conducted at four clinics of the Clinical center of Banja Luka (the second bigest clinical center in Bosnia and Herzegovina). An anonymous questionnaire was distributed to nursing staff dealing with urinary catheters in order to get an overview of their clinical performance. The results showed that in 89% of cases (out of 198 patients with developed catheter-associated urinary infection) were infections caused by gram-negative bacteria's, in 7% caused by gram-positive bacteria's and in 4% caused by candida. The most common bacteria found were E.coli (33,6%), Pseudomonas aeruginosa (14,1%), Proteus mirabilis (13,3%), and Enterobacter (10,5%). The majority of the bacteria's showed extremely high resistance (72-100%) to ampicillin, gentamycin and co-trimoxasole, and in some cases a significant resistance to ciprofloxacine, nalidixic acid, ceftriaxone and ceftazidime. The results obtained by questionnaire showed that nursing staff did not follow the guidelines for medical care of the patients with urinary catheters. It can be concluded that insufficient hygienic and epidemiological measures, as well as the nonrational use of antibiotics, contributed to the uncontrolled development of urinary infection of catheterized patients.

## P - 314

Drug Utilization Analyses in Banja Luka region (North-West Bosnia)

[1]Stojakovic N., [1]Skrbic R., [1]Stoisavljevic-Satara S., [1]Babic-Djuric D., [1]Nezic L., [2]Sabo A.
[1]Department of Pharmacology and Clinical pharmacology, Faculty of Medicine, University of Banja luka, Banja Luka, Bosnia and Herzegovina, [2]Department of Pharmacology, Toxicology and Clinical pharmacology, Faculty of Medicinel, University of Novi Sad, Novi Sad, Serbia & Monte Negro

Using the ATC/DDD methodology, we analysed the utilization of drugs dispensed on prescription in Banja Luka region in 2000 - 2001. A retrospective study on drug utilization, according to ATC classification, was conducted on the basis of data received from "Apotekarska ustanova" (Central City Pharmacy) Banja Luka, and the results were presented in DDD/1000 inhabitants/day. Pharmaco-epidemiological analysis showed that the list of 20 most frequently prescribed drugs in 2000 contained 8 drugs from the cardiovascular drug group, and 6 drugs from the anti-infective drug group. In 2001, among 20 most frequently prescribed drugs, there were 9 drugs from cardiovascular drug group, and 4 from anti-infective drug group. Regarding anti-infective drugs, the most frequently prescribed antibiotics were amoxicillin, doxicillin, co-trimoxazole and gentamicin. The most frequently prescribed drug in 2000 was diazepam (5,33 DDD/1000 inhabitants/day). The use of this drug had a significant increase in 2001 (7,95 DDD/1000 inhabitants/day). Based on the total analysis, it could be concluded that the positive drug list, defined by the Health Insurance Fund, had a significant influence on drug utilization profile, but some drug groups continued to be nonrationally prescribed. It will take a lot of time, efforts and funds for upgrading of prescribing practice among general practitioners including the good pharmacy practice among pharmacists, too.

## P - 315

Therapeutic Approach to the Patients with Coronary Heart Disease; The results of Coronary Prevention Study in Republic of Srpska (ROSCOPS) - Bosnia and Herzegovina

[1]Skrbic R., [2]Vulic D., [3]Lazarevic A., [2]Keric L., [2]Krneta M.
[1]Department of Pharmacology and Clinical pharmacology, Faculty of Medicine, University of Banja luka, Banja Luka, Bosnia and Herzegovina, [2] Center for medical research, Medical Electronics, Banja Luka, Bosnia and Herzegovina, [3]Clinic for Cardiology, Clinical Center of Banja Luka, Banja Luka, Bosnia and Herzegovina

Cardiovascular diseases are the leading cause of death in Republic of Srpska - Bosnia and Herzegovina. Although the cardiovascular mortality decrease in western countries are 2% per year, the figures in our country showed significant increase in cardiovascular mortality from 50% in 1990, to 53,9% in 2000 and 53,4% in 2001. Recently, the National program for prevention of cardiovascular diseases has been introduced with the aim to improve the current trends in cardiovascular morbidity and to put more efforts on cardiovascular prevention and improvement of treatment. The first evaluation study ROSCOPS (Republic Of Srpska Coronary Prevention Study) was done in 2001 and the follow up is planned for this year. The survey was undertaken in five regional centers. Consecutive patients (<70 years, N=430) were identified retrospectively with the diagnoses: coronary artery disease, acute myocardial infarction, and acute myocardial ischaemia without infarction. Data collection was based on prospective interview and examination of patients at the primary health care centers. The results showed that 40% of patients smoked cigarettes, 26% were overweight, 74% had raised blood pressure (systolic BP >140 mmHg, and diastolic BP >90 mmHg), 28% had raised total plasma cholesterol (>5.5 mmol/L) and 24% were diabetic. Medical treatment at interview was: antiplatelet drugs (Aspirin) 45.9%, beta-blockers 22.9%, ACE inhibitors 62.2%, anti-coagulants 5.4%, lipid lowering drugs 5.4%, calcium antagonists 27%, nitrates 59.4% and antidiabetics 10.8%. As a part of national program for cardiovascular diseases, we are putting a lot of efforts on professional education, evidence-based medication, essential drug list rationalization, and health promotion, in order to improve primary and secondary prevention of cardiovascular diseases.

## P - 316

Antibiotic Utilization in Banja Luka Region (North-West Bosnia) During the Past Decade

[1]Stoisavljevic-Satara S., [1]Babic-Djuric D., [2]Vucen M., [1]Skrbic R., [1]Stojakovic N., [1]Nezic L.
[1]Department of Pharmacology and Clinical pharmacology, Faculty of Medicine, University of Banja Luka, Banja Luka, Bosnia and Herzegovina, [2]Apotekarska ustanova, Banja Luka, Bosnia and Herzegovina

An inappropriate use of antibiotics, besides being costly, unnecessarily exposes a patient to the adverse effects of drugs and influences developing of resistance species that are a great therapeutic problem. Using the ATC/DDD methodology, we analysed the antibiotic utilization in Banja Luka region (North-west Bosnia) in the previous ten years. A retrospective study on antibiotic utilization, was conducted on the basis of data received from "Apotekarska ustanova" (City Pharmacy Department) Banja Luka, and the results were presented in DDD/1000 inhabitants/day. Pharmaco-epidemiological analysis showed that the total antibiotic utilisation in 1990 was extremely high, 23.8 (DDD/1000 inhabitants/day), comparing to 4.2 in 1994, 4.9 in 1998, and 8.7 in 2000. Aminopenicillins were most frequently prescribed antibiotics during the period of observation (42.5%-54.1%), followed by cephalosporins (14.7%-23.4%), natural penicillins (6.7%-18.9%), tetracyclines, (2.8%-15.1%), and macrolides (4.6%-8.4%). In the year 1990, oral ampicillin was more frequently prescribed than oral amoxicillin (34.8% vs. 12.7%), while in the year 2000 this proportion was considerably in favour of amoxicillin (9.9% vs. 32.5%). During the war period in Bosnia (in 1994) antibiotics were significantly less used and some were not prescribed at all, eg quinolones. It is important to emphasise that in 1990 all antibiotics were on the positive drug list, during the time of war the list was considerably reduced and thus consisted major antibiotic groups only, while in 2000 the list was qualitatively improved. Moreover, considerable efforts have been put on education of health professionals to improve their prescribing practice.

## P - 317

Protective Role of Glutathione S-transferase P1 (GSTP1) Val105Val Genotype in Patients with Bronchial Asthma

[1,2]Aynacioglu A.Ş., [2]Nacak M., [3]Filiz A., [3]Ekinci E., [1]Roots I.
[1]Institute of Clinical Pharmacology, University Clinic Charité, Humboldt University, Berlin, Germany, [2]Department of Pharmacology, Faculty of Medicine, University of Gaziantep, Gaziantep, Turkey, [4]Department of Pulmonology, Faculty of Medicine, University of Gaziantep, Gaziantep, Turkey

Background: Glutathion S-transferase P1 (GSTP1), the abundant isoform of Glutathion S-transferases (GSTs) in lung epithelium, plays an important role in cellular protection against oxidative stress and toxic foreign chemicals. It has been suggested that polymorphisms in the GSTP1 gene are associated with asthma and related phenotypes. As significant inter-individual and inter-ethnic differences exist in the distribution of xenobiotic-metabolizing enzymes, we have studied the GSTP1 Ile105Val polymorphism in patients with asthma in a Turkish sample.
Methods: GSTP1 Ile105Val polymorphism was determined in 210 patients with asthma (112 extrinsic and 108 intrinsic) and 265 control individuals without lung diseases and without history of allergy or atopy, using PCR-RFLP analysis.
Results: The frequency of GSTP1 Val105 homozygotes was significantly lower in the patients with asthma than in the control individuals (3.8% vs. 12.1%, p=0.01). The odds ratio for GSTP1 Val105 homozygotes versus Ile105 homozygotes was 0.31 (95%CL 0.14-0.69, p=0.03). The distribution of GSTP1 Ile105Val genotypes and the frequency of GSTP1 Val105Val homozygotes (%3,7 vs. %3,9) was not significantly different between extrinsic and intrinsic asthmatics.
Conclusion: These results suggest a significant association between GSTP1 Ile105Val polymorphism and susceptibility to asthma and that the GSTP1 Val105Val genotype may be protective against developing this disease.

## P - 318

Cytochrome P450 2C19 Genotype-Phenotype Correlation Using Omeprazole as a Probe Drug

[1,2]Aynacioglu A.Ş., [2]Ongen H.Z., [1]Bauer S., [1]Roots I., [1,3]Brockmöller J.
[1]Institute of Clinical Pharmacology, University Clinic Charité, Humboldt University, Berlin, Germany [2]Department of Pharmacology, Faculty of Medicine, University of Gaziantep, Gaziantep, Turkey, [3]Institute of Clinical Pharmacology, Faculty of Medicine, University of Göttingen, Göttingen, Germany

Background: Cytochrome P450 2C19 (CYP2C19) metabolizes many important drugs including omeprazole (OMZ). The aim of the study was to identify the CYP2C19 phenotype-genotype relationship by using OMZ as a test drug and whether there are ultra-rapid metabolizers of omeprazole in the Turkish population.
Methods: We phenotyped 118 healthy unrelated subjects using 60 mg OMZ. The plasma concentration of OMZ, its R- and S-enantiomers, 4-hydroxy-omeprazole (OH-OMZ), and OMZ sulfone was quantified by h.p.l.c. CYP2C19 alleles *2 and *3 were analyzed by PCR-RFLP. Rare alleles CYP2C19 *4, *5, *6, *7, and *8 were determined in subjects with genotype-phenotype discrepancy.
Results: Allele frequencies of CYP2C19*1, *2, and *3 were 89.8%, 9.8% and 0.4%, respectively. Mean OMZ plasma concentrations (± SD) at 3 h after dosage were 631±65 ng/ml in carriers of the genotype CYP2C19*1/1; 956±179 ng/ml in CYP2C19*1/2; 2856±296 ng/ml in CYP2C19*2/2; and 1065 ng/ml in CYP2C19*1/3. Mean 3 h concentration ratios of OMZ/OH-OMZ were 2.1 for CYP2C19*1/1; 3.9 for CYP2C19*1/2; 20.0 for CYP2C19*2/2 and 3.0 for CYP2C19*1/3. The rare alleles were not detected in two subjects with phenotyp-genotype discrepancy. Four individuals had a OMZ/OH-OMZ ratio below 0.05 and were considered as ultra rapid metabolizers.
Conclusions: OMZ/OH-OMZ metabolic ratio could be used as an indicator in the in vivo evaluation of the activity of CYP2C19 and relatively high dose of OMZ (60 mg) to detect "ultra rapid" metabolizers for CYP2C19.

## P - 319

Length Of Gambling History as a Predictor Of Treatment Participation

Brands B., Toneatto T., Selby P., Selhi Z., Gorthy L.
Centre for Addiction and Mental Health and Departments of Pharmacology,
Psychiatry and Family and Community Medicine, University of Toronto, Toronto, Canada

Pathological Gambling Disorder (PG) and alcohol disorders co-occur frequently. Naltrexone is effective in reducing alcohol consumption and preliminary data suggests that naltrexone reduces urges to gamble and gambling behaviours. This is a randomized controlled study to evaluate naltrexone as a treatment for concurrent alcohol disorders and PG. We present here the results from the assessment phase. Of 371 telephone contacts, 115 met screening criteria for both disorders. Of the 51% (n=59) who attended their initial assessment, a higher percentage were males (93% vs 88%) and were older (41.7±12.1 vs. 38.1±11.3 yrs) compared to non-attenders (n=56). The attenders had longer gambling histories (14.8±13.0 vs 10.6±9.2 yrs, *p=0.05) despite similar levels of gambling frequency (4.7±2.3 vs. 4.2±2.1 times/week) and weekly cost of gambling ($443±$637 vs. $377±$627/week). Alcohol use histories were similar (19.3±11.9 vs. 18.4±10.3 yrs), as were other alcohol consumption measures, other substance use histories, and previous treatment for gambling and alcohol problems. These findings suggest that in individuals with concurrent PG and alcohol problems the length of gambling history may be a more important determinant of treatment participation than current gambling characteristics, alcohol use histories or previous treatments. Therefore, this is an important component of any brief assessment tool developed for clinical or research purposes in this population.

## P - 320

The Permeability of Haemofilter, Haemodialyzer and Plasma Separator Membranes for Amphotericin B: Implications for Plasma Pharmacokinetics During Haemofiltration and for Investigation of Target Site Pharmacokinetics by Microdialysis

[1]Bellmann R., [2]Joukhadar C., [2]Dehghanyar P., [1]Egger P., [2]Müller M., [1]Wiedermann CJ.
[1]Medical Intensive Care Research Laboratory, Department of Internal Medicine, University of Innsbruck, Austria, [2]Department of Clinical Pharmacology, Division of Clinical Pharmacokinetics, University of Vienna Medical School, Austria

Amphotericin B (AmB) is the standard drug for treatment of systemic fungal infections. Lipid-formulations of AmB are frequently used because of their lower toxicity. The influence of continuous veno-venous haemofiltration on plasma pharmacokinetics and the haemofilter clearance of AmB were studied in critically ill patients who were treated with AmB deoxycholate, liposomal AmB and AmB colloidal dispersion, respectively. Eleven patients required haemofiltration because of renal failure, which was performed with a polysuphone membrane (molecular cut-off 30 kDa). Lipid-formulated AmB and AmB, which has been liberated from its lipid moiety and is protein-bound in the plasma were separattely quantified. Plasma pharmacokinetics of the total and free fraction resembles that of AmB deoxycholate. The elimination of the lipid-formulated fraction is different and differentially affected by haemofiltration. The haemofilter clearance (CLHF) of AmB deoxycholate was 0.42 L/h (8.10% of total CL) and the sieving coefficient was 0.29. During treatment with lipid-formulated AmB, the sieving coefficient of free AmB was about 0.2 and CLHF about 2% of total CL. CLHF of lipid-bound AmB was negligible. The microdialysis technique has been established for the investigation of target site pharmacokinetics of numerous drugs, but not for AmB. Therefore we tested the permeability for AmB of several commercially available haemofilter, haemodialyzer and plasma separator membranes in vitro. Only one polyethylene polymer plasma separator membrane with a molecular cut off 3,000 kDa provided a promising in vitro recovery (17.5%). Thus, using a microdialysis probe equipped with this membrane, microdialysis technique should be applicable for assessment of AmB target site concentrations.

## P - 321

The Influence Of Hemp On CNS Depression Induced By Pentobarbital

Horvat[1] O., [1]Jakovljevic V, [1]Sabo A., [2]Stanojevic Z.
[1]Dept. Pharm. Tox.& Clin. Pharm., Medical Faculty Novi Sad, [2]Dept. Pharm. and Tox., Medical Faculty Kosovska Mitrovica, Yugoslavia.

The aim of the study was to exam the influence of two various types of hemp, commercial one with lower concentration and indian one with higher concentration of THC (tetrahydrocannabinol), on CNS depression induced by pentobarbital. The experiment was done on adult laboratory rats, both sexes, body weight 200-250 g. The animals were divided into 3 groups: the control group received only water ad libidum; the 1st experimental group was treated with infusion of commercial hemp ad libidum chronically during 20 days (3,3 g/l boiling water); the 2nd experimental group was treated with infusion of indian hemp ad libidum chronically during 20 days (3,3 g/l boiling water). Each group was pretreated with pentobarbital (40 mg/kg i.p.) just before the determination of sleeping induction and sleeping time. The time at wich the animals lost right-reflex was registered as sleeping induction. The time interval between the lost and regaining of righting reflex was measured as sleeping time. We concluded that the sleeping time in both experimental groups treated with both types of infusion were significantly increased in relation to control group. The sleeping time of the animals treated with infusion of commercial hemp was longer than of the animals treated with infusion of indian hemp, but without statistical significance. The duration of sleeping induction was the same in every group.

## P - 322

Treatment of Schizophrenic Out-patients with Depot Haloperidol: Impact of CYP2D6 Polymorphism on Pharmacokinetic Parameters and Clinical Outcome.

[1]Holger W. A., [2]Panagiotidis G., [2]Dahl M.L., [2]Sjöqvist F.
[1]Departments of Psychiatry and [2]Clinical Pharmacology, Huddinge University
Hospital, S-141 86 Stockholm, Sweden

Most neuroleptic drugs are metabolised by the polymorphic cytochrome P450 (CYP) 2D6 enzyme. Our study was conducted in 26 schizophrenic outpatients with depot-haloperidol treatment as monotherapy. All patients were stable in their disease and the dosage had been adjusted based on clinical observations. Psychotic symptomatology and extra pyramidal adverse effects were assessed with rating scales ESRS and PANSS. One patient was genotyped as CYP2D6 poor metaboliser (PM), one as ultra rapid metaboliser (UM), eight were heterozygous extensive metabolisers (EM het) and sixteen were homozygous extensive metabolisers (EM hom). The haloperidol dose (calculated per day) ranged 0.4-14.3 mg. The trough-plasma concentrations were gathered in the range 1-20 nmol/L except for one value of 50 nmol/L. The dose corrected plasma concentrations (DCC) showed a significant correlation to the CYP2D6 genotype with the highest DCC in the PM followed by the heterozygous EM, the homozygous EM and the lowest DCC in the UM. ESRS and PANSS ratings showed no significant difference between EM het. and EM hom.

Conclusion: The CYP2D6 genotype influences the plasma levels of haloperidol after intramuscular administration. Dose adjustment by clinical guidance results in a relatively narrow range of plasma concentrations that make it less likely to detect any significant impact of the CYP2D6 polymorphism on the clinical outcome of depot-haloperidol therapy.

## P - 323

Influence of Genetic Polymorphisms on Rifampicin-Mediated Induction of MRP2 (ABCC2) mRNA Expression

Cascorbi I., Haenisch S., Gießmann T., Dazert P., [1]Hecker U., Kroemer HK., Siegmund W.
Peter Holtz Center of Pharmacology and Experimental Therapeutics, [1]Dept. of
Internal Medicine, Ernst Moritz Arndt University, D-17487 Greifswald, Germany

The multidrug resistance protein 2 (MRP2; ABCC2) has an excretory protective role by transporting conjugated endogenous and xenobiotic substrates. It is expressed on the apical domain particularly of hepatocytes and small intestine epithelium and can be induced by rifampicin via PXR binding elements. Some hereditary mutations of the MRP2 gene are linked with the Dubin-Johnson syndrome, however a number of polymorphisms have been identified with yet unknown function. We have genotyped the six most frequent MRP2 SNPs C-24T in the 5'-UTR, G1249 (Val417Ile), C2302T (Arg768Trp) and C2366T (Ser789Phe), C3972T (Ile1324Ile), and G4348A (Ala1450Thr) in 196 German unrelated subjects using conventional PCR/RFLP methods. Intestinal mRNA was isolated from duodenal biopsy specimens of 28 healthy subjects included in drug interaction studies with rifampicin. MRP2 mRNA was quantified using TaqMan rt-PCR. The following allelic frequencies were assessed: C-24T 31.6%, G1249A 44.4%. C3972T 62.2%. C2302T, C2366T, and G4348A could not be confirmed. Basal mRNA levels were not affected by any SNP. 13 samples were induced by rifampicin (3.2-fold, p= 0.013 Wilcoxon test), however a pronounced induction was detectable only in ten carriers of -24CC (2.85-fold) but not in the three carriers of CT (0.73-fold). The induction was 1.5-fold in six 1249GG, but 5.76-fold in six GA, and 5.15-fold in six 3972CC-subjects and 1.36-fold in six CT-genotypes. In conclusion, the SNPs investigated do not have a considerable functional impact on basal MRP2 expression, but possibly on the extent of induction in presence of PXR ligands.

## P - 324

Mutations in the Drug Transporter Genes MDR1 And MRP2 and Pharmakokinetics in Patients Treated with Saquinavir/Lopinavir

Cascorbi I., Breske A., Moecklinghoff C., Stocker H., Kruse G., Sawyer A., Staszewski S., Kurowski M.
Peter Holtz Center of Pharmacology and Experimental Therapeutics, Dept of Internal Medicine, Ernst Moritz Arndt University, Greifswald, Germany.

Recently plasma PI concentrations have been correlated with mutations in the MDR1 gene which codes for the drug transporter P-glycoprotein. PIs have also been shown to inhibit MRP2-mediated transport across membranes in animal models. Thus variations in the drug transporter genes may contribute to the high variability of the pharmacokinetics observed with PIs in patients. In 34 patients treated with either protease inhibitors alone or combinations with nucleosides PCR analysis was performed for MDR1 and MRP2 from lymphocyte preparations. We measured concentrations of the protease inhibitors saquinavir (SQV), ritonavir (RTV) and lopinavir (LPV) over a 24h interval by LC-tandem mass spectrometry. Ctrough, Cmax and area under the curve (AUC) were determined for each PI. PK parameters of wild type, heterozygous and homozygous groups were compared by t-tests. The prevalence of MDR1 mutations were as follows: Exon 21 G2677T (Ala893Ser) GG: 53%, GT: 38%, TT: 9%; exon 26 C3435T: CC: 26%, CT: 56%, and TT18 %. The distribution of MRP2 polymorphisms for C-24T in the 5'-UTR region was CC: 59%, CT: 38%, TT: 3%; for G1249A in exon 10 (Val417Ile) GG: 73%, GA: 18%, AA: 9%, and for C3972T in exon 28 CC: 50%, CT: 41%, TT: 9 %. The comparison of the variants concerning MDR1 showed a significant trend of LPV AUC in dependence of G2677T (p Kruskal-Wallis 0.033. The observed difference in LPV plasma levels among variants of the MDR1 gene suggest a functional impact of the Ala893Ser amino acid replacement and invoke a larger trial in order to test our findings

ORAL

Assessing the Prevalence Of Adverse Drug Reactions in a French University Hospital : A Capture-Recapture Study Using Data From PMSI and the French Pharmacovigilance Database

Lugardon S., Desboeuf K., Fernet P., Montastruc JL., Lapeyre-Mestre M.

Estimation of ADR frequency remains necessary to evaluate the medical, social and economic consequences of ADR. Spontaneous reporting system is limited by underreporting. Computerized medical databases in French hospitals, i.e. PMSI, could also be used to identify ADR. However, several studies using PMSI showed that it underestimates the real frequency of ADR. The aim of this study was to estimate the prevalence of serious ADR treated in Toulouse University Hospital using data from PMSI and the French Pharmacovigilance Database.The study period was the first semester of 2001. From PMSI database, we have selected all hospitalizations summaries including a ICD-10 code corresponding to a potential ADR. From the French Pharmacovigilance Database, we have selected all serious ADR treated in Toulouse University Hospital during the same period. All cases identified in the two databases were analysed in order to check the presence and the seriousness of each ADR. After identification of common cases, the capture-recapture method has allowed to estimate the total number of ADR.Out of 955 hospitalizations initially identified from the PMSI database, 355 were related to a serious ADR. Out of 315 cases of serious ADR indentified in the French Pharmacovigilance Database, 194 were finally included in the analysis : 65 cases were common to the two databases, giving an estimated number of serious ADR of 1060 (CI 95% [869-1250]), i.e. a prevalence of 3% (CI 95% [2.5-3.5]).This study underlines the interest of merging data from different databases to identify the real impact of ADR in University Hospitals. However, the capture-recapture method exibits the lack of exhaustivity of ADR recording whatever the sources of data.

ORAL

Pediatric Counselling in Community Pharmacies : Knowledge of Pharmacists and Pharmacy Technicians About Drug Uutilisation in Children

Pin M., Lapeyre-Mestre M.

Counselling by community pharmacists is becoming an accepted standard for pharmacy practice. However, drugs available in children without prescription form are scarce, and most of the OTC products have not been tested and approved in children. The aim of this study was to investigate attitude and knowledge of community pharmacists about advice and treatment in several common ailments in children. We sent a postal questionnaire to a sample of 176 community pharmacies in the Midi-Pyrénées area (South western France), asking 2 people in the pharmacy (pharmacist and /or technician) what they would give as advice and/or drugs in five clinical situations presented as simulated cases : diarrhoea in an 8-months old baby; fever , common cold and rhinitis in a 5-years old girl; productive cough in a 4 years old girl and non productive cough in a 10 years old boy. Thirty five percent of pharmacies answered, giving 101 exploitable questionnaires. For each clinical situation, we searched in the literature all available evidence-based data and/or guidelines according to the class of age of each simulated case. Counselling of drug registered in children and in the indication was done by 57.6 to 93.4% of responders, depending on the simulated case. Even if an appropriate advice was given by most of the responders, improvements in advice are needed. For example, 77% of responders have recommended a drug for diarrhoea, when only 44% of responders proposed a oral rehydration solution.

P - 325

Perception of The Risk Of Gastro-Intestinal Adrs With Non Steroidal Anti-inflammatory Drugs (Including Coxibs) : Differences Between General Practitioners, Gastro-Enterologists and Rheumatologists

Montastruc J.L., Bongard V., Lapeyre-Mestre M.

A previous study has found major differences in the perception of risk of Adverse Drug Reactions (ADRs) between health professionals and non health professionals The present study was performed in order to compare the perception of risk of Gastro-Intestinal (GI) ADRs with Non Steroidal Antiinflammatory Drugs (NSAIDs) (including coxibs) in General practitioners (GP), Gastro-Enterologists (GE) and rheumatologists (R) from Southwestern France. 69 GP, 45 GE and 58 R were interviewed using visual analogue scales in order to define a score of perceived risk of ADRs associated with each NSAID (ranking from 0 to 10). Among physicians, GP gave the most important mean risk score (4.7) for NSAIDs as a whole followed by GE (4.6) and R (3.3). Indolic derivatives were ranked as the most dangerous NSAIDs (median score : 5.3) followed by oxicams (4.9), arylcarboxylic derivatives (4.8) and coxibs (2.0). There was no significant difference in the median score for indolic derivatives between the 3 groups of physicians whereas significant differences were found for arylcarboxylic derivatives, oxicams and coxibs with higher values of perceived risks given by GE followed by GP and R. This study show major differences in the perception of risks of GI ADRs between physicians. R had the lower perceived risk of GI ADRs whereas perception of GP and R were quite similar. In contrast, the widely demonstrated difference in GI risk between the different groups of NSAIDS (with for example a higher risk for oxicams) are not known by the 3 studied groups of physicians. This example of Social Pharmacology (Therapie, 2002, 57, 420-6) illustrates the differences in the perception of risks of GI ADRs between physicians according to their medical education and kind of medical exercise.

P - 326

Effect of Rifampin on Pravastatin Pharmacokinetics

Kyrklund C., Backman JT., Neuvonen M., Neuvonen PJ.
Department of Clinical Pharmacology, University of Helsinki and Helsinki University Central Hospital, Helsinki, Finland

Background: Rifampicin, a potent inducer of several cytochrome P450 (CYP) enzymes and transporters, decreased the plasma concentrations of simvastatin acid by more than 90% in a previous study. This study was conducted to investigate the effect of rifampicin on the pharmacokinetics of pravastatin using an identical study design as in the previous study to allow comparison of the interaction potentials of simvastatin and pravastatin.
Methods: In a randomized cross-over study with two phases and a washout of 4 weeks, ten healthy volunteers received a 5-day pretreatment with rifampicin (600 mg daily) or placebo. On day 6, a single 40 mg dose of pravastatin was administered orally. Plasma concentrations of pravastatin were measured up to 12 hours by a sensitive LC-MS-MS method.
Results: During the rifampicin phase, the mean total area under the plasma concentration-time curve of pravastatin [AUCtot] was 69% (range 24 to 220%, $P < 0.05$) of the corresponding value during the placebo phase. In five of the ten subjects the AUCtot of pravastatin during the rifampicin phase was 50% or less of that during the placebo phase. Rifampicin had no significant effect on the peak concentration, elimination half-life or renal clearance of pravastatin. The effect of rifampicin on the AUCtot of pravastatin was significantly smaller than its effect on simvastatin acid in the previous study ($P < 0.001$).
Conclusions: Rifampicin had a minor effect on the pharmakokinetics of pravastatin. Thus, pravastatin seems better suited to be used in combination with CYP-inducers than simvastatin and the other statins studied so far. However, in some subjects the effect of rifampicin can be considerable.

## P - 327

Giving Feedback on Prescribing at a Primary Health Care Center - Important Element in Quality Control of Drug Prescribing in Stockholm, Sweden

Nyman K., Wettermark B., Bergman U.
Division of Clinical Pharmacology, Huddinge University Hospital, Stockholm, Sweden

DU90% - the number of Drugs that account for 90% of the Utilization - and adherence to guidelines in this segment was proposed by the Swedish Medical Quality Council as indicators for assessing the quality of drug prescribing. These DU90% profiles were applied at a primary health care (PHC) center in Stockholm with the guidelines issued by the regional drug committee (LÄKSAK) as a reference. The profiles were based on prescriptions purchased at pharmacies October-December each year. These data were also presented as individual DU90% profiles at the center. The adaptation to the EU regulations gradually increases the Swedish drug market. This was also seen for the PHC center (541 drugs in 2001, 577 in 2002). However, the bulk of the prescribing (DU90%) was about the same (158 vs 155). Among the five permanent GPs the number of drugs ranged from 87 to 134. The adherence to the 2002 guideline increased from 66% in 2001 to 73% in 2002, with an individual range from 63-72% to 68-77%. Although the DU90% method neither examines the appropriateness of use nor provides outcome data, it was shown to be an inexpensive, flexible and simple method for assessing the general quality of drug prescribing.

## P - 328

On an Open, One-centre, Comparative, Randomized, Clinical Trial on Efficacy and Safety of Topical Application of Stomatidin (Hexetidine) in Treating Patients Having Catarrhal Pharyngitis and Tonsilopharyngitis

Kapidzic A., Baksic D. D., Cabaravdic A., Resic M.
Clinic for ear, throat and nose, Clinical Centre of University of Sarajevo and Bosnalijek Sarajevo, Bosnia and Herzegovina.

The aim of the research: The aim of this study was to evaluate efficacy and safety of topical application of Stomatidin® in treating patients having catarrhal pharyngitis and tonsilopharyngitis.

Patients and method: The trial included 40 out-patients of both genders, who had catarrhal pharyngitis and tonsilopharyngitis, and were treated at the Otorhinolaryngology Clinic of Clinical Centre at University in Sarajevo, Bosnia and Herzegovina. An average age of patients was 41.8±10.5, including 20 men and 20 women. Stomatidin® manufactured by "Bosnalijek" was topically applied in 1 group, while the second group of patients was treated with Hexoral® manufactured by "Gödecke/Parke-Davis". Both medicines were applied for 30 seconds in the dose of 15 ml 0.1% undiluted solution, twice a day; in the mornings and evenings after meal. Symptoms and signs of the disease were analyzed at the first check-up, on fourth, and eighth day of the treatment. Tolerance of the tested medicament (Stomatidin®) was monitored during the treatment.

Results: Statistical analysis of local signs did not show any significant variations between the groups. Statistic processing of laboratory tests from the beginning and end of the trial did not show any significant differences (Stomatidin® vs. Hexoral®). Conclusion: On the basis of all the results, efficacy and safety of topical application of Stomatidin has been proven. Both medicaments have shown similar acting during the trial.

## P - 329

The Role Of Circadian Rhythm in the Pharmacokinetic of Methotrexate in Sidm Rats

Gumustekin M., Kalkan S., Murat N., Gur O., Hocaoglu N., Gidener S.
Department of Pharmacology, Dokuz Eylul University, School of Medicine, Izmir, Turkey

The aim of this study is to evaluate the role of circadian rhythm in the pharmacokinetic of MTX in streptozotocin-induced diabetes mellitus (SIDM)rats. Dark/light regimen was continued for a minimum of 3 weeks before the iniation of experimental procedures. The studies performed at 6-h intervals, blood samples were collected at 5., 15., 30. and 60. min. after iv infusion of MTX in both groups (SIDM and control). Also, in both groups was treated with dexamethasone one hour before the administration of MTX. We evaluated whether the circadian rhythm's role in the pharmacokinetic parameters of MTX in the SIDDM rats. The value of MTX AUC was significantly increased at 21 HALO( hours after light on, late in the dark phase (31.94±1.82 (1400) , p<0.05) when we compared with the other day periods(17±0.69 (2000) , 22.95±1.07 (0200) ve 19.05±1.79 (0800). The MTX AUC values in diabetic groups were higher than control groups, in all day periods. The endogenous production of corticosterone was supressed by treatment with dexamethasone the MTX blood concentrations were markedly increased at all daytime. These results suggest that the extent of MTX pharmacokinetics in the SIDM rats , varies with the time of day and might be related corticosteron concentrations changes.

## P - 330

Effect of Short-Term Ibuprofen Treatment on Gastroduodenal Mucosa

Tomalik-Scharte D., [1]Goeser T., [2]Sörgel F., [3]Lehmacher W., Jetter A., Szymanski J., [1]Töx U., Fuhr U., [2]Kinzig-Schippers M.
Institute for Pharmacology, [1]Department of Internal Medicine IV, [3]Institute for Medical Statistics, Informatics and Epidemiology, University of Köln; [1]IBMP - Institute for Biomedical and Pharmaceutical Research, Nürnberg-Heroldsberg; Germany

It is well-known that non-selective COX inhibitors may damage the gastroduodenal mucosa. The present study was conducted to quantify this effect following a short-term treatment with ibuprofen as it may occur in the treatment of toothache or other short pain episodes. A commercial immediate release ibuprofen preparation (L-arginin salt) was administered at doses of 400 mg of ibuprofen thrice daily for 10 doses. Fifteen healthy volunteers (3 women, 12 men, age 27 +/- 5 years) were included. Participants underwent a baseline gastroduodenoscopy and a second gastroduodenoscopy exactly 2 hours after the 10th ibuprofen dose. Mucosa damage was assessed in fundus, body, antrum, pylorus and duodenum using a 5-step grading (0: no lesion, 1: one hemorrhage [H] or erosion [E], 2: two to 10 H or E, 3: 11 to 25 H or E, 4: >25 H or E, or an invasive ulcer). The mean overall score significantly changed from 1.00 +/- 0.12 at baseline to 2.47 +/- 0.60 after treatment. One subject had an ulcer after treatment. While 11 of 15 subjects had not more than one lesion at baseline, 14 had 2 or more lesions after treatment. Main lesion sites were body and antrum. In conclusion, even after short-term exposure towards ibuprofen standard doses, extensive damages of gastral mucosa are common.

## P - 331

A Pilot Study Addressing the Role of Renal Function in Phenotyping for Intestinal Transporter Activity Using Oral Marker Substrates

Jabrane W., [2]Kinzig-SchippersM., [2]Malchau G., Tönnes E., Jetter A., Lück H., Hering U., [2]SörgelF., Fuhr U.
Institute for Pharmacology, [1]Clinical Chemistry Laboratory, University of Köln; [2]IBMP - Institute for Biomedical and Pharmaceutical Research, Nürnberg-Heroldsberg; Germany

Phenotyping individuals for the activity of intestinal transporters using oral marker drugs may contribute to recognize drugs as transporter substrates or modifiers. The present study was conducted to assess the role of renal function for phenotyping. In a pilot study, 120 mg of amoxycillin (marker for dipeptide carrier) and 0.5 mg of digoxin (marker for P-glycoprotein) were administered concomitantly to 10 healthy male adults as part of a phenotyping cocktail. Plasma and urine was collected up to 24 hours postdose. Amoxycillin was measured in plasma and urine by LC-MS/MS, plasma digoxin concentrations were determined by ELISA. Noncompartmental pharmacokinetics were calculated. Cmax was used as the metric for transporter activity. Renal function was measured as creatinine clearance. Parameters were compared by linear regression analysis. Mean and SD creatinin clearance was 205 +/- 46 ml/min (range 155-295 ml/min). For digoxin, renal function explained (r squared) 56 % of variation in AUC(0-24h) and 33 % of variation in Cmax. In contrast, renal function explained only 28 % of variation in amoxycillin renal clearance, and 2 % each of variation in amoxycillin AUC and Cmax. Thus, although both marker drugs are mainly eliminated via the kidney, factors other than renal function determine most of the variation in metrics used for transporter phenotyping in healthy subjects. However, taking renal function into account is expected to improve the precision to predict individual p-glycoprotein activity from digoxin Cmax.

## ORAL

Cytochrome P450 2D6 Polymorphism in Patients with Cancer

[1]Babaoglu M.O., [1]Bayar B., [2]Aynacioglu A. S., [3]Abali H., [2]Kerb R., [3]Celik I., [1]Bozkurt A.
[1]Department of Pharmacology, Faculty of Medicine, Hacettepe University, Ankara, Turkey. [2]Pharmacogenetics Laboratory, Epidauros Biotechnology AG, Bernried, Germany. [3]Hacettepe University, Institute of Oncology, Department of Medical Oncology, Ankara, Turkey.

Objective: The genetically polymorphic cytochrome P450 2D6 (CYP2D6) enzyme contributes to the metabolism of about 30% of all drugs. The objective of our study was to investigate the possible role of human CYP2D6 polymorphism in susceptibility to cancer.
Methods: A hundred and one patients with various cancer types, most of which being breast carcinoma, were genotyped for *CYP2D6* alleles by using Taqman analysis. Results: Allele frequencies were calculated as 81.2%, 0.5% and 9.9 % for *CYP2D6*1* (wt), *3 and *4 alleles, respectively. As for the gene multiplication, frequencies were 4.5% for *1x2* type, 0.9% for *1/*4x2* type and 3.0% for *5 (deletion) type alleles. The patients were not genotyped for *2 allele and no subjects were detected to have more than three copies of *CYP2D6* gene or homozygous deletion.
Conclusion: The frequencies of *CYP2D6* genetic variations in subjects with cancer were comparable to those obtained from healthy subjects in a Turkish population reported previously(1). Although not statistically significant, *CYP2D6*5* allele frequency was found to be higher in cancer patients as compared to healthy subjects (3.0 % vs. less than 1.0 %). (1) Aynacioglu AS *et al.*, Clin Pharmacol Ther. 66:185-92, 1999. This study was supported by Tubitak (SBAG-COST B15-2356).

## P - 332

Losartan as a Probe for Phenotyping of Cyp2c9 in a Turkish Population

[1]Babaoglu M.O., [1]Yasar Ü., [1]Dincel A., [2]Eliasson E., [3]Dahl M.-L., [1]Bozkurt Atila [1]Department of Pharmacology, Faculty of Medicine, Hacettepe University, Ankara, Turkey [2]Division of Clinical Pharmacology, Department of Laboratory Medicine, Karolinska Institutet at Huddinge University Hospital, Stockholm, Sweden.
[3]Department of Medical Sciences, Clinical Pharmacology, University Hospital, Uppsala, Sweden

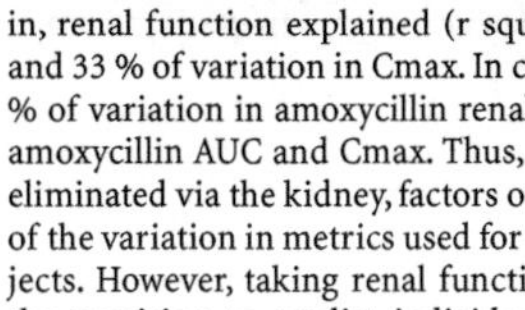


Objective: Cytochrome P450 2C9 (CYP2C9) is a polymorphic enzyme catalyzing the metabolism of several important drugs, such as S-warfarin, phenytoin, oral anti-diabetics and non-steroidal anti-inflammatory drugs. Losartan has recently been suggested as a selective probe for CYP2C9 metabolic activity. The aim of the study was to test losartan as a probe drug for CYP2C9 activity in healthy volunteers in a Turkish population.
Methods: A single oral dose of 25 mg losartan was given to each subject. Concentrations of losartan and its carboxylic acid metabolite, E-3174, were analyzed by HPLC in the urine collected for eight hours (n=80). CYP2C9 genotypes were determined in 26 of the subjects by PCR.
Results: The urinary losartan/E-3174 ratio was significantly higher in the subjects with *CYP2C9*1*3* genotype (2.9±1.5, mean±SD, n=6) compared to the subjects with *CYP2C9*1*1* (1.3±0.8, n=14) and *1*2* (1.0±0.6, n=5) genotypes ($p<0.05$). Conclusion: The distribution of urinary losartan/E-3174 ratio and genotype-phenotype relationship in the Turkish population was similar to a previous report from another Caucasian population (Yasar *et al., Clin Pharmacol Ther*, 2002, 71(1), 89-98). This study was supported by TUBITAK (SBAG-COST B15-2356).

## P - 333

Relationship Between Neonatal Hyperbilirubinemia and Bilirubin UDP-Glucuronosyl Transferase 1A1 Gene Polymorphism

[1]Babaoglu M. O., [2]Yigit S., [3]Aynacioglu A.S., [3]Kerb R., [1]Bayar B., [2]Yurdakok M., [1]Bozkurt A.
[1]Department of Pharmacology, Faculty of Medicine, Hacettepe University, Ankara, Turkey. [2]Hacettepe University Hospital, Department of Pediatrics, Ankara, Turkey. [3]Pharmacogenetics Laboratory, Epidauros Biotechnology Ag, Bernried, Germany

Hepatic microsomal bilirubin uridine diphosphate-glucuronosyltransferase (B-UGT) is the rate limiting enzyme for the conjugation of bilirubin with glucuronic acid in its excretion process into the bile. Variations in B-UGT gene (*UGT-1A1*) have been related to disorders that may cause hyperbilirubinemia. The aim of this study was to investigate whether the number of [TA] repeats in the promoter region of *UGT-1A1* is related to the occurrence of physiologic or prolonged hyperbilirubinemia in neonates.
Fourty-nine neonates were genotyped for their [TA] repeat number in the promoter region of *UGT-1A1* by DNA sequence analysis. Twenty three cases were diagnosed to have indirect hyperbilirubinemia, of which nine had prolonged jaundice. Twenty six cases were age and sex matched healthy control subjects. The frequencies of each genotype are given in the Table.
The frequency of *UGT-1A1* $[TA]_{6/6}$ in subjects with prolonged hyperbilirubinemia seems to be reduced compared to other two groups. Statistical significance was not calculated due to insufficient number of subjects in each group.
This study was supported by TUBITAK (SBAG-COST B15-2356).

| [TA] repeat number | Physiological hyperbilirubinemia (%) | Prolonged hyperbilirubinemia (%) | Control (%) |
|---|---|---|---|
| [TA]6/6 | 64.3 | 44.4 | 57.7 |
| [TA]7/6 | 28.6 | 55.6 | 34.6 |
| [TA]7/7 | 7.1 | 0.0 | 7.7 |

## P - 334

Annual Rhythm of the Acute Neurotoxicity of Sodium Nitroprruside in Mice

[1]Attia M. B., [1]Tchacondo T., [2]Reinberg A. & [3]Boughattas N.A.
[1]Faculté des Sciences de Bizerte, 7021 Zarzouna, Tunisia; [2]Laboratoire de Chronobiologie, Fondation A. de Rothschild, 75940 Paris, France; [3]Faculté de Médecine, 5019 Monastir, Tunisia

The rhythmic organization of biological functions is nowadays, recognized as a fundamental property of all the living beings. Our study aims to investigate the seasonal variation of the acute neurotoxicity of sodium nitroprusside (SNP), used as an hypotensor agent. The 4 seasons of the year (winter, spring, summer, autumn) and 4 circadian times of injection (1, 7, 13 and 19 Hours After Light Onset, HALO) were considered. Experiments were carried out on Albino Swiss male mice (6 mice/dose/circadian time at each experience) aged 7 ± 1 weeks and synchronized by a light-dark cycle (L/D:12/12; L from 07.00 to 19.00 h) for 3 weeks prior i.p. injection of a potentially non lethal dose of SNP (3.6 mg/kg). The motor impairment, as assessed by the horizontal wire test, was used as an index of SNP acute behavior neurotoxicity. Our results show that the percentage of motor impairment varies according to the seasons ($p < 0.001$, Chi-square test). The maximum of this toxicity is observed in autumn, season of weak tolerance of mice to SNP, and minimum in spring, season which corresponded to the optimal tolerance. The acute behavioral toxicity of SNP appeared to be dependent on the season of its administration.

## P - 335

The comparison of the Treatment of Epilepsy in Czech Republic and Sweden

[1]Koristkova B., [1]Grundmann M., [2]Bergman U., [2]Sjöqvist F.
[1]Department of Clinical Pharmacology, University Hospital and Medico Social Faculty University of Ostrava, Ostrava, Czech Republic, [2]Department of Clinical Pharmacology, Huddinge University Hospital, Stockholm,Sweden

The treatment of epilepsy in the University Hospitals in Ostrava and Huddinge was compared. Request forms for therapeutic drug monitoring were used as data source. 2789 blood samples from 1108 in-patients (60% children, mean age 15±15 years, mean body weight 38±25 kg) were analysed during 1995-1999 in Ostrava. 10543 samples from 3232 out- as well as in-patientes (11% children, mean age 43±23, body weight unknown) were analysed in Huddinge. The treatment of epilepsy was very similar. Monotherapy was the most common pattern (Ostrava-Huddinge: 50%-59% samples) followed by combination of two drugs (33%-29%). 60% of patterns involved carbamazepine, valproic acid and phenytoin in monotherapy, and combination of valproic acid or phenytoin with carbamazepine in both hospitals. Phenytoin was more frequent in adult patients, while children were treated more often with valproic acid. Higher ratio of adult patients in Huddinge caused the only difference - higher frequency in usage of phenytoin in Huddinge.

## ORAL

The Anti Doping Hot-Line, A Means to Detect and Prevent the Abuse of Doping Agents in The Swedish Society And a new Service Function in Clinical Pharmacology

Sjöqvist F., Eklöf A.C., Thurelius A.M., Garle M., Rane A.
Department of Clinical Pharmacology,Huddinge University Hospital, Stockholm, Sweden

With the support of the Swedish National Institute of Health a national telephone service was started in 1993 aiming to detect and prevent the abuse of doping agents in the general public. Between October 1993 and December 2000 25.835 calls were received with a peak during spring and autumn. Most calls (12.400) came from non-abusers, 60 % being males. Callers connected with gyms represented the largest group (30 %). Most calls about specific drugs concerned anabolic androgenic steroids (AAS). Other drugs or products included ephedrine, clenbuterol and creatine. The most commonly abused anabolic steroids were testosterone, nandrolone-decanoate, methandienone and stanozolol. The ten most commonly reported ADR:s were aggressiveness (835), depression (829), acne (770), gynecomastia (637), anxiousness (637), potency problems (413), testicular atrophy (404), sleep disorders (328), fluid retention (318) and mood disturbances (302).

## P - 336

Melatonin Protects Against Oxidative Organ Injury in a Rat Model of Sepsis

[1]Toklu H., [1]Şener G., [1]Kapucu C., [3]Kaçmaz A., [3]Tilki M., [2]Yeğen B.Ç.
Marmara University [1]School of Pharmacy, Dept. of Pharmacology; [2]School of Medicine, Dept. Physiology; [3]Haydarpasa Numune Research Hospital, Division of General Surgery; Istanbul, Turkey

Introduction: Recent studies have shown that sepsis is associated with enhanced generation of reactive oxygen metabolites, which lead to multiple organ dysfunction. Based on the potent antioxidant effects of melatonin, we investigated the putative protective role of melatonin against sepsis-induced oxidative organ damage.

Materials and Methods: Sepsis was induced by cecal ligation and puncture in Wistar Albino rats. Sham operated (control) and sepsis group had received saline or melatonin (10mg/kg, ip) 30 minutes prior to and 6 hours after the operation. Sixteen hours after the surgery, rats were decapitated and the biochemical changes were determined in liver and kidney tissues by malondialdehyde (MDA) content -an index of lipid peroxidation-, glutathione (GSH) levels -a key antioxidant- and myeloperoxidase (MPO) activity- an index of neutrophil infiltration-.

Results: Kidney and liver MDA levels in the sepsis group were significantly increased ($p<0.001$) with concomitant decreases in GSH levels ($p<0.01$-$p<0.001$), when compared to control group. Similarly MPO activity was significantly increased ($p<0.001$) in both hepatic and renal tissues. On the other hand, melatonin treatment significantly reversed ($p<0.001$) the elevations in MDA and MPO levels, while reduced GSH levels were increased back to control levels ($p<0.01$-$p<0.001$).

Conclusion: The results of the present study indicate that melatonin demonstrates an antioxidant effect on sepsis-induced hepatorenal injury, by a neutrophil-dependent mechanism. These findings suggest that melatonin could be considered as a useful therapeutic agent in preventing sepsis-induced oxidative organ injury.

## P - 337

Sistemic Apsorption of 2% Lidocaine Hydrochloride Gel after Colonoscopically Examined Patients

Siuc Valkovic D., Vitezic D., Oguic R., Stimac D., Niksic M.
Jadran Galenic Laboratory d.d., Universityof Rijeka Medical School and University Hospital Centre Rijeka, Rijeka,Croatia

Lidocaine hydrochloride is a local anesthetic agent used topically during different endoscopic procedures. The aim of our study was to investigate pharmacokinetics of lidocaine hydrochloride 2% gel in colonoscopically examined patients. We determined lidocaine serum concentrations after drug topical application for anestetic effect during colonoscopy. The study was approved by our local ethical committee and the patients gave their informed consent. We included 15 patients (9 men) and lidocaine (25 ml) was applied 10 minutes before endoscopic procedure. The case record form was used for each patient (i.e. general data, diagnosis, medical history, laboratory data etc.) and lidocaine serum concentrations were determined by TDX apparatus at 0, 15 min and 30 min after the drug application. The serum lidocaine concentrations were measurable 5 min after the application in 3/15 samples with the average value of 0.018 &g/ml. The mean concentrations of the drug 15 min after application were 0.224 &g/ml (measurable values in 13/15 samples) and after 30 min in all 15 samples we had measurable values at the average of 0.491 &g/ml. No adverse effects were noticed in our patients. Our results showed that lidocaine accomplished significant concentrations in the serum after topical rectal application, but the concentrations of the drug were several times lower than the concentrations which could be connected with the increased risk for adverse effects of the drug (levels higher than 5 &g/ml). Therefore, according to our pharmacokinetic results we can presume that lidocaine could be safely applied during colonoscopy.

## P - 338

Influence of CYP2D6 And CYP2C9 Genotypes on Fluoxetine Plasma Concentrations in Psychiatric Patients

[1,2]Llerena A., [1]Dorado P., [1]Berecz R., [1]González A.P., [1]Cáceres M.C.
[1]Department of Pharmacology and Psychiatry, Faculty of Medicine, University of Extremadura, Badajoz, Spain. [2]Department of Medical Sciences, Faculty of Health Sciences, University of Beira Interior, Covilhã, Portugal.

The drug metabolizing enzyme CYP2D6 has been shown to be involved in fluoxetine metabolism in vitro and in vivo, however CYP2C9 has not been studied in humans. The aim of the present study was to evaluate the influence of CYP2D6 and CYP2C9 genotypes on the plasma concentration of fluoxetine and norfluoxetine among sixty-six white European psychiatric patients. The dose corrected plasma concentrations of fluoxetine were related ($p<0.05$) to CYP2D6 genotypes (number of active genes). The fluoxetine/norfluoxetine ratio also correlated ($p<0.01$) with the number of active CYP2D6 genes. Among CYP2D6*1/*1 (n=38), dose corrected plasma concentrations of fluoxetine and the active moiety were ($p<0.05$) higher in the CYP2C9*1/*2 and*1/*3 genotype groups compared to *1/*1 homozygotes. The results show that fluoxetine metabolism is related to CYP2D6 and CYP2C9 genotypes. Since these enzymes are involved in the metabolism of several widely used drugs (antidepressant, antipsychotic, oral antidiabetic, anticoagulant, antiepileptic drugs, etc), interactions with fluoxetine may occur. Thus, in clinical practice, CYP2D6 and CYP2C9 genotyping may help to prevent potentially dangerous side effects.

This study was supported by grants from the Spanish Ministry of Health, Instituto Carlos III (FIS 01/0699) and Junta de Extremadura, Consejería de Sanidad y Consumo (2002/48).

## P - 339

QTc Interval Lengthening and CYP2D6 in Patients Treated with Risperidone

[1,2]Llerena A., [1]Berecz R., [1]Dorado P., [1]de-la-Rubia A., [1]Sanz-de-la-Garza C.
[1]Department of Pharmacology and Psychiatry, Faculty of Medicine, University of Extremadura, Badajoz, Spain. [2]Department of Medical Sciences, Faculty of Health Sciences, University of Beira Interior, Covilhã, Portugal.

The role of drug metabolizing enzymes in cardiotoxicity, such as CYP2D6 for thioridazine, has been suggested. Risperidone has been shown to inhibit the rapid component of the cardiac delayed rectifier $K^+$ channels in vitro, which may be related to a QTc lengthening and to a risk for arrhythmias type torsade de pointes type. CYP2D6 is involved in the metabolism of risperidone to 9-OH-risperidone. The present study was aimed at evaluating the influence of CYP2D6, and plasma concentrations of risperidone and 9-OH-risperidone on the QTc interval in patients under steady-state condition. The influence of CYP2D6 on risperidone and 9-OH-risperidone plasma concentrations was also analysed. Fifty-four European psychiatric patients were studied. The QTc interval was found to be higher ($p<0.05$) in patients treated with CYP2D6 inhibitors compared to those under risperidone monotherapy, it was also related ($p<0.05$) to CYP2D6 genotype. The number of CYP2D6 active genes was related to the dose-corrected plasma concentration of risperidone ($p<0.05$) and the risperidone/9-OH-risperidone ratio ($p<0.05$). The results suggest that CYP2D6 may be related to QTc lengthening during treatment with risperidone.

This study was supported by grants from the Spanish Ministry of Health, Instituto Carlos III (FIS 01/0699) and Junta de Extremadura, Consejería de Sanidad y Consumo (2002/48).

## P - 340

Influence of CYP2D6 ON Haloperidol Plasma Concentration and QTc Interval

[1]Berecz R., [2]de la Rubia A., [1]Dorado P., [1]González I., [1,2,3]Llerena A.
[1]Department of Pharmacology and Psychiatry, Faculty of Medicine, University of Extremadura, Badajoz, Spain. [2]Unit of Research and Clinical Psychopharmacology, Psychiatric Hospital, Mérida. [3]Department of Medical Sciences, Faculty of Health Sciences, University of Beira Interior, Covilhã, Portugal.

The present study was aimed to evaluate the possible inhibition of CYP2D6 during haloperidol treatment, and to determine the effect of CYP2D6 genotype on the plasma concentration of haloperidol and QTc interval. Thirty Caucasian psychiatric patients under haloperidol monotherapy were studied. CYP2D6 activity was evaluated by the debrisoquine metabolic ratio (MR). The number of patients with debrisoquine MR>12.6 was higher comparing to healthy volunteers (13% vs. 6.6%, respectively). Debrisoquine MR was correlated with the dose of haloperidol ($r=0.40$, $p<0.05$), and also with the plasma concentration ($r=0.58$, $p<0.001$). CYP2D6 genotype was not related to the dose or plasma concentration of haloperidol. QTc interval was not related to any of the parameters studied, however the mean of QTc interval was higher among subjects carrying 1 compared to 2 CYP2D6 active genes. The present data support the dose-dependent inhibitory effect of haloperidol on CYP2D6, and the influence of this enzyme activity on haloperidol plasma concentration under steady-state conditions.

This study was supported by grants from the Spanish Ministry of Health, Instituto Carlos III (FIS 01/0699) and Junta de Extremadura, Consejería de Sanidad y Consumo (2002/48).

## P - 341

Thioridazine Plasma Concentrations, CYP2D6 and QTc Interval Lengthening

[1,3]de la Rubia A., [1]Berecz R., [1]Dorado P., [2]Fernández-Salguero P., [1,4]Llerena A.
[1]University of Extremadura, Departments of Pharmacology and Psychiatry and [2]Biochemistry and Molecular Biology, [3]Unit of Research and Clinical Psychopharmacology at Mérida Psychiatric Hospital, Badajoz, Spain; [4]Beira Interior University, Medical School, Covilhã, Portugal.

The present study was aimed at evaluating the influence of the dose, plasma concentration of thioridazine, debrisoquine Metabolic Ratio (MR), CYP2D6 on the QTc interval in psychiatric patients treated at therapeutic doses. QTc intervals, plasma levels of thioridazine and its metabolites, debrisoquine MR were studied among sixty-five Caucasian patients receiving thioridazine. CYP2D6 genotypes were also studied among 63 of them.
QTc interval was correlated with thioridazine daily dose (p<0.01), plasma concentration (p<0.01), as well as with debrisoquine MR (p<0.001) and thioridazine/mesoridazine ratio (p<0.01). However no relationship was found between QTc interval and CYP2D6 genotypes. CYP2D6 active genes (p<0.05) were related to thioridazine dose/corrected plasma concentrations. According to the present results CYP2D6 seems to be related to thioridazine plasma concentration, and thus might be a determining factor for the risk for QTc interval lengthening, and increased risk of sudden death due to torsade de pointes type cardiac arrhythmia.
This study was supported by grants from the Spanish Ministry of Health, Instituto Carlos III (FIS 01/0699) and Junta de Extremadura, Consejería de Sanidad y Consumo (2002/48).

## P - 342

Reproducibility Over Time of the Diclofenac/4'-OH Diclofenac Urinary Ratio Among Different CYP2C9 Genotypes

[1]Dorado P., [1]Berecz R., [1]Cáceres M.C., [1]González I., [1,2]Llerena A.
[1]Department of Pharmacology and Psychiatry, Faculty of Medicine, University of Extremadura, Badajoz, Spain. [2]Department of Medical Sciences, Faculty of Health Sciences, University of Beira Interior, Covilhã, Portugal.

Diclofenac has been used for the evaluation of CYP2C9 activity in vitro as well as in vivo with varying results. The present study was aimed at evaluating the reproducibility of the urine diclofenac/4'-OH diclofenac ratio among different CYP2C9 genotypes in healthy volunteers. The study of CYP2C9 genotypes in a family is also reported. The urinary diclofenac/4'-OH diclofenac ratio was determined on two occasions within a period of 9-12 months, and was found to be correlated (r=0.83, p<0.05). The mean (±SD) of diclofenac/4'-OH diclofenac ratio was 1.5 times higher among subjects carrying CYP2C9*3 allele (CYP2C9*1/*3 and CYP2C9*2/*3 genotypes) (0.91±0.28), compared to CYP2C9*1/*1 subjects (0.60±0.11). The results show that the urine diclofenac/4'-OH diclofenac ratio might be used to study CYP2C9 hydroxylation capacity in humans. The data agree with previous studies showing that the CYP2C9*3 allelic variant seems to cause a decreased CYP2C9 hydroxylation capacity.
This study was supported by a grant from the Spanish Ministry of Health, Instituto Carlos III (FIS 01/0699), and by the Hungarian-Spanish S&T Cooperation Programme (E-45/2001).

## P - 343

Analysis of Debrisoquine and 4-Hidroxydebrisoquine in Human Urine by High-Performance Liquid Chromatography

[1,2]Llerena A., [1]González I., [1]Dorado P., [1]Berecz R., [1]Cáceres M.C.
[1]Department of Pharmacology and Psychiatry, Faculty of Medicine, University of Extremadura, Badajoz, Spain. [2]Department of Medical Sciences, University of Beira Interior Medical School, Covilhã, Portugal.

A high-performance liquid chromatographic method for simultaneous urine analysis of debrisoquine and its primary metabolite, 4-hydroxydebrisoquine is described. A $C_{18}$ extraction column was used with a mobile phase consisting of acetonitrile, 20% potassium dihydrogen phosphate, 5% trietylamine (50 mM) and 40 ml of N,N-dimethyloctylamine, at pH=3.5 at a flow rate of 0.8 ml/min. The peaks of interest were eluted from the column in less than 10 min. The method described was validated for within-day and between-day accuracy and precision for both debrisoquine and 4-hydroxydebrisoquine. Coefficients of variation at all concentrations tested were <3% for both compounds. Based on urine sample volume of 1 ml, the limit of detection of debrisoquine and 4-hydroxydebrisoquine was 0.15 and 0.07 µg/ml respectively.
This study was supported bya grant from Junta de Extremadura, Consejería de Sanidad y Consumo (2002/48).

## P - 344

Frequencies of CYP2C9 Allelic Variants Among Cubans and Spaniards

[1,2]González I., [1]Dorado P., [2]Calzadilla L.R., [3]Pérez B., [1]Llerena A.
[1]Department of Pharmacology and Psychiatry, Faculty of Medicine, University of Extremadura, Badajoz, Spain. [2]Havana Psychiatric Hospital, Cuba. [3]Faculty of Medical Sciences "Calixto García", Havana, Cuba.

The genetic polymorphism of the cytochrome P450 enzymes is one of the major determinants of the interindividual variability of pharmacokinetics and drug response. CYP2C9 seems to be implicated in the metabolism of several important drugs. We have shown the genetic polymorphism of CYP2C9 among Spaniards. Of the various CYP2C9 alleles, CYP2C9*2 and CYP2C9*3 have been reported with altered catalytic activities compared to the wild type CYP2C9*1. Interethnic differences in cytochrome P450 polymorphism might be responsible, at least in part, for the variations in drug disposition between ethnic groups. The present study is aimed to analyze the CYP2C9 polymorphism in a Cuban Population to be compared with a previous studied Spanish population. Differences between Spaniards and Cubans on the CYP2C9 allele frequencies are shown in the Table. No differences was found between white Europeans from Spain and Cuba, however the frequency of CYP2C9*2 was lower among Cuban-Mestizos compared to Cuban-Caucasian (p<0.001).

| Alleles | N | | | Frequency (IC 95%) | | |
|---|---|---|---|---|---|---|
| | White-Cubans | Mestizos-Cubans | Spaniards | White-Cubans | Mestizos-Cubans | Spaniards |
| *CYP2C9*1* | 408 | 213 | 215 | 0.78 (0.75-0.82) | 0.85 (0.80-0.89) | 0.78 (0.73-0.83) |
| *CYP2C9*2* | 61 | 14 | 39 | 0.12 (0.09-0.15) | 0.06* (0.03-0.09) | 0.14 (0.10-0.18) |
| *CYP2C9*3* | 51 | 23 | 22 | 0.10 (0.08-0.13) | 0.09 (0.06-0.13) | 0.08 (0.05-0.11) |

*p<0.01, compared with White-Cubans and Spaniards, using Fisher's exact test.

The authors thank Dr. Eduardo B. Ordaz Ducungé for supporting the present research.

## P - 345

Drug Treatment of Schizophrenia First Episode in Hungary, Spain And Cuba

Llerena A., González I., Berecz R., Cáceres M.C., de la Rubia A., Calzadilla L.
University of Extremadura, Spain. University of Debrecen, Hungary. 3Havana Psychiatric Hospital, Cuba

The present study was aimed at evaluating the international differences of schizophrenia treatment in Cuba, Hungary and Spain. All patients who were diagnosed with schizophrenia in their lifetime during in-patient treatment were studied. All psychiatric beds in the Spanish region of Extremadura and Hajdu-Bihar in Hungary were analysed. Havana Psychiatric Hospital was studied in Cuba for comparisons. The study period was four years in Hungary (1995-98) and Cuba (1998-2001), and five years in Spain (1995-1999). The number of patients studied was 21 in Hungary, 218 in Cuba and 203 in Spain. The data on the use of neuroleptics was collected retrospectively from the patient case records and average prescribed daily doses were calculated for each patient and each hospital. The study revealed, that atypical neuroleptics were frequently used in Hungary. Haloperidol is still frequently used in Spain and Cuba. (Table I). The lack of convincing evidence on greater cost-effectiveness of the new generation of neuroleptics is discussed.

| Debrecen, Hungary | La Habana, Cuba | Extremadura, Spain |
|---|---|---|
| 1. Clozapine (45%, 178 mg) | 1. Haloperidol (18%, 10 mg) | 1. Haloperidol (26%, 9 mg) |
| 2. Risperidone (25%, 4.4 mg) | 2. Clorpromazine (13%, 143 mg) | 2. Risperidone (22%, 6 mg) |
| 3. Haloperidol (8%, 5 mg) | 3. Flufenazine (5%, 16 mg) | 3. Levomepromazin (20%,51 mg) |
| 4. Sulpiride (7%, 340 mg) | 4. Levomepromazine (5%, 30 mg) | 4. Olanzapine (11%, 14 mg) |
| 5. Sertindole (4%, 8.1 mg) | 3. Trifluoperazine (5%, 27 mg) | 5. Clozapine (3%, 234 mg) |

Table I. The ranking of five most often prescribed neuroleptics (per cent from total nr of treatment days and average prescribed daily dose)

The authors thank Dr. Eduardo B. Ordaz Ducungé for supporting the present research.

## P - 346

Anticancer Effects of Aspirin on A549, HeLa, HT-29, MCF-7 Cancer Cells : A Comparative Study with NIH3T3 Fibroblast Cells

Korkmaz S., Öztürk Y.
Anadolu University, Faculty of Pharmacy, Department of Pharmacology, Eskisehir

Aspirin is a well known anti-inflamatuvar, analgesic drug. Recently, aspirin has been shown to have preventive, antiangiogenic and antiproliferative effects against colon cancer. In the present study, anticancer effects of aspirin were investigated by using A549 non-small cells lung adenocarcinoma, HeLa servix adenocarcinoma, HT-29 colon carcinoma and MCF-7 breast carcinoma cell lines comparing to NIH3T3 fibroblasts. These cell lines were preferred as a representative for common cancer types. Being a representative for healthy cells, NIH3T3 fibroblast cell line was used as a control. Aspirin was applied at the doses of 1,6-8-40-200 and 1000 microM/ml and its anti-proliferative effects on cells were by employing MTT proliferation assay measured for four days in a dose- and time-dependent manner. Our findings indicated that low dose aspirin was effective on all cell lines tested with the exception of HeLa. However, aspirin was found to have a relatively shorter duration of antiproliferative action on MCF-7 cells. Taking into account all the findings obtained in the present study, it may be suggested that aspirin may be a clinically useful agent as an adjunct to conventional modalities for cancer therapy.

## P - 347

Attenuation of Ischemia-Reperfusion-Induced Myocardial Infarct Size in Rats by Aminoguanidine

[1]Parlakpinar H., [1]Ozer M.K., [2]Sahna E., [1]Acet A.
[1]Department of Pharmacology, Faculty of Medicine, Inonu University, Malatya, Turkey [2]Department of Pharmacology, Faculty of Medicine, Firat University, Elazig, Turkey

Background: Myocardial infarction is a major complication of coronary diseases. Postischemic reperfusion may profoundly alter cardiac functions. Upon reflow, oxygen radicals are generated in large amounts, overwhelming cellular defenses and inducing oxidative tissue damage. Cardiac myocytes constitutively express the endothelial isoform of NO synthase (eNOS), suggesting a mechanism for modulation of contractility. In addition to eNOS, inducible NO synthase (iNOS) can be expressed in the heart. Thus, cardiac iNOS may play a pivotal role in the progress of myocardial damage in many heart diseases. Therefore, inhibition of cardiac iNOS by aminoguanidine, (AG) a relatively selective inhibitor of NOS, could be useful in reducing ischemia-reperfusion induced myocardial damage in rats.
Methods And Statistic: To produce necrosis, a branch of the left coronary artery was occluded for 30 minutes followed by 2 hours reperfusion. AG (200mg/kg) was given intravenously 10 min before ischemia. Infarction was measured triphenyl tetrazolium staining. The infarct and risk zone, considered to be the area lacking fluorescence under UV light, were traced.
Results: Compared to the control group, AG statistically significantly reduced myocardial infarct size [52.57±3.30 *vs* 36.70±5.25 respectively]in rat model of ischemia-reperfusion.
Conclussion: These result suggest that, AG is an effective antioxidant and free radical scavenger reduced ischemia-reperfusion induced myocardial infarct size in rat model. Thus, AG appears to exert a heart protective activity in ischemia-reperfusion injury. We believe that it could be effectively combination with other cardioprotective agents.

## P - 348

Protective Effect of Aminoguanidine Against Cardiotoxicity Induced by Doxorubucin In Rats

[1]Parlakpinar H., [1]Ozer M.K., [2]Sahna E., [3]Ciğremiş Y., [1]Acet A.
[1]Department of Pharmacology Faculty of Medicine, Inonu University, Malatya, Turkey, [2]Department of Pharmacology Faculty of Medicine, Firat University, Elazig, Turkey [3]Department of Biology Faculty of Art and Science, Inonu University, Malatya, Turkey

Background:Doxorubicin (Dox) is a broad spectrum anthracycline antibiotic that has cardiotoxicity as a major side effect. One mechanism of this toxicity is believed to reactive oxygen radical species (ROS) generation. Aminoguanidine (AG) acted as an antioxidant and free radical scavenger in vivo, preventing ROS formation and lipid peroxidation in cells and tissues preventing oxidant-induced injury. It has been proposed that antioxidant maintain the concentration of reduced glutathione (GSH) and may restore the cellular defense mechanisms and block lipid peroxidation thus protecting against the toxicity of wide variety of cardiotoxic chemicals. We investigated effects of AG on Dox-induced related changes of malondialdehyde (MDA) a lipid peroxidation product and GSH. Methods and statistic:We used 21 adult female Wistar rats. The rats were divided into three groups equally: I) injected with vehicle; II) injected with Dox (ip) 20 mg/kg at a single dose; III) injected with Dox plus AG (ip) 200 mg/kg 1 h before the administration of Dox for 3days.The heart MDA and GSH levels of rats were measured by spectrophotometrically. Results are expressed as nmol/g tissue. Results:According to control, Dox administration to rats further increased MDA [42.6±0.4 *vs* 56.9±1.8, respectively] and decreased GSH levels [335±14.8 *vs* 186.7±7.3, respectively]. AG administration significantly decreased MDA [22.3±2.1] and increased GSH levels[323±9.5] in the Dox treated rats heart compared to levels in rats treated with Dox only.
Conclusion:Our results suggest that AG is an effective antioxidant and free radical scavenger reduced Dox-induced MDA and increased GSH levels. Therefore, AG could protect the heart tissue against free radical injury..

## P - 349

Reduction of Amikacin-Induced Nephrotoxicity in Rats by Caffeic Acid Phenethyl Ester (CAPE)

[1]Parlakpinar H., [1]Ozer M.K., [2]Sahna E., [3]Gaffaroglu M., [1]Acet A.
[1]Department of Pharmacology, Faculty of Medicine, Inonu University, Malatya, Turkey [2]Department of Pharmacology, Faculty of Medicine, Firat University, Elazig, Turkey, [3]Department of Biology, Faculty of Art and Science, Inonu University, Malatya, Turkey

Background: Amikacin (AK)-induced nephrotoxicity may be the consequence of oxidative stress. Caffeic acid phenethyl ester (CAPE) was recently shown to have free radical scavenging ability and it reduces lipid peroxidation. CAPE could be useful in reducing AK nephrotoxicity.
Methods: The rats were distributed into three groups: I) injected with vehicle; II) injected (i.p) with 1,2 g/kg AK at a single dose; III) injected (i.p) with AK plus 10 µmol/kg CAPE and continued for 3 days. Two hundred mg kidney tissue was homogenized in ice-cold 150 mM KCL for determination of MDA, a lipid peroxidation product. The MDA content of homogenates was determined spectrophotometrically by measuring the presence of thiobarbituric acid reactive substances.
Results: Results are expressed as nmol/g tissue. MDA levels were found to be higher in rats given AK than control [90±8 *vs* 45±3, respectively]. CAPE administration 1 hour before AK injection caused significant decrease in MDA levels [68±2].
Conclussion: Increased MDA levels as a result of AK induction lead us to propose that free radicals may have a critical role in this injury. AK plus CAPE group was significant decrease in MDA levels. Thus, CAPE appears to exert a renal protective activity in AK induced renal injury by inhibiting lipid peroxidation.

## P - 350

Effects of Captopril and Losartan on Ischemia-Reperfusion-Induced Myocardial Infarct Size in Rats

Parlakpinar H., Ozer M.K., Acet A.
Department of Pharmacology, Faculty of Medicine, Inonu University, Malatya, Turkey

Background: Myocardial infarction is the underlying event in the majority of deaths from cardiovascular diseases. Angiotensin II (Ang II) elicits several physiological effects that exacerbate ischemia-reperfusion (IR) injury. Consequently, the cardioprotective efficacy of strategies that decrease Ang II receptor stimulation has been investigated in models of IR injury. Although angiotensin converting enzyme (ACE) inhibitors and receptor antagonists are beneficial during myocardial ischemia, their effects on reperfused myocardium remain controversial. The aim of this study was to examine the effects of ACE inhibitor captopril, and Ang II type 1 ($AT_1$) receptor blocker losartan on ischemia-reperfusion induced myocardial infarct size in an *in vivo* rat model. Methods: To produce necrosis, a branch of the left coronary artery was occluded for 30 minutes followed by 2 hours reperfusion. Captopril (3mg/kg) and losartan (2mg/kg) were given intravenously 10 min before ischemia and continued during ischemia by infusion pump. Infarction was measured triphenyl tetrazolium staining. Results: Compared to the control group [%55.62±4.00] both captopril and losartan statistically significant reduced myocardial infarct size [%30.50±3.26 and %37.75±4.44, respectively]in rat model of ischemia-reperfusion.
Conclussion: These result suggest that, Ang II plays a major role in IR-induced myocardial injury.. The therapeutic success of these drugs is related to their unique pharmacological profile involving both a reduction of plasma and tissue Ang II concentrations and blockage of Ang II harmful effects by $AT_1$ receptor.

## P - 351

Psychopharmacological Issues in Latin America

Pacheco Hernandez A.
Central University Of Venezuela

Psychopharmacology in Latinamericans patients is a young clinical and research issue. Although the use of psychotropic medication to treat hispanic patients was already reported in the 1930s, scientifically rigorous clinical research in this area did not appear until the 1970s. Broad based enthusiam among practitioners for psychopharmacological treatment in patients did not really emerge until the beginning of the 1980s. Most psychiatrists assume that primary and secondary effects of medication are similar across races and cultures. This paper will review the scientific literature and sound clinical and ethical standars that appears to show that the use of psychopharmacological drugs is related with a diversity of cultural issues in Latinamerican countries. Prescribing and adherence to treatment are influenced by particular cultural factors. To be sensitive about these aspects will result in a better acceptance of treatment and better quality of psychiatric care.

## P - 352

Higher Methadone Maintenance Doses are Associated with a Longer Stay in Methadone Maintenance Therapy

[1]Dickinson G.L., [1]Rostami-Hodjegan A., [2]Pratt P., [1]Lennard M.S.
[1]Molecular Pharmacology & Pharmacogenetics, University of Sheffield, [2]Community Health Sheffield (CHS) Substance Misuse Services, Sheffield

Background: The average methadone maintenance (MMT) dose is currently around 50mg/day in the UK. However, it has been shown that a higher dose is associated with increased effectiveness and retention in treatment. The latter is associated with a decreased chance of a return to illicit opioid use. This study aimed to explore a possible link between the length of time in MMT (LTMMT) and dose, by analysing a large database of methadone prescriptions. Methods: For the purpose of this study, we used the Community Health Sheffield (CHS) Substance Misuse Service to identify patients who entered and left the service during the six year period (5,085 prescriptions, 301 patients) using Microsoft Access®. The relationship between the various measures of dosage and LTMMT was investigated by correlation analysis using Microsoft Excel®. Results: The dosage measures correlated significantly with LTMMT ($r = 0.15 - 0.33$, $p < 0.01$). The best correlation was with the "maximum dose". The regression between the "average dose" and LTMMT indicated that for every extra mg of methadone given, the patients had remained on MMT for an additional 2.7 days (95% CI = 1.6 - 3.8 days). The corresponding value for the "maximum dose" was 3.3 days (95% CI = 2.2 - 4.4 days). Discussion and Conclusions: A higher dose was shown to be associated with a longer stay in MMT. However, as only 11% of the variation in the length of stay is related to methadone dose, the importance of the other aspects of treatment (counselling/rehabilitation etc) should also be considered for the successful maintenance of patients[6].

## P - 353

Reversal of the Oxidative Organ Damages and Dysfunction Due to Chronic Nicotine Administration by Melatonin in the Rat

[1]Şener G., [1]Kapucu C., [1]Paskaloğlu K., [1]Ayanoğlu-Dülger G., [2]Alican İ.
Marmara University [1]School of Pharmacy, Dept. of Pharmacology; [2]School of Medicine, Dept. Physiology; Istanbul/ Turkey

Introduction:Nicotine, a major toxic component of cigarette smoke, has long been recognized to result in oxidative stress by inducing the generation of reactive oxygen species. Based on the potent antioxidant effects of melatonin, we investigated the putative protective role of melatonin against nicotine-induced oxidative organ damage. Materials and Methods: Wistar Albino rats were injected i.p. with nicotine hydogen bitartarate (75 g/kg daily for 21 days) or saline. Melatonin (10 mg/kg, i.p.) was administered alone or with nicotine injections for 21 days. After decapitation penis and thoracic aorta were dissected. Corporeal tissues and aorta were used for contractility studies and for the measurement of malondialdehyde (MDA); an index of lipid peroxidation and glutathione (GSH); a key antioxidant, levels. Results: In control rats phenylephrine added cumulatively caused a concentration dependent contraction in corpus cavernosum strips and aorta rings precontracted with KCl, and acetylcholine added to the same tissue precontracted with phenylephrine caused dose dependent relaxation response. In nicotine treated group, the contraction and relaxation response of both tissues decreased significantly compared with controls. Melatonin treatment reversed these responses. Aorta and corporeal MDA levels in the nicotine group were significantly increased ($p<0.001$) with concomitant decreases in GSH levels ($p<0.01$-$p<0.001$), when compared to control group. On the other hand, melatonin treatment significantly reversed ($p<0.001$) the elevations in MDA levels, while reduced GSH levels were increased back to control levels ($p<0.01$-$p<0.001$).
Conclusions: The results of the present study indicate that melatonin, by its antioxidant effect, prevented the nicotine-induced oxidative damage and reversed the low contractile / relaxant responses of rat corporeal and aortic tissues.

## P - 354

Studies Concerning the Gastric Damage Induced by Alendronate Sodium and Protective Effects of Melatonin and Omeprazole Against This Damage

[1]Şener G., [2]Gören F., [1]Ayanoğlu-Dülger G.
[1]Marmara University, School of Pharmacy, Department of Pharmacology, Haydarpaşa, & [2]Eczacıbaşı Drug Company, Turkey

Introduction: Alendronate(AL) is a commonly used bisphosphonate against bone resorption,but causes adverse GI effects. In this study we aimed to investigate if free radicals have any role in the damage induced by AL and if melatonin (Mel) or Omeprazole (Omp) are protective against this damage. AL was administered orally and ip to determine if the gastric damage is a result of local irritation or if there is another reason for the damage. Materials and Methods: Wistar albino rats of either sex were administered, following an overnight fast, 20mg/kg AL by gavage for 4 days either alone or following treatment with Mel or Omep. Study was performed on 6 groups of animals; 1.Control, 2. Starvation 3.AL (po) 4.Mel(10 mg/kg,ip)+AL(po), 5.Omep( 20 M/kg, po)+AL(po), 6.AL (ip), On the last day of the study, following drug administration, pilor ligation was performed and 2h later, rats were killed stomachs removed, gastric acidity and tissue ulcer index values, as well as lipid peroxidation (LPO), glutathione (GSH) levels and myeloperoxidase (MPO) activity of the tissues were determined. Results: Chronic oral administration of AL induced significant gastric damage, and LPO and MPO increased while tissue GSH levels decreased significantly. Treatment with Omep, or Mel prevented this gastric damage as well as the increases in LPO and MPO and the decrease in GSH levels. However, ip administration of AL did not appear to cause much gastric irritation, and did not increase the acidity.
Conclusion: The present study suggests that AL induces gastric damage mainly by a local irritant effect,and that Mel and Omep are protective against this damage by their antioxidant properties.

## P - 355

Investigation of the Effects of Melatonin Treatment on Streptozotocin (STZ)-Induced Diabetic Rat Corpus Cavernosum in Vitro

Paskaloglu K., Şener G., Ayanoğlu-Dülger G.
Marmara University, School of Pharmacy, Department of Pharmacology, Haydarpaşa, Istanbul, Turkey

Introduction: Diabetes Mellitus is a contributing cause of erectile dysfunction which is associated with increased reactive oxygen species (ROS). This study was designed to determine the possible protective effect of melatonin (Mel) and/or insulin (Ins) treatment on the functional and biochemical changes caused by hyperglycemia induced oxidative damage in the corpus cavernosum of STZ diabetic rats.
Materials and Methods: Wistar albino rats of both sexes were subjected to streptozotocin (STZ, 65 mg/kg ip) to induce diabetes. Mel (10 mg/kg ip) and /or Ins (6U/kg sc) were administered for 8 weeks.
Results: Endothelium dependent relaxations induced by acetylcholine (Ach 10-8-10-3M) in the corpus cavernosum precontacted with phenylephrine were significantly attenuated in the diabetic group, but the relaxations induced by sodium nitroprusside and papaverin were not changed. Phenylephrine (10-8-10-3M) induced contractile responses of the corpus cavernosum were also reduced. Impaired relaxation and contractile responses were restored by treatment with the combination treatment whereas Mel or Ins alone have provided limited protection. GSH levels which significantly decreased in diabetes were elevated to control levels in the group treated with Mel and Ins combination, and the Mel group, whereas treatment with Ins alone provided only a limited protection. The increase in MDA levels observed after diabetes were also prevented by treatment with the Mel and Ins combination or the Mel group.
Conclusion: Diabetic state enhances the generation of free radicals and both Mel and Ins treatment reduce this oxidative stress. Thus our results suggested that supplementing diabetic patients with adjuvant therapy of melatonin may have some benefit for controlling diabetic complications.

## P - 356

A Population Model of Dexecadotril and Racecadotril Pharmacokinetics in Healthy Adults and Children with Diarrhoea.

[1]Dartois C., [2]Ben Becher S., [3]Pons G., [4]Thebault J.J., [5]Denis E., [5]Robert P., [5]de Paillette L., [6]Tod M.
[1]Pharmacy, Avicenne Hospital, [2] Pediatric Hospital, Tunis, [3]Pharmacology, Cochin-St-Vincent de Paul Hospital, [4]Aster Institute, [5]Bioprojet, [6]Pharmacy, Cochin-St-Vincent de Paul Hospital, AP-HP, Paris, France.

Until now Tiorfan®, an enkephalinase inhibitor, was used under racemic form (racecadotril), as an intestinal antisecretory agent for treating acute diarrhoea. Dexecadotril, the most specific enantiomer, is under development. A study was performed in children and adults to compare dexecadotril and racecadotril pharmacokinetics. Children ($n = 25$, 3 months to four years, body weight 4.9 to 15 kg) with diarrhoea were treated per os with 1.5 mg/kg of a solution of racecadotril or dexecadotril. Adult healthy volunteers ($n = 24$) received a 100 mg capsule of racecadotril and a 150 mg tablet of dexecadotril in cross-over. A population pharmacokinetic modelling approach allowed to describe adequately drugs disposition by a one-compartment model with two absorption phases, two lag-times and the same absorption rate constant for both phases. The absorption rate was the same for both drugs when given as a solution, greater for racecadotril capsule and even greater for dexecadotril tablet. Their median apparent clearance (CL/F) were in the reverse order (5.13, 2.88 and 1.50 l.h-1.kg-1 respectively). This may be due to differences in F due to drug formulation (tablet > capsule > solution) or physiological status (lower F in case of diarrhoea) but also to a larger CL in children than in adults. Consequently, the mean AUC of racecadotril and dexecadotril for a 1.5 mg/kg dose in children with diarrhoea were similar (903 and 807 nM.h respectively) but lower than that in healthy adults. Clinical efficacy of the two drugs in children was not significantely different. Hence, dexecadotril doses of 1.5 mg/kg in children and 75 mg in adults seem appropriate.

## P - 357

A Pharmacokinetic-Pharmacodynamic (PK-PD) Study of Racecadotril and Dexecadotril in Healthy Adults

[1]Dartois C., [2]Pons G., [3]Denis E., [4]Thebault J.J., [3]de Paillette L., [5]Tod M.
[1]Pharmacy, Avicenne Hospital, [2]Pharmacology, Cochin-St-Vincent de Paul Hospital, [3]Bioprojet, [4]Aster Institute, [5]Pharmacy, Cochin-St-Vincent de Paul Hospital, AP-HP, Paris, France

Racecadotril (Rac, [R,S] acetorphan, Tiorfan®) is an enkephalinase inhibitor used as an intestinal antisecretion drug in acute diarrhoea. The most specific enantiomer dexecadotril (Dex, [R]acetorphan) is under development. Twenty-four adult volunteers were treated in 4- way cross over with a 100 mg capsule of Rac or a 37.5, 75 and 150 mg tablet of Dex per os. Concentrations of the active metabolites ([R,S] or [R] thiorphan) and % inhibition of enkephalinase in plasma were measured until 24h after dosing. A population modelling approach allowed to describe jointly PK and PD using NONMEM. A one-compartment model with two absorption phases, two lag-times and the same absorption rate constant for both phases was the most adequate. The kinetics of Dex were found to be linear in the dose range studied. The absorption rate of Dex was twice larger than that of Rac. The median V/F and CL/F of Dex were 1.56 times lower than that of Rac, probably owing to a larger bioavailability of Dex tablets. A Hill effect model was fitted to PD data. The effect-vs-plasma concentration relationship was the same for the two drugs (median IC50: 128 nM, interindividual CV 31%). The maximal effect was reached in 0.5 to 2h and half the maximum 2 to 3h later. Based on the mean & SD 0-8h area under effect vs time simulated curve at steady state (the most clinically relevant parameter), 100 mg of Rac were equivalent to 75 mg of Dex (430 & 106 vs 426 & 99 %.h).

## P - 358

The Effect of Methadone on Mood State is Shorter Than its Effect on Subjective Opiate Withdrawal Score in Patients Undergoing Methadone Maintenance Therapy (MMT)

[1]Shiran M.R., [1]Rostami-Hodjegan A., [1]Lennard M.S., [2]Iqbal M.Z., [2]Lagundoye O., [2]Seivewright N., [1]Tucker G.T.
[1]Molecular Pharmacology & Pharmacogenetics, University of Sheffield, [2]Community Health Sheffield (CHS) Substance Misuse Services, Sheffield, UK

Background: The "Total Mood Disturbance" (TMD) scale and the "Subjective Opiate Withdrawal Scale" (SOWS) have both been used to assess the pharmacodynamic effect of methadone. The main aim of this study was to compare the time profile of these scores following daily methadone dosage. In addition, the correlation between SOWS and the "Objective Opiate Withdrawal Scale" (OOWS) was investigated.
Methods: MMT patients (17 Male, 14 Female; 27-49 y; 29 Caucasian; daily dose 20-130 mg) completed the relevant scoring sheets on five occasions (1 before and 4 after methadone dosage) over 10 h. A specialist registrar completed the data sheet for OOWS up to 5 h post dose. TMD, SOWS and OOWS scores were calculated and compared with baseline values (paired t-test, SPSS ver.10). Results: Significant decreases ($p<0.04$) were observed in TMD, SOWS and OOWS scores following methadone dosage up to 5 h. The TMD score returned to the baseline by 10 h after the dose while the SOWS score remained significantly below baseline ($p = 0.001$). There was no significant correlation between individual SOWS and OOWS.
Discussion and Conclusions: The observation of a significant mood change in MMT patients after methadone dosage is similar to previous findings. However, the duration of this effect was shorter than the effect of methadone in stabilising withdrawal symptoms. Thus, once daily dose of methadone, may not be adequate to improve mood disturbances in some patients. The lack of correlation between the SOWS ( reflecting the patient's experience ) and the OOWS ( reflecting the view of the independent observer ) indicates the need for simultaneous assessment of both components as part of patient evaluation in opiate withdrawal.

## ORAL

Lamivudine Combined with Corticosteroids in Prolonged Acute Hepatitis

Kosseva B.O., Jelev D., Spasova Z., Avramova B., Krastev Z.
University Hospital St. Ivan Rilski, Clinic of Gastroenterology, Sofia, Bulgaria

Lamivudine is the nucleoside analog and potent inhibitor of HBV - replication. We report the use of lamivudine combined with corticosteroids in two patients with acute hepatitis B, with prolonged progression, persistent high aminotransferase levels - 15 times above the norm, severe hyperbilirubinemia and progressive deterioration of both clinical and biochemical features. They received 100 mg lamivudine daily and short term administration of corticosteroid in gradually tapered doses. The patients tolerated the therapy well. Liver function tests/LFT/ normalized within 9 weeks and HbeAg seroconvestion took place. During the 9 months follow up after the end of lamivudine therapy in one of the patients HbsAg was negative and all liver tests were normal. In the other patient till the end of 4 month all LFT were in referent ranges. Transaminases increased 1,5 time above the norm during the 5 and 6 month and again were normal in 7-9 months. In all controls HBV DNA was undetectable. Our report indicate that combined antiinflamatatory and antiviral short therapy might be a promising therapeutic approach in selected patients with acute hepatitis B. Further observations are needed.
Key words: acute hepatitis B, lamivudine, corticosteroids.

## ORAL

The Impact of Unlicensed and Off-Labeled Drug Use on Adverse Drug Reactions in Pediatric Patients

Neubert A.
Department of Experimental and Clinical Pharmacology and Toxicology, University Erlangen, Germany

Objective : Many drugs used to treat children are either not licensed for use (unlicensed) or prescribed outside the terms of the product license (off-labeled). The incidence of adverse drug reactions (ADRs) associated with the use of such drugs remains to be established. The present study investigates the impact of unlicensed and off-labeled drug use on ADRs on a pediatric ward.
Design and settings : An 8-month prospective pharmaco-epidemiological survey was conducted on a 10-bed pediatric ward. All patients were intensively monitored for ADRs by a pharmaco-epidemiological team. All drug administrations were evaluated retrospectively as to unlicensed or off-labeled use on the basis of the product information. Results : A total of 178 patients was included in the study. 156 patients received 740 drugs (i.e. 3 per patient). In 198 cases (27.7% of all prescriptions) drugs were used in either an unlicensed (3) or off-labeled (195) manner. Within this study population a total of 46 ADRs was observed in 31 patients (17.8%). ADRs were associated with 29 (5.6%) of the 519 licensed drug prescriptions and with 12 (6.1%) of the 198 unlicensed or off-labeled drug prescriptions. ($p<0.05$) The majority of ADRs caused by unlicensed or off-labeled drugs were recognized by the attending physician.
Conclusion : In summary, the present study shows a high incidence of ADRs in pediatric patients with no significant difference in the incidence rates caused by licensed or unlicensed and off-labeled drugs

## P - 359

The Economic Impact of Adverse Drug Reactions and Readmissions in Medical Gastroenterology

Dormann,Harald
Department of Medicine I University Hospital Erlangen-Nuremberg, Erlangen, Germany

Recent studies show that nearly half of the hospitalized patients are readmitted within six month from discharge. No data exist about the relationship between adverse drug reactions and readmittance.
Methods A cohort based, prospective, 18 month survey was conducted in the department of gastroenterology at the University Hospital of Erlangen. All ADRs were intensively monitored by a team of physicians and pharmacists and classified by WHO-ART. During a 6 month period ADR-positive patients were matched to non ADR patients applying diagnosis-related group categorization (DRG) in order to measure the impact of ADRs on the duration and frequency of hospitalization, Results Of 1000 admissions 424 patients had single admissions and 206 patients had recurrent readmissions (min 1, max 9). The prevalence of readmissions was 37 % (n=370). In 145 (23 %) out of 630 patients 305 ADRs were observed. ADRs caused hospitalizations in 5.7 % of first admissions and in 2.9 % of readmissions. According to the Schumock algorithm 135 (44.3 %) ADRs were found to be preventable. The ADR incidence was similar in first admissions and readmissions. ADRs had not been found to predict further readmissions and lack of ADRs had not been found to preclude readmissions. The occurrence and numbers of ADRs per admission were found to prolong hospitalization period significantly ($r=0.48$; $r=0.51$; $p<0.001$; $n=135$). Out of 9107 treatment days 11 % (>973 days) were caused by preventable ADRs in admissions and readmissions. Conclusions Intensified drug monitoring is essential for early detecting and prevention of ADRs and saving hospital resources.

## P - 360

Pharmacokinetics of Gabapentin in Neonates and During Lactation

[1]Öhman I., [1]Vitols S., [2]Tomson T.
Department of Medicine, divisions of [1]Clinical Pharmacology and [2]Clinical Neuroscience, Karolinska Hospital, Stockholm, Sweden

Purpose: To investigate the pharmacokinetics of gabapentin (GBP) in the neonatal period and during lactation.
Methods: GBP concentrations in plasma and breast milk were analysed with high-performance liquid chromatography (HPLC) in two women with epilepsy treated with gabapentin, and in their offspring. Samples were obtained at delivery, the first days after birth and at breastfeeding at two weeks or three months postpartum.
Results: Maternal GBP plasma concentration in the first patient was 30 µmol/L at delivery. GBP plasma levels in the newborn declined rather rapidly. At 24 h the concentration was 45 % lower than the GBP level at 6 h postpartum. At sampling before dose intake two weeks after delivery the milk/plasma concentration ratio was 0.7. In the second patient, GBP level in the umbilical cord was 61 µmol/L and the concentration in the neonate was 5 µmol/L at 48 h postpartum. Three months after parturition maternal plasma level was 45 µmol/L before nursing and a simultaneously taken milk sample was 51 µmol/L. The milk/plasma concentration ratio was 1.1. The infant's plasma concentrations were below the quantification limit.
Conclusions: Our limited observations suggest extensive excretion of GBP into breast-milk and that newborns seem to have a reasonable capacity to eliminate GBP. No adverse effects were observed in the infants.

## P - 361

Allele and Genotype Frequencies of Polymorphic CYP2C9 and CYP2C19 in the Beninese and Belgian Populations

Allabi A.C., Gala J.L., Desager J.P., Heusterspreute M., Horsmans Y.
Clinical Pharmacology Unit, St Luc University Hospital (UCL), Brussels, Belgium

AIMS This study was carried out to investigate the distribution of cytochrome P450 CYP2C9 and CYP2C19 in the Beninese population and to compare it with the distribution in the Belgian Caucasian population. METHODS 111 Beninese and 121 Belgian Caucasians were genotyped for CYP2C9*2, CYP2C9*3, CYP2C9*4, CYP2C9*5, CYP2C9*11, CYP2C19*2, CYP2C19*3. Genotyping was performed by using either the single- tube tetra-primer PCR assay method (CYP2C9*2, CYP2C19*2 and CYP2C19*3) and by sequence analysis (CYP2C9*3, CYP2C9*4, CYP2C9*5 and CYP2C9*11 alleles). RESULTS In the Beninese and Belgian subjects, distribution of the CYP2C9 alleles was as follows: CYP2C9*1: 95.5 vs 82.2%; CYP2C9*2: 0 vs 10%; CYP2C9*3: 0 vs 7.4%; CYP2C9*4: 0 vs 0%; CYP2C9*5: 1.8 vs 0%; and CYP2C9*11: 2.7 vs 0.4%; respectively. CYP2C19*2 alleles was found in 13 vs 9.1%, respectively whereas the CYP2C19*3 allele was found neither in the Beninese nor in the Belgian group. CONCLUSIONS These data highlight the distribution of CYP2C9 and CYP2C19 alleles in the Beninese population. Significant differences are observed between the Beninese and Belgian groups for the CYP2C9*2, *3, *5 and *11. No significant difference is observed for CYP2C9*4 nor for the CYP2C19*2 and *3. Such differences could have important clinical implications with regards to numerous drugs.

## ORAL

Incidence of Cytochrome-P450-polymorphisms in Geriatric Patients and Their Association with Adverse Drug Reactions

Tobias E.
Institut of Pharmacology and Toxicology, Erlangen, Germany

Objective: It has been established that 1-23 % of the population, according to ethnic background, has genetically determined differences in metabolizing drugs through the cytochrome-enzymes CYP2C9, CYP2C19 and CYP2D6. Limited data exist about these polymorphisms and their relationship to adverse drug reactions (ADRs) in geriatric patients.
Main Outcome Measures: In a prospective 6-month cohort study of 243 patients of a geriatric rehabilitation ward, mean age 80.0±7.2 yrs. ADRs were identified by a pharmacoepidemiological team, consisting of pharmacists and physicians by intensive monitoring. Out of these 243 Caucasian patients 125 were genotyped for polymorphisms of CYP2C9, CYP2C19 and CYP2D6 by TaqMan-polymerase chain reaction. Genotype frequencies were compared in ADR-positive and ADR-negative patients.
Results: Patients received an average of 14 drugs during hospitalization which led to 251 ADRs in 144 of 243 patients (59.1%). Genotype frequencies of CYP2C9 were 25.9% Intermediate Metabolizers (IM) (n=29) and 2.7% Poor Metabolizers (PM) (n=3). For the enzyme CYP2C19 26.8% IMs (n=33) and 0.8% PMs (n=1) were detected. CYP2D6-IMs occurred in 24.1% (n=26), -PMs in 3.7% (n=4). The genotype did not differ significantly in ADR-positive and ADR-negative patients.
Conclusion: Geriatric patients show a high ADR-incidence in this survey. However, no association between the ADR-rate and the patients´ genotype could be found, which may be most commonly due to the low amount of blood samples. Otherwise the genotype frequencies detected in this survey are typical for the Caucasian population.

## P - 362

The Relative Sensitivity of the Metabolic Ratios of CYP2D6 Probes (Debrisoquine (DB), Dextromethorphan (DM) And Metoprolol (MP)) to Urine pH.

[1]Özdemir M., [1]Aktan Y., [2]Rostami-Hodjegan A., [2]Crewe K.H., [2]Tucker G.T.
[1]Dept. Pharmacology, Faculty of Medicine, Osmangazi University, Eskişehir, Turkey [2]Molecular Pharmacology & Pharmacogenetics, University of Sheffield, UK

Background: Urinary drug/metabolite ratios (MR) of DB, DM and MP are used to assess CYP2D6 activity non-invasively in vivo. However, these indices are potentially confounded by the effect of renal function. The aim of this study was to assess the effect of changes in urinary pH on the MRs of DB (polar base) and DM and MP (lipophilic bases).
Methods: Three groups of healthy volunteers each comprising 12 individuals were given either DB (10mg), DM (25mg) or MP (100mg). The probe drugs were administered on 3 occasions separated by 10 day intervals - when the urine was acidified by taking ammonium chloride, when it was alkalinized by ingestion of sodium bicarbonate and when urine pH was uncontrolled. A randomized cross-over design was used. Results: The geometric mean MR for DB was not significantly different in any of the study arms while those for MP and DM were significantly different under acidified or alkalinised urine conditions compared to control ($p < 0.005$, see Table).
Discussion: Under conditions of uncontrolled urine pH the ability to mark CYP2D6 activity accurately with DM and MP may be compromised. Variability in urine pH may also confound genotype-phenotype correlation within subtypes of extensive metabolisers2. Being polar, DB is not subject to pH-dependent renal reabsorption and may be a more robust marker of CYP2D6 than DM or MP.

Table- Relative MR values (95% CI) compared to uncontrolled urine (* significantly different from 1)

| | DB | MP | DX |
|---|---|---|---|
| Acidified Urine | 1.3 (0.9 – 1.8) | 0.4 (0.3 – 0.5)* | 0.13 (0.05 – 0.35)* |
| Alkalinized Urine | 1.3 (0.9 – 2.0) | 3.4 (1.6 – 7.1)* | 4.5 (2.4 – 8.7)* |

## P - 363

The Role of Nitric Oxide in Iron-Induced Rat Renal Injury

Kadkhodaee M., Gol A., Keshavarz M., Shams S., Aryamanesh S.
Department of Physiology, Faculty of Medicine, Tehran Medical Sciences University, Tehran, Iran

Iron overload and enhanced hydroxyl radical formation have been implicated as the causative factors of oxidative stress in different organs. Both prooxidant and antioxidant properties have been reported for nitric oxide (NO) in iron-mediated oxidative stress. To determine the contribution of NO to iron-induced renal injury, 8 groups of rats (8 in each group) were studied as follows: Control (normal saline), L-Arg (l-arginine as a substrate of NO synthase, 400mg/kg), L-NAME (an inhibitor of NO synthase, 8mg/kg), Fe (iron dextran, 600mg/kg), DFO (deferroxamine as a chelator of iron, 150mg/kg), Fe+L-Arg, Fe+L-NAME, DFO+L-Arg. 24 hours after the injections, blood samples were taken and kidneys removed for biochemical analysis and histological assays. Plasma creatinine and urea were used to stimate renal function. Renal tissue and plasma vitamin E levels, the most important endogenous fat soluble antioxidant, were measured by HPLC and UV detection. In this study, renal function was markedly reduced in Fe group compared to controls (creatinine, 1.02 ±0.05 mg/dl vs 0.78 ±0.04 $p<0.05$; urea, 49.59±1.69 mg/dl vs 40.75 ±0.86, $p<0.01$). Vitamin E levels were significantly lower in Fe group compared to controls (plasma $p<0.01$; tissue $p<0.05$). L-NAME increased iron toxicity significantly while L-Arg showed no effects on both control and Fe-treated groups. As a conclusion, NO synthase blockade enhances iron-mediated renal toxicity in this model.

## P - 364

A Randomized Comparison of Venlafaxine and Fluoxetine For Anxiety Side Effect in the Early Stage of Antidepressant Therapy

[1]Sağlam E., [2]Mırsal H., [2]Beyazyürek M., [3]Sur H.
[1]Maltepe University, Faculty of Medicine, Department of Pharmacology and Clinical Pharmacology, [2]Maltepe University, Faculty of Medicine, Department of Psychiatry, [3]Marmara University, Faculty of Healt Education, Department of Healt Management

Introduction: Within 2-3 weeks after starting the therapy with antidepressant drugs, the level of the receptors responsible for the antidepressant effects of the drug shows adaptive changes in a true manner. At the same time, the acute effects of the antidepressant drugs specially in synaptic gap cause anxiety side effects. In this trial our aim was to make a comparative study between venlafaxine (serotonin -norepinephrine reuptake inhibitor-SNRI) and fluoxetine (selective serotonin reuptake inhibitor-SSRI) concerning their anxiety side effects, which usually occur in the early stage of the therapy.
Methods: The outpatietns who met DSM-IV criteria for major depressive disorder were given (n=20 venlafaxine: 75 mg/day, n=20 fluoxetine: 20mg/day). The patients were randomly assigned. The antidepressant effects and anxiety side-affect outcome measures were the final ratings on Hamilton Rating Scala for Depression (HAM-D) and Hamilton Rating Scala for Anxiety (HAM-A). These tests were applied when a patient visited the clinic for the first time and later on at the end of first, second, and third weeks.
Results: In our study, both venlafaxine and fluoxetine are significantly increased anxiety in the first three weeks. When compared with each other, the anxiogenic side effect of venlafaxine group was found significantly lower fluoxetine group.

## P - 365

Application of a Modified Two-Portion Absorption Model to Famotidine Plasma Concentrations with Double Peaks or Irregular Shaped Single Peaks

[1]Yin O.Q.P., [2]Tomlinson B., [1]Chow A.H.L., [1]Chow M.S.S.
[1]School of Pharmacy and [2]Dept. of Medicine & Therapeutics, Faculty of Medicine, The Chinese University of Hong Kong, Shatin, N. T., Hong Kong

Purpose: The pharmacokinetics of oral drugs exhibiting erratic or double absorption peaks cannot be adequately characterized by using conventional compartmental models. We have previously proposed a modified two-portion absorption model based on physiological and biopharmaceutical considerations to describe the double-peak concentration-time curve of ranitidine. The present study is to further evaluate the utility and applicability of this model.
Methods: The model assumes that a given oral dose of drug is absorbed sequentially in two portions due to delayed gastric emptying and variable gastrointestinal motility, thus a gut compartment was incorporated in addition to the conventional two (central and peripheral) compartments. Plasma famotidine concentrations (PFC) from 26 subjects following a single 40 mg oral dose were utilized for model testing.
Results: All plasma famotidine data of the 26 subjects that exhibited double peaks and irregular shaped single peaks were well described by the model. The PFC predicted by the model correlated with the observed values, with R averaging 0.994 ± 0.004 and 0.991 ± 0.005 for the double and single peaks respectively. The model generated parameters $t_{1/2\beta}$, CL/F, Vc/F and Vss/F were in agreement with the literature values, and the estimates of $C_{max}$, $t_{max}$ and AUC were also close to those calculated by standard non-compartmental method.
Conclusions: Our proposed modified two-portion absorption model is versatile and useful for describing plasma drug concentrations with either distinct double peaks or irregular shaped single peaks.
Key words: modified two-portion absorption model, double-peak, famotidine

## P - 366

Antibiotics Consumption in Hungarian Hospitals 1996-2002

Matuz M., Nagy G., Soos Gy.
University of Szeged, Department of Clinical Pharmacy, MIS Consulting Ltd,Budapest, Hungary

Background:.The introduction and maintenance of rational antibiotic policy needs continuos critical analysis. In Hungary, similarly to the other Euoropean countries in the last couple of years many efforts were made to improve the antibacterial treatment. This countrywide survey intends to show the potential changes on hospital antibiotics consumption in the last seven years, to assess the effectiveness of the interventions.
Method: According to the WHO ATC/DDD methodology the drug use was expressed in DDD/100 bed-day unit. The raw consumption data were given from a wholesaler database, the source of patient's turnover data is the national health statistics.
Results: The continuous slight decreasing tendency (19,92 vs.18,65) could be seen during the investigated period with important alteration of the used drug groups. Decreasing consumption was found in the next groups: J01A:2,85 vs.091 -tetracyclines-, J01DA: 3,4 vs.2,91 -cephalosporins-,J01E: 2,86 vs.1,43 -sulfonamides and trimethoprim-, J01G: 1,14 vs.0,57 -aminoglycosides -, but in the other groups - J01C penicillins,J01DH carbapenems,J01FA macrolides, J01FF lincosamid, J01M quinolones and J01XA glycopepides - increasing tendency could be seen. Assessing the effect of the antibiotic policy of the university teaching hospitals on the sorrounding geographical area the consumption of four questionable counties was compared with the national average level.Two of them were regularly higher, the other two lower than the comparator. Discussion/conclusion: The Hungarian hospital antibiotic use seems lower than was found by other authors in similar settings (Croatia, Czech Republic, Karolinska Hospital, Smolensk etc.), but it should be emphasised that our results reflected to the national average. This general picture is positive, but it may cover hidden bias.

## P - 367

Phenytoin Metabolic Ratio (PMR) Correlates with Formation Clearance of (S)-7-OH-Warfarin

Adar L., Bialer M., Blotnick S., Caraco Y.
The Hebrew University of Jerusalem, Tel Aviv, Israel

The response to warfarin (W) and its pharmacokinetics are characterized by marked interindividual variation. Genetic polymorphisms in the gene encoding for CYP2C9, the isoform responsible for the formation of W major metabolite, (S)-7-OH-warfarin (S7OHW), account for much of this variability. CYP2C9 is also the major enzyme involved in phenytoin (PHT) metabolism and PMR defined as the ratio of 5-(4-hydroxyphenyl)-5-phenylhydantoin (p-HPPH) content in a 24 hours urine collection to mid-interval plasma PHT concentration has been validated as a useful marker of CYP2C9 activity in-vivo. The aim of this study was to examine correlation between PMR and formation clearance (CLf) of S7OHW in order to evaluate future use of PMR as a mode to predict W maintenance dose. CYP2C9 activity was evaluated by way of PMR in a cohort of patients prior to W initiation. Once stable anticoagulation was reached, the patients were required to collect urine over 24 hours and S7OHW CLf was derived from the ratio of S7OHW cumulative amount excreted in urine to plasma (S)-W concentration at the mid interval point after normalization to the body weight. Preliminary results indicate that PMR was significantly correlated with S7OHW CLf ($R=1$; $P<0.001$; $n=8$).In conclusion; CYP2C9 activity as evaluated by PMR is predictive of W oxidation to S7OHW. It remains to be evaluated weather W induction based on PMR may enhance the safety and efficacy of W loading. A.L. deeply acknowledges a partial travel grant by the David R. Bloom Center for Pharmacy at the Hebrew University of Jerusalem, in support of her participation in this conference.

## P - 368

Use of Antibiotics in Estonian Children Under 4 Years of Age

[1]Rootslane L., [2]Kiivet R.A., [3]Irs A.
[1]Department of Pharmacy, [2]Department of Public Health, [3]Division of Clinical Pharmacology, University of Tartu

The growing antibiotic resistance of pathogenic bacteria is an emerging problem worldwide, including Estonia. Misuse of antibiotics is one of the major determinants in its development. Overuse of antibiotics is a major problem in children. Upper respiratory tract infections are a common reason for an antibiotic prescription, in spite of the fact that most of these infections are of viral origin. The aim of the study was to analyse the use of antibiotics in the treatment of children under 4 years of age in Estonia. Antibiotics' prescription data of 2001 for children under 4 years old were obtained from the Estonian Health Insurance Fund database. Antibiotics covered more that 40% of all prescriptions of children. The most often prescribed antibiotic was amoxicillin, counting for about one third of all studied prescriptions for antibiotics, followed by the medicines containing erythromycin and combination of trimethoprim and sulfamethoxasol. The cephalosporins were used often, counting for 15% of all antibiotic prescriptions, but penicillin was used in negligible number of cases. The use of antibiotics was highest during the last quarter of the year and differed threefold between months. The average total consumption of antibiotics was similar in all counties of Estonia, but the choice of medicinal products differed slightly. To conclude, antibiotics were the most often prescribed medicines for children less than 4 years of age and broad-spectrum penicillins were the most widely used preparations.

## P - 369

Safety of Propiverine Hydrochloride in Patients with Glaucoma

Gatchev E., Petkova N., Rankova C., Vlahov V., Braeter M., de Mey C.
Dept.Clin.Pharmacol.Ther., Univ. Hospital Queen Giovanna, Sofia, Bulgaria

Introduction & objectives: Propiverine hydrochloride (PRO) is widely used for the treatment of overactive bladder. The ocular and systemic safety of PRO was investigated in patients with stable primary open-angle (POAG, treated with topical ?-blockers) and angle-closure glaucoma (PACG treated with pilocarpine ± previous laser therapy of glaucoma surgery). Material & methods: In each study, 24 patients, 38-75 years of age were investigated according to a randomised, placebo-controlled, double-blind, parallel-group study design, receiving either PRO (15 mg t.i.d) or placebo (PL / PRO:PL= 15:9) for one week. Intra-ocular pressure (IOP) and pupil diameter (PUD) were investigated throughout. Results In POAG-patients, PRO-treatment yielded a median systemic exposure of 241 ng/mL (range: 99-509) at 3:00 h after the 18th dose led to an increase in PUD (PRO-PL: 0.79 mm, 95% CI: 0.28 to 1.31) with no change in IOP (PRO-PL: 0.14 mmHg, 95% CI: -1.51 to 1.79). In PACG- patients , PRO yielded a median systemic exposure of 222 ng/mL (range: 104-419) led to a discrete non-significant rise in PUD (PRO- PL: 0.39 mm, CI: -0.23 to 1.01) with no change in IOP (PROP- PL: 0.42 mmHg, CI: -0.45 to 1.29) shortly after pilocarpine; at times of less pilocarpine penetration, a more distinct rise in PUD was seen (PRO-PL: 0.56: CI: 0.01 to 1.11), but a gain without rise in IOP (PRO-PL: -1.30, CI: -1.98 to 0.38). There were no signs or symptoms of glaucoma and no effects on visual acuity and accommodation at any time.
Conclusions: Treatment with PRO is safe and well tolerated in patients with stable POAG and PACG.

## P - 370

A New Ontology for Computerized Detection of Adverse Drug Reactions

Dormann N.
Dept. of Medicine I and Dept of Clinical and Experimental Pharmacology FAU Erlangen, Germany

Background and Aim: Using computerized methods for improving quality of drug therapy is limited due to missing standardization of patients data in hospital information systems and availability of non standardized medical knowledge only.
Methods: A computerized monitoring system (CMS) for the systematic detection of adverse drug reactions (ADRs) by abnormal laboratory tests (ALS) coded in LOINC (Laboratory Object Identifiers and Codes - international standard) was refined by implementation of a new drug database containing standardized information on ADRs expressed in 156 LOINC for 700 generic substances mapped to ATC. To apply patients laboratory tests to potential ADRs a novel ontology including the standardized drug database was implemented. Data collected on a prospective 6-month pharmacoepidemiological survey on a medical ward at the University Hospital Erlangen were used for the evaluation of the CMS.
Results: A total of 109 ADRs were detected in 474 admissions by intensive ADR monitoring. Out of 32861 laboratory tests 9043 ALS were observed. Using the novel ontology the amount of laboratory signals was reduced by CMS automatically to 3203 ALS of which 1340 were associated ADRs. The sensitivity of the CMS was 76 % - out of 76 ADR positive admissions 58 were identified by generated ALS - and the specificity was 53 % - out of 398 non ADR admissions in 211 cases no signal was generated by CMS.
Conclusion: This study shows that CMS enhanced by standardized drug database implemented in hospital information system could be a useful tool for the systematic detection of ADRs.

## P - 371

Epitestosterone Crucial in Doping Tests. Genetic Cause of Large Variation?

Jakobsson J., Ekström L., Garle M., Björkhem I., Rane A.
Department of Laboratorial Medicine at Karolinska Institute, Division of Clinical Pharmacology, Huddinge University Hospital, Stockholm, Sweden

Background : Epitestosterone (EpiT) is a naturally occurring 17α-hydroxy epimer of testosterone (T). To detect T abuse the urinary T/EpiT ratio is measured. According to the International Olympic Committee, a ratio above 6 is a strong indication of abuse of certain androgens including T. However, large inter-individual and inter-ethnic differences in this ratio have been detected. Occasionally constitutional T/EpiT ratios >6 have been found in Caucasian individuals. Asian people generally have lower T/EpiT ratios (< 0.5) than Caucasians (around 1). These differences are important to investigate since it has major implications for the interpretation of anti-doping test results. Androstenedione is a weak androgen that is converted to T in the body. In a few Caucasian individuals and in the majority of Asians, androstenedione administration is associated with an increase of EpiT levels in the urine. 3-Hydroxysteroid dehydrogenase (3α-HSD), an enzyme that plays a central role in steroid metabolism, is a likely candidate for this reaction. There are three types of 3α-HSD. They have similar (>80 %) amino acid sequences but different substrate specificities and tissue distribution.
Results : We have identified four polymorphisms in the 3α-HSD II gene, one in the promoter, two in exon 2 and one in the intron between exons 8 and 9. One of the mutations in exon 2 leads to a change of a glutamic acid to a glycine. The allele frequency of that mutation is 20 % in Caucasians and 1 % in Asians. The different phenotypes are currently investigated in bioassays and may be related to the observed difference in formation of EpiT.

## P - 372

Nonesterified Fatty Acids Induce Alterations of Haemodynamics in Humans

[1,2]Stojiljkovic M.P., [1]Mitchell J.M., [2]Zhang D., [2,3]Lopes H.F., [2]Lee C.G., [4]Goodfriend T.L., [2]Egan B.M.
[1]Department of Pharmacology and Toxicology, Military Medical Academy, Belgrade, Serbia and Montenegro; [2]Departments of Pharmacology & Medicine, Medical University of South Carolina, Charleston, SC, USA; [3]Unidade de Hipertensao-Heart Institute (InCor), HCFM-USP, Sao Paulo, Brazil; [4]Departments of Medicine and Pharmacology, William S. Middleton Veterans Memorial Hospital, University of Wisconsin, Madison, WI, USA

Nonesterified fatty acids (NEFAs), along with hypertension, dyslipidemia, abdominal obesity, glucose intolerance, hyperinsulinemia and non-insulin dependent diabetes mellitus play an important role in the cluster of risk factors for various cardiovascular disease, such as hypertension and atherosclerosis.
A group of 31 volunteers underwent a four-hour-long infusions of either 20% Intralipid or saline at 0.8 ml/m2/min and heparin (200-U bolus, followed by 1000 U/h) to raise plasma NEFAs. Heparin is a plasma phospholipase A2 activator that increases liberation of NEFAs from Intralipid.
Two and four hours after starting the infusions, plasma NEFAs increased by 134% and 111% in those receiving Intralipid and heparin, whereas plasma NEFAs did not change in the those volunteers who received saline and heparin. The infusion of Intralipid and heparin induced a significant increase in systolic (13.5 - 2.1 mmHg) and diastolic (8.0 - 1.5 mmHg) blood pressure (BP) as well as heart rate (9.4 - 1.4 bpm). In contrast, BP and heart rate did not change in same volunteers during a four-hour infusion of saline and heparin.
These data raise the possibility that lipid abnormalities associated with insulin resistance contribute to the elevated BP and heart rate observed in subjects with the cardiovascular risk factor cluster. It also might suggest that in some patients effective treatment of these lipid abnormalities could contribute to the overall success of antihypertensive therapy.

## P - 373

Comparison the Effects of Steroidal Therapy by Measuring Exhaled Carbon Monoxide (CO) in Bronchial Asthma and COPD.

[1]Bicak M., [2]Gul H., [1]Ozkan M., [2]Yildiz O., [1]Ekiz K., [3]Saygı Ş., [1]Demirci N.
Gülhane Military Medical Academy, Faculty of Medicine, [1]Department of Respiratory Medicine and [2]Pharmacology, [3]Toxicology 06018 Etlik, Ankara, Turkey

Background: Endogenous exhaled CO (ECO) concentrations may be clinically useful in the management and monitoring of oxidation and inflammatory mediated lung injury. ECO could be useful to evaluate the response to anti-inflammatory treatment in asthma. We evaluated the beneficial effects of steroidal therapy in bronchial asthma by measuring exhaled CO.
Methods: Twenty patients with bronchial asthma (BA) exacerbation and twenty with asthma in remission were treated with oral and/or inhaled steroidal therapy. CO was also measured in a group of healthy (smoking and non-smoking) and patients with chronic obstructive pulmonary disease (COPD). CO was measured by means of a chemical analyzer.
Results: CO values were higher in COPD and BA patients (either with exacerbation or not) than nonsmoking healthy individuals significantly (5.05±0.18, 5.15±0.17 and 2.12±0.07 ppm, respectively) ($P < 0.05$). In smoking healthy individuals, exhaled CO values were the highest (9.49±0.57, $P < 0.05$). After steroidal therapy, CO values were significantly reduced in BA groups ($P < 0.05$) but not in COPD patients. Forced expiratory volume-1 (FEV1) values were reduced in BA and COPD patients, but it was higher in BA groups than COPD ($P < 0.05$).
Conclusions: These results showed that exhaled CO values were a valuable method for assessing the beneficial effects of steroidal therapy in BA. Beneficial effects of steroidal therapy in COPD disease was minimal and not significant. Therefore, exhaled CO can be used for the monitoring of the treatment and in choosing of the drugs in BA. Measurement of exhaled CO concentrations may also be useful as a simple method in discrimination of the BA and COPD disease.

## P - 374

### A New Role for Application of Botulinum Toxin (BT) Injection in Patients with Idiopathic Chalasia:A Case-Control Study

Mikaeli J., Yaghoobi M., Montazeri G., Nouri N., Malekzadeh R.
Achalasia Research Unit, Digestive Disease Research Center, Tehran University of Medical Sciences, Iran

The role of BT in the treatment of achalasia is unclear. In this study we aimed at evaluating this role in enhancing the efficacy of PD with 30 mm balloon.Patients treated with BT before PD with 30 mm balloon as well as age and sex-matched controls treated only with PD were enrolled in the study. Symptomatic scores before and one month and each 6 months after PD were measured. Whenever the score exceeds more than 50% of the initial one, it was considered as a relapse.

12 cases [4 males, 8 females, mean age: 40.3 (10-70) yrs] and 12 sex and age-matched controls were enrolled. At the end of the follow-up period, one of the patients in the case group relapsed after 30 months after PD but the others were in remission. In control group all the patients relapsed after the mean period of 12.6 months and needed a 35 mm balloon dilatation. The cumulative remission rate was significantly higher in case group as compared to control group ($p<0.01$). The mean symptom score had a 76% decrease in case group ($p<0.001$) and 53% in controls ($p<0.01$) at the end of first month. Among the factors evaluated at the initial presentation (age, sex, duration of symptoms and severity of symptoms), none were predictive of response to treatment.

It seems that BT is a meaningful enhancing factor in the long-term efficacy of PD. PD with 30 mm balloon after a BT session could resolve the need for the future higher grade PD to some extent and reduce the perforation risk in procedures with higher-diameter balloons.

## P - 375

### Adverse Events after 24 Month Treatment with Betaferon in Patients with Multiple Sclerosis

[1]Kostadinova I., [2]Manova M., [2]Vasileva T., [2]Trenova A.
[1]Department of Pharmacology, Clinical Pharmacology and drug toxicology, [2]Department of neurology - Medical University, Plovdiv

A prospective, non-randomized, open trial study of adverse events /AE/ during Betaferon treatment was carried out on patients with Relapsing-Remitting Multiple sclerosis. /RRMS/. The aim was to assess AE that have been described up to the 24 month of the treatment with Betaferon. A total of 35 / 22 female, 13 male, average age - 35,97±1,6/ patients were studied, all of them selected in accordance with the criteria for Betaferon treatment eligibility. Betaferon 8 MIU was applied SC in the morning, following the presented pattern: 1st week - three applications - 25 % of the daily dose; 50% of the daily dose; a normal daily dose - 8 MIU. From the second month onward: regular applications of 8 MIU - day on - day off. According the type and length of AEs Paracetamol, Ibuprofen, Pentoxyphyllin /Trental/, Prednisolone- alone and in combination were applied when needed. Expanded Disability Status Scale /EDSS/, Lymphocytes, ASAT, ALAT, erythema in injection places, flu-like symptoms at the end of 1st, 6th, 12th and 24th were monitored. A significant decrease in local reactions was discovered from 42,85% at the end of the first month, to 20 % at the end of the 24th month. Flu- like symptoms were decreased from 37,14% at the end of the first month to 2,86% at the end of the 6ht month and eventually disappear and are not found after 12 and 24 months of treatment. The periodic checks on the liver function tests showed no abnormalities during the period of application of Betaferon.

## ORAL

### Inequivalence Between 2 Reference Drugs

[1]Bakracheva N., [2]Koytchev R., [1]Vlahov V.
[1]Dept. Clinical Pharmacology and Therapy, Medical University of Sofia, Bulgaria, [2]CCDRD Berlin, Germany

Two reference drugs from 2 different clinical studies on the bioequivalence of metformine were compared. The reference drugs contained metformine 1000 mg and were produced by different firms. Both studies were based on the same design: open randomized, cross-over clinical trial in 24 healthy volunteers. The first study was carried out in July 2000 and the second study was carried out in august, 2002. The reference drugs were administered orally with 240 ml tap water.

The results were as follows:

| | AUC0-¥ of Reference Drug 1 (ng.h/ml) | AUC0-¥ of Reference Drug 2 (ng.h/ml) |
|---|---|---|
| Mean | 889.19 | 1246.36 |
| SD | 348.14 | 238.71 |
| Median | 839.00 | 1157.00 |
| Minimum | 467.00 | 928.00 |
| Maximum | 1626.00 | 1597.00 |

The difference between both reference drugs was significant according to the Student-Fisher t-Test ($p<0.05$). In conclusion, it is very important to chose precisely the reference drug, when performing bioequivalence studies.

## P - 376

### Effect of Vitamin C on Body Lead Levels in Children

Gilani A.H., Tariq S.A., Shah A.J., Zaidi S.A.H., Butt S.A.H., Ghayur M.N.
Department of Biological and Biomedical Sciences, The Aga Khan University Medical College, Karachi, Pakistan.

Environmental lead exposure adversely affects human health especially in children. This preliminary study describes that Vitamin C removes lead from the bodies of children.

Pre-treatment urine and hair samples were collected from 8 school children (7 -12 years). One 500 mg Vitamin C tablet was given orally after dinner daily for 24 days. Late night and early morning urine was collected daily and 3 days samples were pooled (because of low urinary lead concentration). Hair samples were recollected 24 days post-treatment. Weighed hair samples were heated with 10 ml of 65 % concentrated nitric acid. Urine samples were digested similarly at 110°C, reduced below 50ml volume, and then cooled to room temperature. Lead concentrations were determined using a Perkin Elmer Analyst 300 Atomic Absorption Spectrometer, located at the Geological Survey of Pakistan, Karachi.

Post-treatment lead concentration (3.9±3.5 mg l-1; mean ± s.d.) was much lower ($P< 0.05$, paired t-test) than the control value (12.7±6.6). Pre-treatment urinary lead concentration was < 0.1 mcg g-1. Post-treatment lead in 1st three days pooled sample (4.5 ± 3.2 mcg g-1) was at least 45 times higher. Subsequent three samples (collected weekly) showed reduction to 0.07±0.03, 0.08±0.01 and 0.09±0.02 mg l-1 respectively, which are close to control values.

These data indicate that Vitamin C treatment reduces body lead level through urinary excretion probably by forming water-soluble complex (lead-ascorbate). This study, which has important public health implications, is in progress.

## P - 377

Population Pharmacokinetic Modeling in Evaluating Comparative Average Bioavailability of Two Oral Preparations of Ampicillin

Terziivanov D., Christov E., Bozhinova K., Atanasova I.
Clinic Ther Clin Pharmacol, Univ Hosp «St. I. Rilsky», Sofia, Bulgaria

Objectives: To explore the combined ability of population pharmacokinetic (PK) modeling and D-optimal strategy in assessing the comparative average drug bioavailability and disposition. Design: Single-dose, balanced, two-period, two-treatment, crossover study with a 7-day washout period. Participants:. 18 healthy Bulgarian Caucasian volunteers (9 men and 9 women, between 18 and 45 years with normal renal and liver functions). Methods: Participants received single doses of ampicillin 500 mg p.o. as Ampicillin (Biovet, Bulgaria)[test] and Standacillin(r) (Biochemie, Austria)[reference]. Plasma samples for measuring ampicillin concentrations were taken at time points according to D-optimality. A two steps population PK analysis was performed based on nonparametric expectation maximization (NPEM) algorithm. Step 1 involved development of population PK models of ampicillin for the test and reference formulation based on two types of parameterization: with absorption and elimination rate constants, KA and KEL, and volume of distribution, VOL, and with plasma drug clearance, CL, instead of KEL. Step 2 consisted in comparing the predictive performance of the population models for the test and reference product in Bayesian forecasting of ampicillin levels generated by the counter formulation.
Results: The mean amount of information, provided by ampicillin concentrations generated by both formulations, was between 161 and 217% for structural PK parameters. There was no statistical difference between NPEM average estimates of ampicillin population PK parameters for the test and reference population models. The 2 population models demonstrated comparable accuracy and precision. Conclusions: Collectively, the results show that the NPEM method combined with D-optimal strategy is a suitable and relevant one for comparing average bioavailabilty of two oral drug preparations when limited sampling is advisable in special target populations.

## P - 378

Polymorphisms of CYP1A1 Gene: Susceptibility for Uro-Genital Cancers

Seremak-Mrozikiewicz A., Drews K., Semczuk A., Mrozikiewicz P.M.
Department of Perinatology and Gynaecology, Division of Perinatology, Karol Marcinkowski University of Medical Sciences, Poznan, Poland Department of Gynaecological Surgery, Lublin School of Medicine, Lublin, Poland Institute of Medicinal Plants, Poznan, Poland Institute of Clinical Pharmacology, Humboldt University of Berlin, Berlin, Germany

The polycyclic aromatic hydrocarbon-inducible cytochrome P-450 1A1 (CYP1A1) plays important role in carcinogenesis - it transforms procarcinogens, including many of those contained in cigarette smoke, to potentially carcinogenic metabolites. The aim of our study was to prove possible roleof CYP1A1 mutations as susceptibility factors in female genital cancers. We have analysed two groups of women with endometrial (71 subjects, age range 44-80 years, mean 44.0 +/- 8.7) and ovarian cancer (39 subjects, age range 30-78 years, mean 52.0 +/- 10.7), and 132 healthy women (age range 24-64 years, mean 44.1 +/- 11.4). CYP1A1 alleles were detected by PCR/RFLP assays. The frequencies of mutated CYP1A1 aleles *2A and *2B were similar in all investigated groups. We have determined the overrepresentation of *4 allele in cancer groups (2.5% and 2.8% vs. 1.1%, odds ratios, 2.2 and 2.5 for ovarian and endometrial cancer, respectively). The overrepresentation of CYP1A1*4 alleles in the both, ovarian and endometrial cancers, could indicate a role of CYP1A1 activity in the pathogenesis of genital cancers.

## ORAL

C3435T Polymorphism of the MDR1 Gene is Correlated with Endometrial Cancer

Seremak-Mrozikiewicz A., Drews K., Semczuk A., Mrozikiewicz P.M.
Department of Perinatology and Gynecology, Division of Perinatology, Karol Marcinkowski University, Poznan, Poland Department of Gynecological Surgery, Lublin Medical School, Lublin, Poland Institute of Medicinal Plants, Poznan, Poland Institute of Clinical Pharmacology, Humboldt University, Charité, Berlin, Germany

The human multidrug-resistance (MDR1) gene encodes an integral cell membrane protein, P-glycoprotein (PGP). Its physiological role is to generate the ATP-dependent cellular transport of numerous substances. PGP could increase the transport of metabolites, toxic substances, and xenobiotics from cells and in this way protect them from the death. Recent investigations have shown that the polymorphisms (the most functional of them is the C3435T point mutation in exon 26) could influence the activity of MDR1 and suggested its role in development of several cancers. We have studied the frequency of C3435T mutation of MDR1 in the group of 99 women with endometrial cancer (mean age 64.0 +/- 8.7 years). Our results were compared to the previously studied healthy controls from the Polish population. The genotypes were determined real-time PCR assay on Light Cycler (Roche). We have detected the overrepresentation of mutated homozygous genotype 3435T/T (31.3% vs. 24.4%) and subsequent overrepresentation of mutated allele 3435T (58.1% vs. 51.1%) in endometrial cancer group. The overrepresentation of mutated 3435T allele detected in our study suggest that MDR1 polymorphism could influence inter individual susceptibility to develop endometrial cancer. Our observation could also indicate the possible role of MDR1 polymorphism in other uro-genital cancers.

## P - 379

Vitamin D Receptor Polymorphism in Women with Low Bone Mineral Density

Seremak-Mrozikiewicz A., Drews K., Mielcarek S., Kopyra P., Mrozikiewicz P.M.
Department of Perinatology and Gynaecology, Division of Perinatology, Karol Marcinkowski University of Medical Sciences, Poznan, Poland Institute of Medicinal Plants, Poznan, Poland

Osteoporosis is a multifactoral disease caused from the hormonal, environmental and genetic factors. Candidate gene for osteoporosis susceptibility is the gene encoding for vitamin D receptor (VDR). VDR polymorphism was associated with bone mineral density (BMD) and mutated variants could be involved in the earlier onset of osteoporosis. The goal of our study was to determine the role of BsmI polymorphism of VDR gene in the group of postmenopausal women from middle-west Poland. We have studied 34 postmenopausal women (mean age 58.2 +/- 7.2 years) with low BMD (mean 0.854 +/- 0.1, range 0.621 - 1.072). Last period mean age 47.5 +/- 5.1 years. As a controls we have analysed 40 healthy women (mean age 57.7 +/- 5.4 years). BMD measurements at the lumbar spine (L2-L4) were performed by dual-energy X-ray absorptiometry (DXA). The VDR polymorphism was determined using polymerase chain reaction/restriction fragment length polymorphism (PCR/RFLP) assay. We have determined statistically significant overrepresentation of the heterozygotic Bb genotypes (85.3% vs. 32.5%) and the statistically significant lower number of the bb genotypes in the group of women with low BMD (8.8% vs. 42.5%). The distribution of genotypes were: 5.9 : 85.3 : 8.8% for BB : Bb : bb, respectively. We have observed the higher frequency of B allele in the group of women with low BMD (48.5% vs. 41.2%) and lower frequency of b allele in the group of women with low BMD if compered to the controls (51.5% vs. 58.8%). Observed lower frequency of bb genotype in the investigated group postmenopausal women with low BMD suggests the protective role of this genotype against osteoporosis.

## P - 380

### Rapid Detection of MDR 1 Mutations Using Fluorogenic Hybridization Probes in the Sample from Polish Population

Mrozikiewicz P.M., Niewinski P., Nowakowski-Gashaw I., Roots I.
Institute of Clinical Pharmacology, Humboldt University of Berlin, Berlin, Germany Institute of Medicinal Plants, Poznan, Poland Department of Clinical Pharmacology, Wroclaw Medical University, Poland

The human multidrug-resistance (MDR1) gene encodes an integral membrane protein, P-glycoprotein (PGP), whose function is the energy-dependent cellular transport. Many drugs are substrates of PGP. Therefore, expression and functionality of the MDR1 gene product can directly affect the therapeutic efficacy. We have developed a rapid method for genotyping of the MDR1 polymorphisms which combines rapid-cycle PCR and fluorescent probe melting point analysis on the LightCycler (Roche). Fluorescent melting point analysis is a technique that detects mutations by differences in the melting temperature of fluorescent oligonucleotides hybridized to different alleles. Primers and fluorescent probes were designed on the basis of thermodynamic double-strand DNA stability calculations. Our assay was optimised for -1G/A, T12C, A61G, G1199A, C1236T, G2677T/A, C3435T, and C3396T mutations. The protocol developed allows fluorescence genotyping of MDR1 mutations in 32 samples in less than 40 min without need for enzyme digestion or electrophoresis. In investigated 262 individuals of Polish origin most frequent was C3435T variant with allelic frequency of 51.1 % (3435T). Other mutated alleles variants detected as follows: 2.7 % (12C), 7.4 % (-1A), 15.3 % (61G), 4.0% (1199A), 39.1 (1236T), 42.2 (2677T), and 3.2 (2677A).No mutation 3396T was found. Observed frequencies were in accordance with those obtained for other Caucasian populations. Routine determination of MDR1 mutations is accurate, rapid, reliable, and low-cost methods. Knowledge of an individual's MDR1 mutations can help in avoiding adverse reactions or therapeutic failure and thus enhance therapeutic efficiency.

## ORAL

### NSAIDs, Inflammatory Mediators and on Cartilage Changes in Osteoarthritis

K.D. Rainsford, P.A. Revell, S. Rashad, F.S. Walker (deceased), R. Seabrook, R.A.D. Bunning, Biomedical Research Centre, Sheffield Hallam University, Sheffield, S1 1WB.

Prostaglandins (PGs) are important regulators of proteoglycan (PrGn) and other macromolecules in cartilage and some NSAID's may exert a detrimental effect on the synthesis or turnover of PrGns in cartilage. The suggestion that inhibition of PG production could regulate production of proinflammatory cytokines could be related to cartilage changes or that some NSAIDs could inhibit production of tissue destructive oxyradicals , nitric oxide or metalloproteinases could be significant in affecting the integrity of cartilage in OA.
Early studies with indomethacin and azapropazone provided evidence that the reduced cartilage PrGns in the hip joints of OA patients who had undergone arthroplasty and who had received long-term treatment with these NSAIDs might be related to differences in inhibitory effects of these drugs on PrGn synthesis. Studies have found that the changes in PrGn's were linearly correlated with PG concentrations. This suggests that inhibition of PrGn production might be related to potency of PG inhibition by unselective COX-1/COX-2 inhibitors. Increase in production of pro-inflammatory cytokines (IL-1 and TNFα) by some NSAIDs (e.g. indomethacin) in response to PG inhibition may account in part for the acceleration of cartilage destruction by NSAIDs by negative control by PGs of PrGn turnover. Some drugs (e.g. oxaprozin) do not affect synovial production or actions of pro-inflammatory cytokines [IL-1, TNFα] and some (e.g. nimesulide ) reduce their production. These data suggest that reduction in PG's by potent inhibitors of COX's may lead to a range of biochemical changes, eg. increase in pro-inflammatory cytokine production inhibition of NO and oxyradicals so affecting either positively or negatively the acceleration of cartilage destruction in OA.

## P - 381

### A Study on the Rational Use of Antibacterial Means Under Special Regime of Prescription and Usage at St Anna University Hospital, Varna

[1]Georgieva M., [2]Eliseev V.
[1]Department Of Preclinical And Clinical Pharmacology And Biochemistry, Mu-Varna, [2]"St. Anna" University Hospital, Varna

Monitoring of the use of antibiotics of strategic importance was carried out at the clinics of urology, neurosurgery and vascular surgery and at the emergency department of St Anna University Hospital, Varna, for the period of July and August 2002.
Aim of the study: 1) to identify the indications for usage; 2) to assess the frequency of usage - DDD/100 beds; 3) to assess retrospectively the rationality of the choice and the usage of the following antibiotics of strategic importance: cephalosporin IIIrd and IVth generation, glycopeptides, carbapenemes, fluconazole (all under special regime of prescription and usage).
Methods used: 1) quantitative analysis with standard and statistical approaches; 2) qualitative analysis of medicinal use.

## P - 382

### Goitrogenic Effects of P-Coumaric Acid in Rats

[1]Taha R.A., [2]Touhami F.K., [1]Badary O.A., [3]Lezzar A., [1]Hamada F.M.
[1]Al-Azhar University, Cairo, Egypt; [2]Mentouri University, Constantine, Algeria; [3]University hospital Iben Bades, Constantine, Algeria

The effects of three phenolic acids (caffeic, ferulic and P-coumaric acids) on the rat thyroid were examined in a 3-week oral treatment study. Forty male Wistar albino rats, divided into groups of ten rats each and fed Purina iodine-rich diet. They were administered by gastrointestinal tube saline (control), caffeic, ferulic or P-coumaric acid at a dose level of 50 mg/kg/day for 3 weeks. The mean absolute and relative thyroid weights in caffeic, ferulic or P-coumaric groups were significantly increase to 127 & 132% or 146 & 153% or 189 & 201%compared to control value, respectively. Histological examinations of the thyroids of P-coumaric acid group revealed marked hypertrophy and/or hyperplasia of the follicles with rich colloid and formation of a fibrous capsule. Caffeic or ferulic acid groups showed slight to moderate thyroid enlargement. Thyroid lesions in P-coumaric acid group was associated with significant increase in cellular proliferation as indicated by the rate of [H]thymidine incorporation. In addition, the goitrogenic effect of P-coumaric acid was further confirmed by significant decreases (50%) in serum tri-iodothyronine (T3) and thyroxine (T4) and a parallel increase (90%) in serum thyroid stimulating hormone (TSH) compared to control group. These results indicate that administration of P-coumaric acid at relatively high doses induces goiter in rats and this may be due to its antithyroid effect.

## ORAL

The Waste of Drugs Among Families Living in Ankara

Gulmez S. E., Tulunay F. C., Ergun H.
Medical School of Ankara University, Department of Pharmacology and Clinical Pharmacolgy, Ankara, Turkey

BACKGROUND: Drugs, either prescribed or OTC, but unused by the patients causes an economically important problem.
METHOD: A questionnaire was planned to find out the drug storage profile in 329 families living in central Ankara. The questionnaire had two parts, the first included the general demographic properties of the families, such as their social medical security, monthly income, number of the family members, number of working people, number of doctor visits a year for the whole family. The second part included for any drug found in their house, the active compound and generic names of it, its pharmaceutical form, the size of the package, the unused amount of the drug, and its expire date.
RESULTS: % 90 of the families receive the drugs with a medical social security. Average monthly income was between 120-240 Euros (% 30,9). The average family number was 4, the average number of working people was 1. The average number of yearly doctor visits was 12. Total number of drug boxes counted was 4460 and the mostly found pharmaseutical form was tablets (% 49,1). The mostly found three drugs were Aspirin® (acetyl salicilic acid), Vermidon® (paracetamole), and Mesulide® (nimesulide). When ingredients were analized, the three mostly found active compounds were paracetamole, multivitamin preparates, and acetyl salicilic acid. % 12 of all drugs expired, and the expire dates of % 7 was not known. The most wasted pharmaceutic form was syrup. The drugs with the biggest amount of the package were the most wasted. This survey shows that an important amount of drugs in houses are wasted and kept even if they are expired.

## P - 383

Prescription Knowledge of Turkish Medical Doctors

Ergun H., Gulmez S. E., Tulunay F. C.
Medical School of Ankara University, Department of Pharmacology and Clinical Pharmacology, Sihhiye, Ankara, Turkey

BACKGROUND: Doctors prescibe drugs with their brand names in Turkey. There are many brand names for a known active compound, so it is up to the doctor which one will be prescribed. A questionnaire was planned to evaluate the prescription knowledge of Turkish doctors.
METHODS: 25 of the most prescribed 40 drugs were chosen, and asked 204 doctors, who were randomly chosen from different departments of different University Hospitals, Health Minister Hospitals, Social Insurance Associate Hospitals, and general practicioners, if they know the active compound of the preparate.
RESULTS: Ingredients of % 57,08 of the prescribed drugs were known by Turkish doctors, and this ratio rised up to % 59,44 in the group aged below 30. % 60,44 of the general practitioners, and % 53,02 of the doctors from University Hospitals knew the active compound they prescribed. According to the departments, the first three were general practitioners (% 61,81), surgeons (% 58,85), and internal medicine (% 53,13). This study shows that almost half of the doctors don't know the ingredients (generic name) of the prescripted drugs.

## P - 384

Effects of Armagnac or Vodka on Platelet Aggregation in Healthy Volunteers: A Randomized Clinical Trial.

[1]Umar A., [1]Depont F., [1]Jacquet A., [1]Lignot S., [1]Bégaud B., [2]Segur M.C., [3]Boisseau M., [1]Moore N.
[1]Département de Pharmacologie, Université Victor Segalen, 33076 Bordeaux, France, [2]BNIA, Eauze, France, [3]Departement d'Hématologie, Université Victor Segalen, Bordeaux, France

Background: The "french paradox", has been attributed to the regular use of wine, and to its polyphenols. Ellagitannins, which also have antioxidant properties, are found in wood-aged spirits such as armagnac, most used in Southwest France where the paradox is maximal. In previous studies, we found that freeze-dried alcohol-free armagnac extract could inhibit in vitro human ADP-induced platelet aggregation and in vivo thrombosis in the rat.
Method: randomized control trial comparing five-year old armagnac (30 ml/day for two weeks) to same alcoholic degree vodka, in 20 healthy volunteers, on platelet aggregation induced by ADP, collagen, and thrombin, weekly, during consumption and for two weeks after, bleeding time, partial thromboplastin time (PTT) and plasma lipids.
Results: After 14 days, ADP -induced platelet aggregation was inhibited more in armagnac (-31±3.2% compared to pretreatment values, $p<0.01$) than in vodka (-11.0 ± 6.8%, NS) users ($p<0.05$, armagnac vs vodka). A rebound increase of aggregation was found two weeks later in vodka but not in armagnac users. The same pattern was found for thrombin-induced aggregation, including post-treatment rebound. No effect was found on collagen-induced aggregation, bleeding time, PTT, or plasma lipids.
Conclusion: The chronic ingestion of moderate quantities of armagnac altered platelet aggregation in healthy volunteers. The difference with the effects of same alcohol degree vodka is in favour of an effect of the polyphenols or other constituants in the effects of armagnac, rather than just alcohol. Armagnac could also be involved in the French Paradox. All spirits may not be equal for cardioprotection.

## P - 385

The Treatment of Acute Migrane Attacks with Dipyrone (Novalgin®): A Double-Blind, Cross Over, Randomized, Placebo-Controlled Multi-Center Pilot Study

[1]Tulunay F. C., [1]Ergun H., [1]Gulmez S. E., [2]Ozbenli T., [3]Ozmenoglu M., [3]Boz C., [4]Erdemoglu A. K., [4]Varlikbas A., [5]Goksan B, [6]Inan L.
[1]Medical School of Ankara University, Department of Pharmacology and Clinical Pharmocology, Ankara, [2]Medical School of 19 Mayıs University, Department of Neurology, Samsun, [3]Medical School of Black Sea Technical University, Department of Neurology, Trabzon, [4]Medical School of Kırıkkale University, Department of Neurology, Kırıkkale, [5]Istanbul University, Cerrahpasa Faculty of Medicine, Department of Neurology, Istanbul, [6]Ankara Hospital, Department of Neurology, Ankara, Turkey

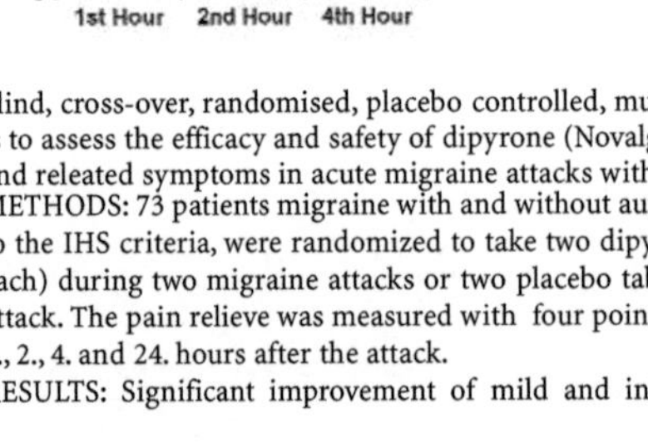


BACKGROUND: Dipyrone (Novalgin®) is an effective analgesic, anti-pyretic and anti-spasmotic agent. It is used in acute treatments of migraine and other types of headache in many countries.
OBJECTIVES: The aim of this double-blind, cross-over, randomised, placebo controlled, multi-center pilot study is to assess the efficacy and safety of dipyrone (Novalgin®) tablets on pain and releated symptoms in acute migraine attacks with and without aura.
METHODS: 73 patients migraine with and without aura, selected according to the IHS criteria, were randomized to take two dipyrone tablets (500 mg each) during two migraine attacks or two placebo tablets in one migraine attack. The pain relieve was measured with four point analgesic scala at 0., 1., 2., 4. and 24. hours after the attack.
RESULTS: Significant improvement of mild and intermediate pain was

achieved with dipyrone 1-4 hours after the attack compared with placebo. Both patients and doctors evaluation were significantly in favor of dipyrone. Side effects were minimum and trivial in both cases.
CONCLUSION: This study shows that dipyrone is an effective, safe and low price drug for the relief of mild and intermediate acute migraine pain and releated symptoms.

## P - 387

Drug Use in Pharmacies in Novi Sad, Serbia And Monte Negro. Comparison Between State and Private Pharmacies

Sabo A., Vukmirovic A., Jakovljevic V., Papuga M.
Department of Pharmacology, Faculty of medicine, Novi Sad, Serbia and Montenegro

Although law in Serbia and Montenegro prohibits sale of the drugs without prescription (with exception OTC) in private pharmacies there is still possibility to buy drugs without prescription. Patients, who buy drugs in private pharmacies without visiting the doctors probably lack informations about the drug proper dosing of d4rrugs and adverse effects. There are short informations about the most drugs insight the drug box, but no all patients understand the terms describing the adverse effects. The purchasing the antibiotics and the drugs with effects on CNS was at the time of investigation also very easy, and no prescriptions were needed in private pharmacies. Therefore we conducted the investigation with the aim to analyze the prescription pattern in pharmacies and the knowledge about the drugs obtained by the doctors. The investigation was performed in state and private pharmacies. During the one-week the drugs obtained were counted and patient were asked about administration and adverse effects of the drugs they were purchasing. The most often purchasing drugs were from cardiovascular system and Alimentary tract in both pharmacies. There were not statistical difference between the purchasing the drugs for CNS and antibiotics. Knowledge of the patients about administration schedule was satisfying, but they did not known much about adverse effects and drug interactions, despite the fact that all patients red he leaflets about the drugs. Changing in law control, drug information and patients attitudes towards the drugs are needed.

## P - 386

The Pre-emptive Analgesic Efficacy of Dipyrone (Novalgin®) During Removal of Nasal Packings After Septal Surgery

[1]Tulunay E. O., [2]Tulunay F. C, [2]Gulmez S. E., [2]Ergun H., [1]Demireller A.
[1]Medical School of Ankara University, Department of Otorhinolaryngology, Ankara, [2]Medical School of Ankara University, Department of Pharmacology and Clinical Pharmacology, Ankara

BACKGROUND: Septoplasty is one of the most common nasal operations performed in the otorhinolaryngological practice. After the operation, most surgeons place nasal packings and remove them after 48-72 hours. The removal of the packings may be very painful. This study was planned to see if pre-emptive analgesia will help the patient to deal better with this painful procedure. METHOD: The study was performed on 38 patients undergoing septal surgery at the Department of Otorhinolaryngology, Ankara University. Twelve patients did not get any analgesic treatment during removal. Ten patients received 4 ml of intramuscular (I.M.) physiological saline solution, and served as the second control group. Sixteen patients were pretreated with 1 gr of intramuscular (I.M.) dipyrone (Novalgin®) 45 minutes prior to the removal of the nasal packings. The patients were asked to express their pain on visual analog scales, and by using the percentage system and verbal scales. The scales were filled out prior to the procedure, just after the packings were removed (0 minutes) and then at 5, 10, 15, 20, 30, 60, 120 minutes after removal. The groups were compared by one way ANOVA.
RESULTS: No significant difference in pain was found between the 3 groups before the procedure started. On the other hand, at «0., 5. and 10. minutes», the dipyrone group showed significant pain relief when compared to the control groups.
CONCLUSION: Dipyrone (Novalgin®) was found to be effective in reducing pain in the first 10 minutes after removal. We conclude that dipyrone pretreatment for the removal of nasal packings is effective for postprocedure pain relief.

## P - 388

Inducible Nitric Oxide Synthase Expression in Prostatic Pathologies

[1]Tulunay O., [2]Baltacı S., [1]Orhan D., [2]Goguş C., [2]Turkolmez K., [2]Goguş O.
Departments of [1]Pathology and [2]Urology. University of Ankara, School of Medicine, Ankara, Turkey

Nitric oxide (NO) synthase (NOS) exists as three different isoforms. Inducible NOS (iNOS) expression is induced by endotoxins and/or cytokines and this enzyme provides a sustained release of NO.
The purpose of the present study was examine iNOS activity immunohistochemically in prostatic intraepithelial neoplasia (PIN) lesions and compare it with the activity in benign prostatic hyperplasia (BPH) and malignant tissues, as iNOS may play a role in the development of BPH and/or prostatic carcinoma (PC).
Immunoreactivity for iNOS was examined in 30 samples each of BPH, PIN and PC.
iNOS expression was detected in all samples from all patients: iNOS expression was detected in both basal and luminal cells of the glandular epithelium. The immunoreactivity for iNOS was more intense in PIN and PC samples than BPH.
The results show that iNOS is expressed in BPH, PIN and PC. More intense iNOS reactivity in PIN and PC suggests a role for iNOS in tumorigenesis. Further studies are needed to determine the exact role of iNOS in the pathogenesis of PC.

Printing and Binding: Stürtz AG, Würzburg

GPSR Compliance

*The European Union's (EU) General Product Safety Regulation (GPSR) is a set of rules that requires consumer products to be safe and our obligations to ensure this.*

*If you have any concerns about our products, you can contact us on ProductSafety@springernature.com*

In case Publisher is established outside the EU, the EU authorized representative is:

Springer Nature Customer Service Center GmbH
Europaplatz 3
69115 Heidelberg, Germany

**Batch number: 10684239**

Printed by Printforce, the Netherlands